JOB TRAI

MEDICAL OFFICE PRACTICE

JOB TRAINING MANUAL

MEDICAL OFFICE PRACTICE

8th Edition

Diane R. Timme, RN, BS

Phillip Atkinson, PhD
Professor Emeritus
Baruch College of the
City University of New York

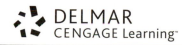
DELMAR
CENGAGE Learning

Australia • Brazil • Japan • Korea • Mexico • Singapore • Spain • United Kingdom • United States

DELMAR
CENGAGE Learning™

Title: Medical Office Practice, Eighth Edition

Authors: Diane R. Timme and Phillip Atkinson

Vice President, Career and Professional Editorial:
Dave Garza

Director of Learning Solutions: Matthew Kane

Senior Acquisitions Editor: Rhonda Dearborn

Managing Editor: Marah Bellegarde

Senior Product Manager: Sarah Prime

Editorial Assistant: Lauren Whalen

Vice President, Career and Professional Marketing:
Jennifer Baker

Marketing Director: Wendy Mapstone

Senior Marketing Manager: Nancy Bradshaw

Marketing Coordinator: Erica Ropitzky

Production Director: Carolyn Miller

Content Project Manager: Thomas Heffernan

Senior Art Director: Jack Pendleton

Technology Project Manager: Erin Zeggert

For product information and technology assistance, contact us at
Cengage Learning Customer & Sales Support, 1-800-354-9706

For permission to use material from this text or product, submit all requests online at **www.cengage.com/permissions.**
Further permissions questions can be e-mailed to
permissionrequest@cengage.com

Library of Congress Control Number: 2010933457
ISBN-13: 978-1-4354-8143-5
ISBN-10: 1-4354-8143-7

Delmar
5 Maxwell Drive
Clifton Park, NY 12065-2919
USA

Cengage Learning is a leading provider of customized learning solutions with office locations around the globe, including Singapore, the United Kingdom, Australia, Mexico, Brazil, and Japan. Locate your local office at: **international.cengage.com/region**

Cengage Learning products are represented in Canada by Nelson Education, Ltd.

To learn more about Delmar, visit **www.cengage.com/delmar**
Purchase any of our products at your local college store or at our preferred online store **www.CengageBrain.com**

NOTICE TO THE READER
Publisher does not warrant or guarantee any of the products described herein or perform any independent analysis in connection with any of the product information contained herein. Publisher does not assume, and expressly disclaims, any obligation to obtain and include information other than that provided to it by the manufacturer. The reader is expressly warned to consider and adopt all safety precautions that might be indicated by the activities described herein and to avoid all potential hazards. By following the instructions contained herein, the reader willingly assumes all risks in connection with such instructions. The publisher makes no representations or warranties of any kind, including but not limited to, the warranties of fitness for particular purpose or merchantability, nor are any such representations implied with respect to the material set forth herein, and the publisher takes no responsibility with respect to such material. The publisher shall not be liable for any special, consequential, or exemplary damages resulting, in whole or part, from the readers' use of, or reliance upon, this material.

Printed in the United States of America
1 2 3 4 5 6 7 12 11 10

Contents

Date	Job		

Welcome to Medical Office Practice!

The jobs and materials chosen for inclusion in this medical office simulation will help you learn as if you were actually employed. After completing *Medical Office Practice,* Eighth Edition, you will be able to:

1. Organize, prepare, and maintain administrative files and patient records.
2. Understand and apply HIPAA concepts to the medical office practice.
3. Revise a patient information brochure.
4. Perform all aspects of computerized patient scheduling and appointment book scheduling.
5. Perform alphabetic filing.
6. Complete computerized patient registration.
7. Process Release of Medical Information forms.
8. Transcribe office-style dictation.
9. Interpret and process telephone messages.
10. Recognize and respond to ethical situations in the medical office.
11. Make a referral to a specialist.
12. Use the Internet to research information on prescription drugs, travel, and medical supplies.
13. Create a travel itinerary.
14. Proofread and prepare final copy from rough draft.
15. Prepare occupational exposure incident report.
16. Order office supplies and prepare a purchase order.
17. Post daily financial transactions on a Day Sheet.
18. Perform computerized procedure and payment postings, including adjustments and refunds.
19. Compute office payroll from a work record.
20. Understand the components of the Material Safety Data Sheet (MSDS).
21. Process and submit managed care insurance claims electronically.
22. Identify appropriate community resources.
23. Schedule admission to a hospital and prepare patient for procedure.
24. Create or update resume and prepare for job interview.

New to this Edition

Medical Office Practice, Eighth Edition features many new enhancements and jobs:

- Medical Office Simulation Software is included for users to gain proficiency in working in simulated Practice Management software.
- A flash drive is included with forms and transcription files and for users to save finished work.
- There is no separate location for forms; all materials and forms are included within the Job Training Manual. Additionally, all forms are provided electronically on the accompanying flash drive.
- New jobs that utilize MOSS: Jobs 3, 5, 6, 7, 11, 13, 18, 25, 26, 29, 30 and 33

- New Job 4: Filing procedures with alphabetic filing guidelines from the Association of Records Managers and Administrators (ARMA)
- New Job 6: Scheduling patient appointments electronically
- New Job 7: More scheduling practice and creating new patient records electronically
- New Job 10: Reviewing telephone messages and using critical thinking skills to determine the appropriate action to take
- Revised Job 11: Looking up patient appointments and making reminder calls for appointments
- New Job 12: Responding to ethical scenarios in a professional and appropriate manner
- New Job 13: Scheduling outpatient appointments
- New Job 18: Blocking the physicians' schedule

- New Job 25: Computerized procedure posting with practice management software
- New Job 26: Computerized payment posting with practice management software
- New Job 27: Computing employee payroll
- New Job 28: Learning about Material Safety Data Sheets (MSDS)
- New Job 29: Posting Adjustments, Credits, and Processing Refunds
- New Job 30: Creating prebilling worksheets and submitting claims electronically
- New Job 31: Coding practice for CPT and ICD-9 codes
- New Job 32: Identifying community resources
- New Job 33: Scheduling a hospital admission
- New Job 35: Creating a resume

Organizational chart for Douglasville Medicine Associates

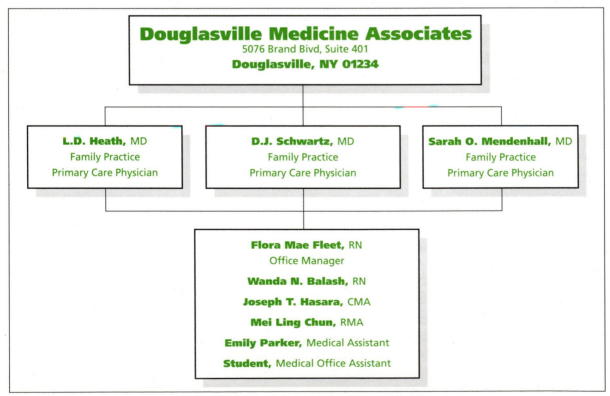

Welcome

For the next five weeks, you will simulate the experience of actual employment. You have been employed as a medical office assistant (in training) by Douglasville Medicine Associates, a medical office in Douglasville, New York. An organizational chart for Douglasville Medicine Associates is displayed below.

You have been hired because you have a basic understanding of the medical profession and the requirements and responsibilities of a medical office assistant. With us, you will gain experience not easily attained except in real employment, and as a new employee, you will be introduced gradually to the work and routines of Douglasville Medicine Associates. As your employers, we want you to be successful in this job, and we want to feel we made the right decision in hiring you.

We ask that all new employees learn the policies and procedures of our practice. This means learning how to do things according to the specific routines of Douglasville Medicine Associates. We realize that you may be familiar with other ways to perform administrative tasks; however, we ask that you follow the instructions presented in our manual in order to complete your training.

For the first few jobs in this simulation, you will be assigned tasks that are easy to do with sufficient instructions. Then, as your knowledge of our office routines increases, you will be assigned to new tasks, but you will be expected to be more self-reliant. Your assignments in the later jobs provide fewer instructions, calling for you to rely upon your resourcefulness to supply missing information from the files and documents you have previously handled.

Employment at Douglasville Medicine Associates

Douglasville Medicine Associates offers medical care for private patients and participates in six different insurance plans, including Medicare and Medicaid, which will be discussed later.

There are three physicians in our office: Sarah O. Mendenhall, MD; L.D. Heath, MD; and D.J. Schwartz, MD. All three physicians offer consultations for private patients, and all three are identified as **primary care physicians (PCP)** in Signal HMO. A Primary Care Physician is a general practitioner who is skilled in handling a broad range of medical problems and who guides patients, as necessary, to consultations with network specialists. All three doctors, on rotation, provide on-side care for patients in the nearby Retirement Inn Nursing Home.

Mrs. Fleet, our office manager, is responsible for your training and is the person from whom you will receive most of your instructions.

Our office is a modern four-story building dedicated to the medical professions. We are at one end of the fourth floor. Out suite of offices begins with a waiting room and a front office where the business activities are carried out and where you will work. Each of our doctors has a private office for contemplation, research, and consultation. We have five examination rooms that are equipped with examination tables and heart monitoring machines. There is a lounge room where the staff keep personal belongings and where they congregate for lunch or at break times. We also have a lab for taking urine and blood specimens. We have a contract with an outside lab, BioPace Laboratories, to pick up and treat the specimens we collect. We also contract with a diagnostic testing group to conduct mammography tests in our office on a regular schedule. We do not do surgery in our offices, and we have no overnight facilities for patients.

Several specialists are also located in this building: Quali-Care Clinic is on the third floor. The physicians in this clinic specialize in orthopedics, oncology, and gastroenterology. You will find their office staff listed in the Appendix A: Reference Materials on page 113. Other medical offices in the building include a physical therapy center on the second floor and a pediatrician's office on the first floor.

Occasionally we refer patients to an outside facility located in Douglasville known as

Midway Specialty Associates, which employs three physicians. Their specialties include obstetrics/gynecology, neurology, and cardiology. Their information is also listed in Appendix A: Reference Materials on page 113.

Insurance

The physicians at Douglasville Medicine Associates participate in several different insurance plans. All three physicians participate in Signal HMO, a **Health Maintenance Organization (HMO)** plan, which requires that patients use in-network providers in order to be "covered" for services. Patients who have Signal HMO must choose a primary care physician (PCP), who serves as their main physician and manages their care by being the "gatekeeper" of other medical services requiring referrals. For example, if a patient requires services that her PCP was not qualified to handle, she would need a referral from her PCP to a specialist in order to obtain those services. With an HMO, patients do have the option to choose physicians who are not "in-network" physicians; however, the patient will have to pay out of pocket, as those services are not reimbursable.

Drs. Heath and Mendenhall participate in Flexihealth PPO, a **Preferred Provider Organization (PPO)** plan. PPOs are somewhat less restrictive than HMOs in that patients are able to choose specialists on their own without going through the "gatekeeper" (their PCP). It is still of benefit to patients to choose "in-network" physicians in order to keep costs down, since physicians who participate in PPOs work on a reduced fee schedule, and choosing physicians out of network means increased cost to the patient.

Drs. Heath and Mendenhall also participate in Medicare, which is a government-funded health insurance program for people over the age of 65. Medicare also serves some people under age 65 who have disabilities, as well as people with end-stage renal disease. There are two parts to Medicare: Part A is hospital insurance, which covers inpatient care, skilled nursing facilities, hospice care, and some home health; Part B is medical insurance, which helps pay for physician services, outpatient care, some preventative services, and other medical services that are deemed medically necessary. Most people do not have to pay for Part A Medicare benefit and are enrolled automatically at age 65. However, most people pay a monthly premium for Part B, which is based on income, and must enroll in Part B in order to have the benefit.

Century SeniorGap is a type of supplemental insurance policy sold by a private insurance company to fill in the "gaps" in a patient's Original Medicare coverage (Part B), since Original Medicare only pays 80% of the approved charges and the beneficiary pays the other 20%. (There is also a deductible with Medicare Part B that must be met every year before benefits are reimbursed, which changes annually.) Douglasville Medicine Associates serves several patients with Century SeniorGap.

Finally, Dr. Mendenhall participates in Medicaid, which is another government-funded health insurance plan for people with limited income who are financially unable to pay for some or all of their medical care.

Your Job Duties

To make your experience with *Medical Office Practice* as realistic as possible, all the patient problems and histories, correspondence, and dictation have been selected from the files of practicing physicians. For confidentiality, all names, dates, places, and any other identifiable characteristics of physicians and patients have been carefully deleted or changed. All forms are replicas of forms in current use.

Though your employer, Douglasville Medicine Associates, does not exist, everything possible has been done in this simulation to help you feel you are working in a real medical office. You will, however, be asked to do some things for expediency because you are, in reality, working in a classroom and only simulating the experience of working in a real medical office. The unrealistic experiences have to do with handling patient files, working with files that are incomplete, and discussing your work with others. Additionally, you will notice that the appointment schedule is empty. In a real office, the appointment schedule would be almost full for the months of October and November (the months you will be working at Douglasville Medicine Associates). You will be scheduling patients into the computer system, but there are limited active patient accounts at the beginning of your training session.

For this simulation, you will have patient files in your possession. You may even carry them out of the classroom. In a medical office, you would not have patient files in your possession. You would certainly not carry them out of the office. Patient files are confidential and remain in the office under the strictest kind of confidentiality.

You will also create original documents that you sometimes keep in your possession. In a real medical office, you might keep a photocopy for your use, but the original would be routed away from your desk immediately. You will not make duplicate copies; therefore, your patient files may be incomplete. Finally, because you are learning to deal with new problems, you and your "fellow workers" and instructor are free to discuss the

patients and the doctors and their procedures. In real employment, you would do nothing to upset physician-patient confidentiality.

Scheduling

The activities in *Medical Office Practice* cover approximately five weeks in October and November, as shown below.

Reference Section

A complete section of reference material has been included in Appendix A: Reference Materials to help you with additional material you may need to complete some of the jobs. The material includes valuable information on the office staff, patients, common abbreviations, transcription and document preparation suggestions, plus accounting and insurance information. You will be referred to each section of these references within specific jobs as needed. For a complete list of the reference section contents, refer to page 113.

Flash Drive and Computer Usage

Medical Office Practice has incorporated the use of the computer into as many jobs as possible, thus simulating current medical office practice. The flash drive in this package contains all of the electronic files necessary to complete the simulation. It includes:

- *Audio dictation files for transcription jobs.* These files are all contained in the "Transcription Folder" on the flash drive and saved by Job name. These files include a variety of transcription jobs for common medical reports used today. A few of the jobs include ethnic dictation to help familiarize you with the accents of foreign-born physicians. You will see headphone icons in the Supplies and Materials section when a job has an audio dictation file.

- *Electronic versions of all forms in this Job Training Manual.* The user has a choice of completing most forms in hard copy or

Medical office practice time period

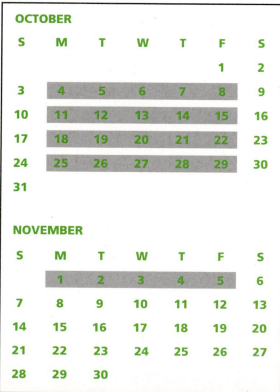

OCTOBER						
S	M	T	W	T	F	S
					1	2
3	4	5	6	7	8	9
10	11	12	13	14	15	16
17	18	19	20	21	22	23
24	25	26	27	28	29	30
31						

NOVEMBER						
S	M	T	W	T	F	S
	1	2	3	4	5	6
7	8	9	10	11	12	13
14	15	16	17	18	19	20
21	22	23	24	25	26	27
28	29	30				

Source: Delmar/Cengage Learning

electronically. The forms are all grouped together on the flash drive in the "Electronic Files Folder" and saved by Job and form name. The electronic forms are writable, meaning that they can be completed electronically and printed or saved. In some cases, you will only use an electronic file to complete a job. You will see forms icons throughout this Job Training Manual indicating when you will need to use a form.

- *Templates to complete jobs.* All document templates from Appendix A: Reference Materials are included on the flash drive in the "Reference Materials Folder," saved by Job and form name.

All work can be saved on the same flash drive. It is recommended that you create a folder on the flash drive named "Completed Work" to save completed forms, documents, etc.

Additionally, there are jobs that require the use of the Internet, and this is indicated in the Materials and Supplies section of each job. (For an at-a-glance overview of what is required for each job in terms of MOSS, Internet, or flash drive, please refer to Appendix B: Job Utilization Chart on page 143.)

Using the Transcription Files

As mentioned above, the audio files to complete transcription jobs (Jobs 9 and 14 and 19) are found on the flash drive, in a "Transcription Folder." The files can be identified by Job name and are provided in mp3 format. A "Transcription Help" file is included on the Flash Drive to assist with any questions in using these audio files.

Medical Office Simulation Software (MOSS)

Medical Office Simulation Software (MOSS) 2.0 (single-user version) is included in this package. MOSS is generic

practice management software designed to help you prepare to work with any commercial software used in medical offices today. With a friendly, highly graphical interface, MOSS allows you to learn the fundamentals of medical office software packages in an educational environment. Installation instructions and information on using MOSS is found in Appendix C: Using Medical Office Simulation Software. Jobs which utilize MOSS are indicated by the MOSS icon in the Materials and Supplies section.

Forms

All forms required to complete *Medical Office Practice* are printed at the end of this Job Training Manual, as well as provided electronically on your flash drive. You will see these icons throughout this Job Training Manual indicating when you will need to use a form.

Icons Key

When You See:	The Job Requires:
	Your Flash Drive.
	One or more Forms.
MOSS	Medical Office Simulation Software (MOSS)
	Audio transcription files from your Flash Drive.
	Folders from the Medical Office Practice package.
A	Alphanumeric File Labels from the Medical Office Practice package.
JAN	The Appointment Schedule from the Medical Office Practice package.
$	The Daysheet from the Medical Office Practice package.

Acknowledgments

I would like to express my sincere gratitude and appreciation to Jeannie Bower and Nicole Vance for contributing their knowledge and expertise to this edition. Thank you also to Amy Kaehler for being my unofficial student editor, who worked diligently through the jobs in an effort to "work out the kinks."

Many thanks to all the individuals at Delmar Cengage Learning who assisted in the revision of this edition. A special thanks to Sarah Prime, Senior Product Manager, whose encouragement, collaboration, and technical expertise throughout this project was invaluable to me.

Most importantly, thank you to my children, Zach and Jordan, and to my family and friends, who have been constant pillars of love and support.

Diane Timme

REVIEWERS

The author and publisher would like to thank the following reviewers for their valuable input, feedback, and accuracy checking:

M. Jeannie Bower, BS, HIS
Adjunct Professor
Central Pennsylvania College
Summerdale, PA

Lela Delaney, BSE, M.Ed
Instructor, Medical Office Technology
Northwest Mississippi Community College
Lafayette-Yalobusha Technical Center
Oxford, MS

Barbara Desch, LVN, CPC, AHI
Program Director, Medical Office Assisting
San Joaquin Valley College
Visalia, CA

Brian Dickens, MBA, RMA, CHI
Medical Assistant Program Director/Instructor
Keiser Career College/Southeastern Institute
   Main Campus
Greenacres, Florida

Sharon M. Goucher-Norris, BS, CCS-P,
   NCICS, HIA, ALCH
Lead Instructor, Medical Insurance Billing
   and Coding
Everest College
Vancouver, WA

Judy Hurtt, M.Ed
Instructor, Business Office and Medical
   Office Technology
East Central Community College
   Decatur, MS

Amy B. Mori, MBA
Dean of Student Services
Bryant & Stratton College
Albany, NY

Lisa Nagle, BS.Ed, CMA(AAMA)
Medical Assisting Program Director
Augusta Technical College
Augusta, GA

Donna Otis, LPN
Medical Instructor
Metro Business College
Rolla, MO

Getting Started: Administrative Functions

MATERIALS AND SUPPLIES

- 5 file folders
- Form: Welcome Letter

TIME ALLOTMENT

30 minutes

OCTOBER 5, 2010

Today is your first day as a new employee of Douglasville Medicine Associates. As your first task, you will organize the supplies and other materials given to you today.

Your *Medical Office Practice* package of materials includes:

- Job Training Manual—Medical Office Practice
- 1 folded Appointment Schedule
- 1 folded Daysheet
- 10 File Folders
- 1 sheet of alphanumeric file labels
- Flash Drive
- Medical Office Simulation Software (MOSS), version 2.0 CD-ROM

Four of the file folders are for your convenience in storing your work. You will create files for the following: Supplies, Work in Progress (in which to keep your unfinished work), Completed Work, and Encounter Forms. You will use the other six file folders for filing patient records. You will want to examine the materials so that you remember what you have and where you have put things.

INSTRUCTIONS

1. Create four working folders by clearly printing one file name on a label for each file: Supplies (see figure below), Work in Progress, Completed Work, and Encounter Forms.

File folder for supplies

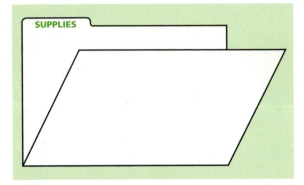

Source: Delmar/Cengage Learning

2. Enclosed is a letter to you from your employers, Douglasville Medicine Associates. When you read it, feel the welcome it conveys to you as a newcomer to the office. Keep it in your *Medical Office Practice* package.

3. Place the folded appointment schedule and daysheet (11" × 17" forms) in your Supplies folder.

4. File the four folders alphabetically in your *Medical Office Practice* package with the file names facing forward.

5. Return unused materials, leftover file folders, file labels, flash drive, and MOSS CD-ROM to the *Medical Office Practice* package until needed.

JOB 1
Introduction to HIPAA and Signing a Confidentiality Statement

MATERIALS AND SUPPLIES

- Form: Job 1—HIPAA Privacy Module
- Form: Job 1—Confidentiality Statement

TIME ALLOTMENT

30 minutes

OCTOBER 5, 2010

As a student medical office assistant of Douglasville Medicine Associates, you will be working with patient files, which must be treated with strictest confidentiality in order to uphold patient privacy.

Today Mrs. Fleet has asked you to familiarize yourself with the **HIPAA (Health Insurance Portability and Accountability Act)** Privacy Module, which outlines important confidentiality guidelines for the practice and delineates your specific roles and responsibilities as an employee in protecting patient health information. After you have finished reading the Module, Mrs. Fleet will answer any questions you may have. She has also requested that you sign a Confidentiality Statement, acknowledging that you have received HIPAA training and agreeing that you will abide by the HIPAA Privacy Regulations.

INSTRUCTIONS

1. Read the HIPAA Privacy Module for Douglasville Medicine Associates in its entirety. (Your instructor may wish to discuss specific details of the Module with you and your fellow "workers.")

2. Using the reading as a guide, answer the following questions:
   a. Who should have access to a patient's protected health information (PHI)?
   b. What are some examples of PHI?
   c. What are "covered entities" under HIPAA? Who is included in that category?
   d. Using the glossary, define a health care clearinghouse.
   e. Who must sign a Notice of Privacy Practices at Douglasville Medicine Associates?
   f. When it is necessary to get a signed authorization form from a patient?

3. If you have no further questions, read and complete the Confidentiality Statement. (Flora Mae Fleet, RN, would witness your signature by signing and dating the form as well; however, since this is a simulation, you can ask one of your classmates to sign and date your form.)

4. File the Confidentiality Statement and the answers to the above questions in your Completed Work folder. File your HIPAA Privacy Module information in your Supplies folder for future reference.

JOB 2
Concepts of Effective Communication—Revising a Patient Information Brochure

MATERIALS AND SUPPLIES

- Flash Drive
- Form *on the flash drive*: Job 2—Patient Information Sheet
- Form *in Job Training Manual*: Job 2—Patient Information Sheet

TIME ALLOTMENT

45 minutes

OCTOBER 6, 2010

Due to recent practice changes, the physicians have asked that the Patient Information Sheet be updated. Additionally, the staff members have suggested that the Patient Information Sheet be turned into a brochure to modernize the look and create a more portable way to share information. Mrs. Fleet would like you to use your creativity to design a brochure that includes the revised information in the old Patient Information Sheet. She also has given you the liberty of adding pictures, borders, or color, as long as they are professional, practice related, and in good taste.

INSTRUCTIONS

1. Retrieve the following form from your flash drive: Job 2—Patient Information Sheet.
2. Remove the out-of-date copy of the Patient Information Sheet from the Forms section in this *Job Training Manual*; the Job number is indicated on it).
3. Read the form carefully; the information in it will be helpful to you in the days to come.
4. Check the changes for correct spelling and for where the insertions are to be placed.
5. Prepare your brochure.
6. Proofread and make your copy correct.
7. Save your work on your flash drive.
8. Print out and place the finished brochure in your Completed Work folder. (Always file your rough drafts with your finished pages for reference should your finished work be questioned.)

 It is very important that you save your finished work on your flash drive for this job and all future jobs.

JOB 3
Administrative Functions—Blocking the Schedule Using MOSS

MATERIALS AND SUPPLIES

- Medical Office Simulation Software (MOSS)
- Revised Patient Information Brochure from your Completed Work Folder

TIME ALLOTMENT

75 minutes

OCTOBER 7, 2010

Mrs. Fleet has approved your changes to the Patient Information Brochure, and now you are ready to incorporate those scheduling changes into the office computer system for October and November 2010. This is a very important step since those changes will directly impact patient scheduling. However, Mrs. Fleet has outlined the directions for you below and will be working with you directly today to accomplish this task. It will be important for you to follow her directions carefully in order to ensure that each physician's schedule is blocked off correctly in accordance with his or her obligations.

INSTRUCTIONS

Since this is the first job that requires MOSS software, follow the instructions in Appendix C to install and open MOSS on your computer. If you are using the single-user version, your name and password are already populated for you, and you can click OK at the password prompt. You should now be in the program, at the Main Menu screen. **Network Version Note: If you are using MOSS 2.0 Network Version to complete this activity, your login name and password will be provided by your instructor.**

1. From the Main Menu, click on Appointment Scheduling. The Practice Schedule appears. On the bottom of the Practice Schedule, click on the Block Calendar button (Figure 3-1).

2. A prompt will ask if you wish to create a new calendar block. Click Yes.

3. Now you must complete the block calendar input window, Fields 1 to 9. We will start with Dr. Mendenhall.

   a. Field 1 is the description of the block and will appear on the schedule once saved. Dr. Mendenhall will be out of the office because she will be on rounds at the New York County Hospital. In Field 1, type "Rounds @ NYCH." (You will have to abbreviate—New York County Hospital does not fit into the field.)

   b. Fields 2 and 3 require start and end dates for the block. You will note from the updated physician schedule that Dr. Mendenhall only rounds at New York County Hospital on Fridays, and the first Friday in October is October 1. Type the date 10/01/2010 in Field 2. The last Friday in November is November 26. In Field 3, type 11/26/2010. (You are using these dates for the purposes of this simulation only. In a real practice, you would block out dates for as long as necessary.)

   c. In Field 4, enter 9:00 a.m., the time Dr. Mendenhall will begin her rounds at New York County Hospital.

FIGURE 3-1

The Block Calendar button on the practice schedule

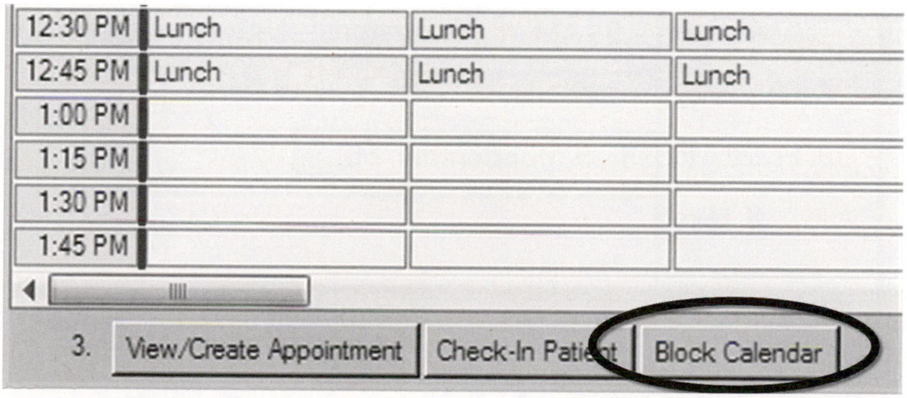

Source: Delmar/Cengage Learning

d. Field 5 requires that you enter the time Dr. Mendenhall will continue her rounds (IN MINUTES). Therefore, you must figure out how many hours Dr. Mendenhall will be on rounds and multiply that times 60 to find the minutes. (Dr. Mendenhall will be on rounds from 9:00 a.m. until 12:00 noon, which is 3 hours. So, $3 \times 60 = 180$ minutes.) Use the drop-down menu to select 180 in Field 5.

e. Field 6 indicates frequency, which means that you are indicating how often this block will occur—whether this is a one-time event, a weekly event, monthly event, and so on. Dr. Mendenhall rounds every week. Use the drop-down menu to select "Weekly."

f. Field 7 is automatically computed based on the information you entered in Fields 2, 3, and 6.

g. In Field 8, use the drop-down menu to select Dr. Mendenhall's name, since she is the physician for whom you are blocking the schedule.

h. Field 9 gives you space to make notes, if necessary. You will leave that blank.

i. Check your work with Figure 3-2, and then click Save.

4. A pop-up menu will indicate that the break information has been posted. Click OK. Now click the Close button to return to the Practice Schedule.

5. You can check to see if Dr. Mendenhall is blocked out by navigating to any Friday in October or November 2010. To navigate to October 1, 2010, use the calendar in the upper right corner of the Practice Schedule. Use the Y− and Y+ buttons to move back and forward between years. Use the M− and M+ to move forward and back between months (see Figure 3-3). Then, click in the calendar to go to a specific day. Alternately, you can type in a specific date (10/01/2010) in the field next to "Go To," located below

FIGURE 3-2
Check your work for Step 3

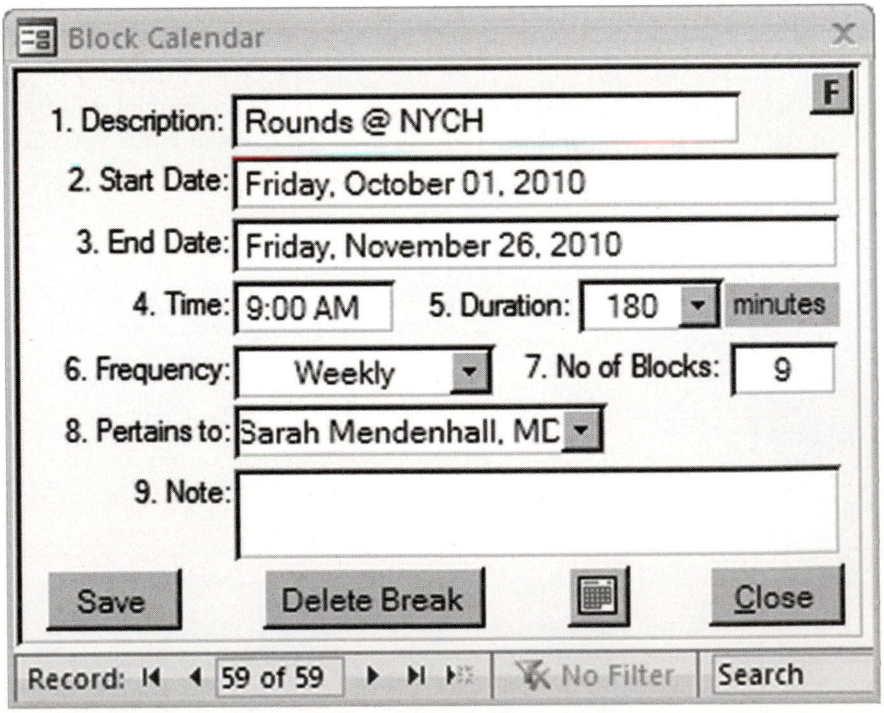

Source: Delmar/Cengage Learning

FIGURE 3-3
Using the calendar to navigate to a specific day in the practice schedule

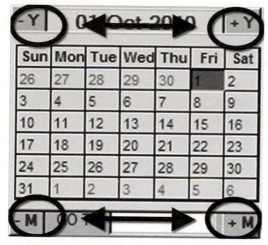

Source: Delmar/Cengage Learning

the calendar. Figure 3-4 shows Dr. Mendenhall's block on Friday, October 1, on the Practice Schedule.

6. Next, you will be blocking off Dr. Mendenhall's schedule from 5:00 p.m. to 6:00 p.m. every day, since she is finished seeing patients at 5:00 p.m. Click on Block Calendar at the bottom of the Practice Schedule. (If you are not already in the Practice Schedule, start by clicking Appointment Scheduling from the Main Menu, and then Block Calendar at the bottom of the Practice Schedule.) Click Yes when prompted to create a new block.

a. Since Dr. Mendenhall is off from 5:00 p.m. to 6:00 p.m., you will type "OFF" in Field 1.

FIGURE 3-4
The appointment schedule block for Dr. Mendenhall as it appears on the practice schedule

Time	HEATH	SCHWARTZ	MENDENHALL
9:00 AM			Rounds @ NYCH
9:15 AM			Rounds @ NYCH
9:30 AM			Rounds @ NYCH
9:45 AM			Rounds @ NYCH
10:00 AM			Rounds @ NYCH
10:15 AM			Rounds @ NYCH
10:30 AM			Rounds @ NYCH
10:45 AM			Rounds @ NYCH
11:00 AM			Rounds @ NYCH
11:15 AM			Rounds @ NYCH
11:30 AM			Rounds @ NYCH
11:45 AM			Rounds @ NYCH
12:00 PM	Lunch	Lunch	Lunch
12:15 PM	Lunch	Lunch	Lunch
12:30 PM	Lunch	Lunch	Lunch
12:45 PM	Lunch	Lunch	Lunch
1:00 PM			
1:15 PM			
1:30 PM			
1:45 PM			

Source: Delmar/Cengage Learning

b. The start date (Field 2) will be Friday, October 1, 2010, and your end date will be Tuesday, November 30, 2010 (Field 3), to include all off October and November.

c. In Field 4, enter 5:00 p.m.

d. The duration (Field 5) is 60 minutes (1 hour = 60 minutes).

e. The frequency is Daily, since she is off every day at the same time.

f. Field 7 is automatically populated after you select the frequency.

g. Use the drop-down menu in Field 8 to choose Dr. Mendenhall.

h. Leave Field 9 blank.

i. Check your work with Figure 3-5 and click Save. A pop-up menu will indicate that the break information has been posted. Click OK. Now click the Close button to return to the Practice Schedule. (You may double-check your work by clicking on any date in October and November through the appointment schedule calendar and viewing Dr. Mendenhall's schedule from 5:00 p.m. to 6:00 p.m.)

Correcting Mistakes in Block Scheduling: If you make a mistake in blocking off the schedule and you have already saved your work, follow the steps below to correct it:

■ Click on Appointment Scheduling in the Main Menu (if you are not already there).

■ Single click on any time slot within your "error" time. (For example, if you blocked off time past 5:00 p.m., and you should have only blocked off time UNTIL 5:00 p.m., click anywhere within that time frame and then click on "Block Calendar.") This should bring up that particular blocking information that you wish to edit.

■ Click Delete Break. This will delete the current information from the calendar and allow you to insert the correct information into the system.

■ Be sure to click on "Save" when you are through entering the correct information and double-check your work in the calendar when you are finished.

FIGURE 3-5
Check your work for Step 6

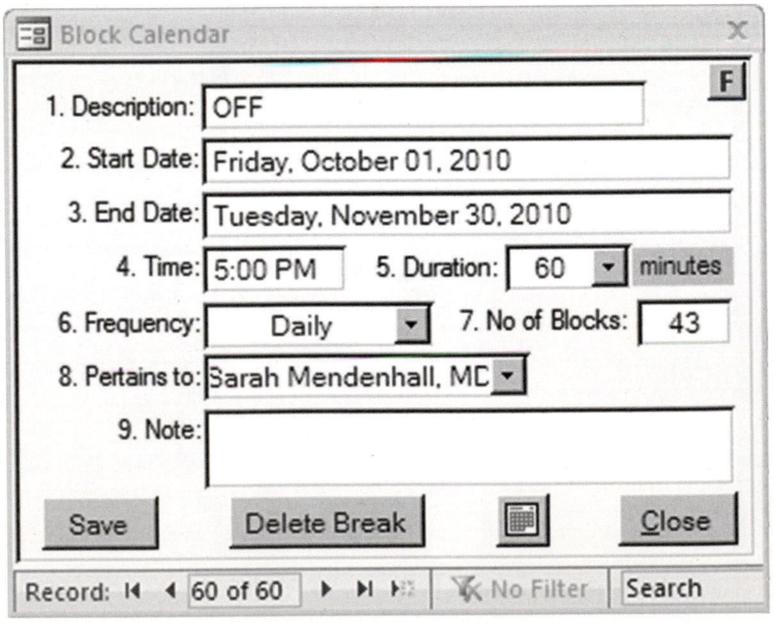

Source: Delmar/Cengage Learning

7. Finally, Dr. Mendenhall is off on Friday afternoons from 1:00 p.m. to 5:00 p.m. Using the steps used in the previous two examples, block off Dr. Mendenhall's schedule appropriately. You may compare your screen with Figure 3-6 before saving, and then check your work by looking at Dr. Mendenhall's schedule. Click on any Friday during the months of October or November to verify.

8. Dr. Heath will be on rounds at Retirement Inn every Wednesday from 1:00 p.m. to 6:00 p.m. Use the calendar to determine start and end dates, and block off his schedule for October and November. Use "Retirement Inn" as your description in Field 1. Compare your screen with Figure 3-7 before clicking Save.

9. Dr. Schwartz will be on rounds at the Community General Hospital every Tuesday from 10:00 a.m. to 12:00 noon. Use the calendar to determine start and end dates, and block off his schedule for October and November accordingly. Use "Rounds @ Comm Gen" as your description for Field 1.

Compare your screen with Figure 3-8 before clicking Save.

10. Dr. Schwartz does not begin office hours until 10:00 a.m. Therefore, you must block off his schedule daily from 9:00 a.m. until 10:00 a.m. Additionally, Dr. Schwartz leaves the practice at 5:00 p.m. You will need to block off his schedule from 5:00 p.m. to 6:00 p.m. daily. Using the steps learned in the previous examples, block off his schedule appropriately for the months of October and November 2010.

11. All three physicians are off for the Thanksgiving holiday, which falls on Thursday, November 25, 2010. You will need to block all three physicians out on this day. Begin by blocking out Dr. Mendenhall from 9:00 am to 12:00 noon and then again from 1:00 p.m. to 5:00 p.m. (You cannot block out the lunch hours as they are set up as part of the practice hours in the software. They will need to remain as is.) The description will be HOLIDAY. Block Dr. Heath out from 9:00 a.m. to 12:00 noon and then again from

FIGURE 3-6

Check your work for Step 7

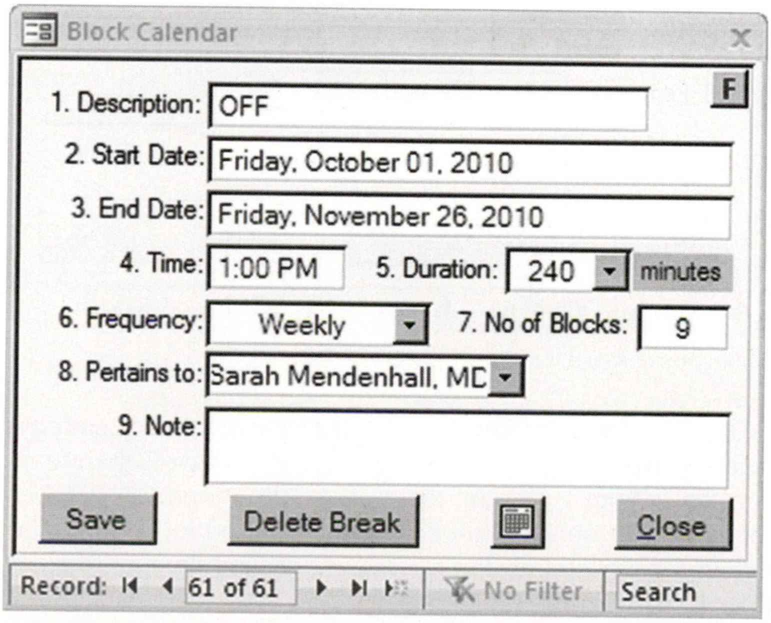

Source: Delmar/Cengage Learning

FIGURE 3-7

Check your work for Step 8

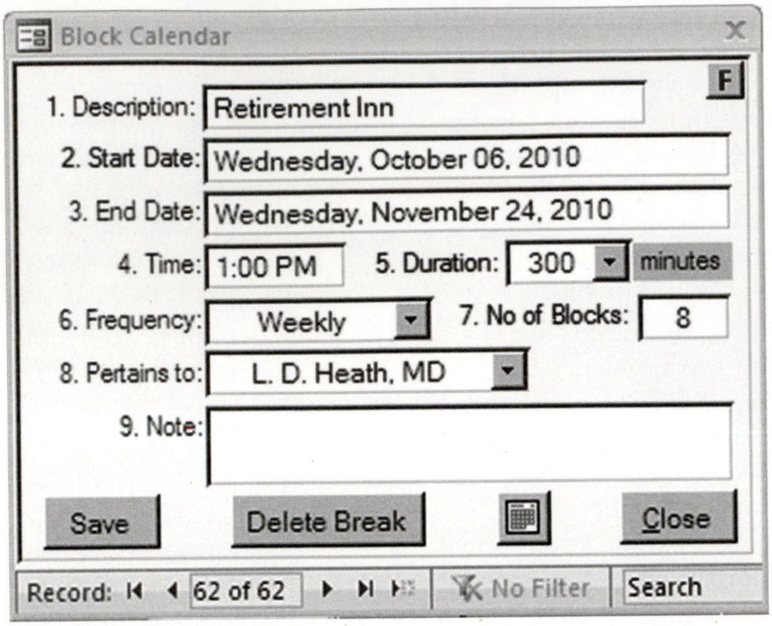

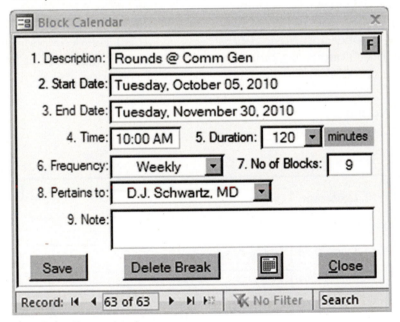

Source: Delmar/Cengage Learning

FIGURE 3-8

Check your work for Step 9

Source: Delmar/Cengage Learning

1:00 p.m. to 6:00 p.m. Dr. Schwartz will be blocked out from 10:00 a.m. to 12:00 noon and then from 1:00 p.m. to 5:00 p.m. When you are finished, the Practice Schedule for November 25, 2010, should look like Figure 3-9.

12. Finally, Drs. Heath and Mendenhall each have separate meetings during the month of October and will need to be blocked out on the Practice Schedule. On Tuesday, October 19, 2010, Dr. Heath has a dinner meeting

FIGURE 3-9

The practice schedule for November 25, 2010

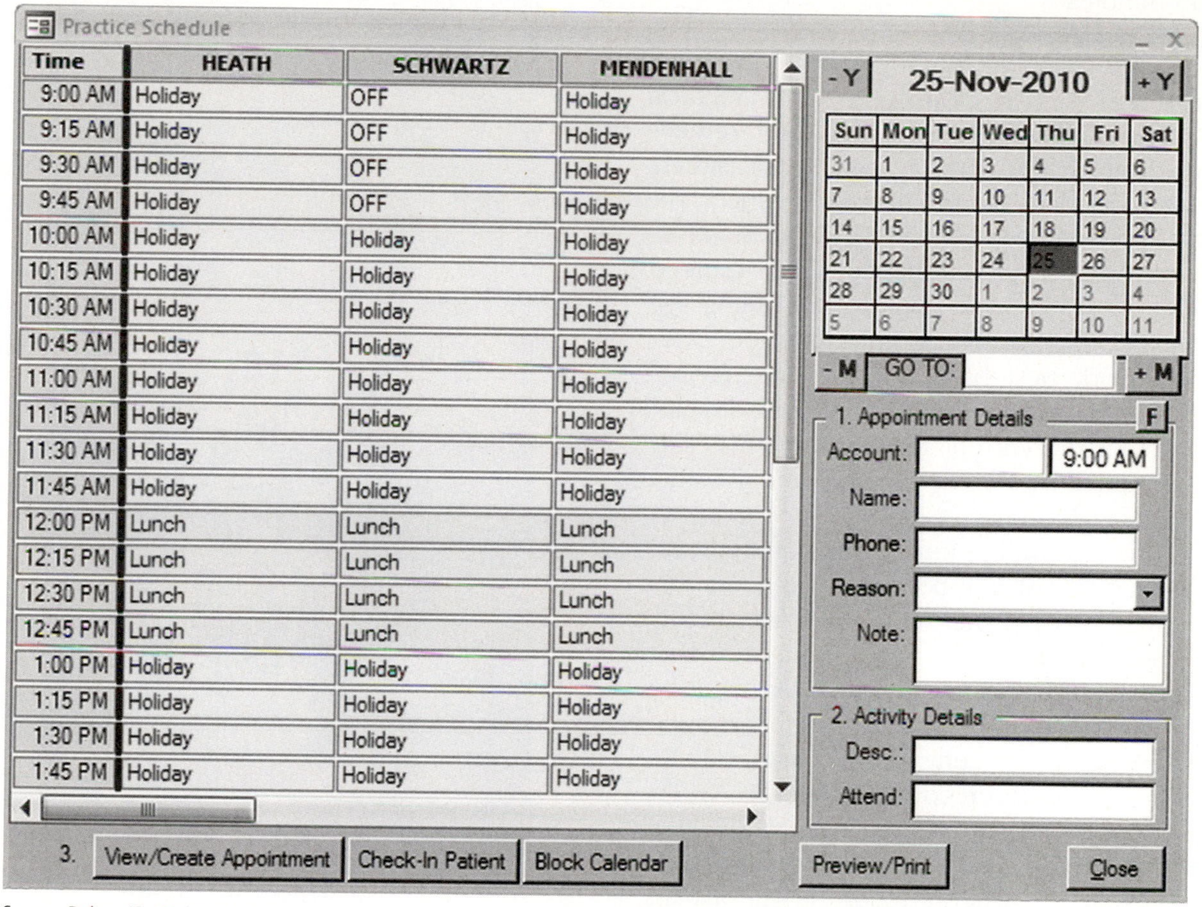

Time	HEATH	SCHWARTZ	MENDENHALL
9:00 AM	Holiday	OFF	Holiday
9:15 AM	Holiday	OFF	Holiday
9:30 AM	Holiday	OFF	Holiday
9:45 AM	Holiday	OFF	Holiday
10:00 AM	Holiday	Holiday	Holiday
10:15 AM	Holiday	Holiday	Holiday
10:30 AM	Holiday	Holiday	Holiday
10:45 AM	Holiday	Holiday	Holiday
11:00 AM	Holiday	Holiday	Holiday
11:15 AM	Holiday	Holiday	Holiday
11:30 AM	Holiday	Holiday	Holiday
11:45 AM	Holiday	Holiday	Holiday
12:00 PM	Lunch	Lunch	Lunch
12:15 PM	Lunch	Lunch	Lunch
12:30 PM	Lunch	Lunch	Lunch
12:45 PM	Lunch	Lunch	Lunch
1:00 PM	Holiday	Holiday	Holiday
1:15 PM	Holiday	Holiday	Holiday
1:30 PM	Holiday	Holiday	Holiday
1:45 PM	Holiday	Holiday	Holiday

25-Nov-2010

Sun	Mon	Tue	Wed	Thu	Fri	Sat
31	1	2	3	4	5	6
7	8	9	10	11	12	13
14	15	16	17	18	19	20
21	22	23	24	25	26	27
28	29	30	1	2	3	4
5	6	7	8	9	10	11

- M   GO TO: + M

1. Appointment Details

Account: 9:00 AM

Name:

Phone:

Reason:

Note:

2. Activity Details

Desc.:

Attend:

3.   View/Create Appointment   Check-In Patient   Block Calendar   Preview/Print   Close

Source: Delmar/Cengage Learning

with a drug company representative beginning at 4:00 p.m. You will need to block out his schedule from 4:00 p.m. until the end of his workday. On the same day, Dr. Mendenhall has her quarterly quality assurance meeting at New York County Hospital from 1:00 p.m. to 5:00 p.m. Using the steps learned previously, block these two times on the Practice Schedule.

13. When you are completely finished with this exercise and have saved your work, file the Patient Information Brochure back in your Completed Work folder. You are now ready to schedule patients using MOSS.

JOB 4
Administrative Functions—Filing Procedures

MATERIALS AND SUPPLIES

- Form: Job 4—Alphabetic Filing Guidelines
- Form: Job 4—Filing Worksheet

TIME ALLOTMENT

45 minutes

OCTOBER 8, 2010

Part of your responsibility as a medical office professional is to file and retrieve medical records using the proper system determined by your physician's office. The two main systems of filing used in physicians' offices are alphabetic and numeric. There are pros and cons to both filing systems, and each office must consider what will work best based on multiple factors, such as ease of retrieval, confidentiality and whether the current manual system is supplemented by a computerized medical office practice.

For example, numeric filing systems utilize a series of numbers as a way to identify each patient. Patient numbers are usually generated randomly from a computer when the patient arrives to the office for his or her first visit to the practice. This number becomes the patient identification number (PIN) or medical record number (MRN). The MRN can be anywhere from 3 digits to 9 digits. Tabs are also color coded so that it is easy to see when a record is out of place (see Figure 4-1). The records are then filed in sequential order from 000 to 9999.

Benefits of numeric filing include ease of filing (everyone knows how to count from 0 to 9, so little training is involved); increased confidentiality (since there are no names included on the medical record tabs, it is more difficult to identify a patient's chart); consistency (there is only one way to file records in numeric sequence); and ease of purging (the oldest records have the lowest numbers).

Drawbacks of numeric filing include double numbers (when one patient has two medical record numbers). This causes a lot of confusion within the system and can be very difficult to correct. When a patient checks in as a "new patient," always remember to check to see if the patient is in the current system. It may be that he or she was a patient many years ago at another practice

FIGURE 4-1

Color-coded tabs on file folders in a numeric filing system

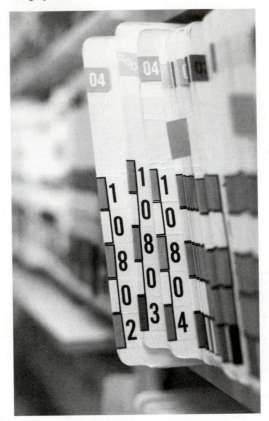

Courtesy of istockphoto.com

location and may still be in the computer. It may also be that a patient is in the system under a previous or maiden name. You would be unable to recognize this if you did not check first. This can be done by entering the patient's social security number rather than the patient's name. In the case of a numeric filing system, if you forget to check, you may generate another number for this patient.

Other drawbacks of numeric filing include transposing numbers when placing the stickers on the chart (giving the patient a chart with the number 073456 when the computer-generated number is actually 073465) or filing the chart in the wrong section due to transposing numbers (i.e., filing chart number 09696 under 09669). However, in the second example, the chart should noticeably stand out due to the color blocking system that is in place. Finally, numeric files must always be cross-referenced with patient names in another location (such as a paper filing system). If the computer system goes down and you must locate John Smith's chart for an emergency appointment, you will need to reference the paper file to determine his chart number in order to pull his chart.

Alphabetic filing systems utilize letters in sequence to make record retrieval and filing simple. Color blocking is used to assist in ease of retrieval, as well as to identify when a chart is out of place.

Benefits of an alphabetic filing system include rapid retrieval (a chart on patient John A. Smith can be easily be located by looking through the "S" tabs until you locate the "Smi" charts and then continuing until you locate the correct patient). Medical records are typically filed using the first three letters of the patient's last name (see Figure 4-2). Another benefit of alphabetic filing system includes having the same names together (instant reference rather than having to cross-reference a number with a name as in numeric filing).

Drawbacks of an alphabetic filing system include increased training (there must be consistency with filing rules and interpretations); files with patient names misspelled; transposition of letters causing misfiling; and increased filing time.

Douglasville Medicine Associates uses an alphabetic filing system, which will remain in place for the medical records that are still in paper form (and for those records that are inactive) until all data are put into the computerized medical office system. Mrs. Fleet would like to make sure that you are familiar with the proper filing procedures.

The Association of Records Managers and Administrators (ARMA) has published general guidelines and simplified filing rules to follow to provide and maintain consistency

FIGURE 4-2

Alphabetic filing systems typically use the first three letters of the patient's last name

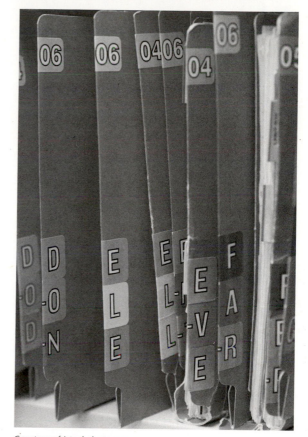

Courtesy of istockphoto.com

throughout this process, and Mrs. Fleet has given you a quick reference guide (Form: Job 4—Alphabetic Filing Guidelines) to use based on their recommendations.

INSTRUCTIONS

1. Review the guidelines in Form: Job 4—Alphabetic Filing Guidelines and then complete Form: Job 4— Filing Worksheet.

2. When you have finished, file the worksheet (Form: Job 4—Filing Worksheet) in your Completed Work folder.

JOB 5
Administrative Functions and Managed Care/Insurance— Preparing Patient Files

MATERIALS AND SUPPLIES

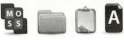

- Medical Office Simulation Software (MOSS)
- 6 File Folders
- Alphanumeric File Labels
- 6 Patient Information Forms: Job 5—Patient Information Forms for Patients Prosser, Nolte, Lingard, Richard, Alvarez, and Wittmer
- 1 Progress Note Form: Job 5— Progress Note for Patient Prosser
- 3 History and Physical Forms: Job 5—H&P for Patients Alvarez, Wittmer, and Prosser

TIME ALLOTMENT

60 minutes

Note: Due to the simulation aspect of this job, you will be creating patient files similar to files in a real medical office. You will need these to file patient documents throughout the remainder of this medical office simulation experience, even though Douglasville Medicine Associates is in the process of moving toward a computerized electronic medical records (EMR) system. With the EMR system, all patient information is stored in the patient's computerized medical file— from the Patient Information Form, which includes basic demographic information that is obtained on the first new patient visit, to the actual medical history and physical and chart notes, to the patient's medication history. Douglasville Medicine Associates is in the beginning stages of the EMR process,

and part of your job responsibility will be updating Dr. Mendenhall's patients into the computer system as they come in to the office over the next few weeks. Patients for Drs. Heath and Schwartz have already been updated into the system; however, it will be important to verify each patient's demographic data (i.e., address, telephone number, and insurance information) since the information in the patient files and the information initially keyed into the computer system may have changed since the patient's last visit. Finally, keep in mind that some medical offices are still utilizing charts in the office that are filed either alphabetically or numerically. In this job, you will be using an alphabetical filing system.

PRIOR TO COMPLETING TASKS FOR JOB 5:

Prepare six patient file folders for Harold M. Prosser, Theresa F. Lingard, Raymond A. Nolte, Julia T. Richard, Francisco B. Alvarez, and John J. Wittmer in which to keep their documents for the remainder of this simulation experience. To begin, retrieve the file folders from your *Medical Office Practice* package. Label the top, left horizontal edge of the folder with the last two digits of the current year using the numeric file labels (see Figure 5-1). Leave a little space and print the patient's last name, first name, and middle initial. Finally, using the alphabetical file labels label the top right horizontal edge of the folder with the first three letters of the patient's last name. For example, for Harold Prosser, use the "P," "R," and "O" stickers (refer to Figure 5-1 again). Complete this process for all five patients before moving on to the next phase of this job. Also, since Julia Richard, Francisco Alvarez, and John Wittmer will not be seen today, you may file their Patient Information Forms in their files for future reference.

OCTOBER 8, 2010

Today Mrs. Fleet has assigned you to the front desk to assist Mei Ling Chun, RMA, with check-in. You will be performing

FIGURE 5-1
Open folder showing placement of patient name, information form, and progress note

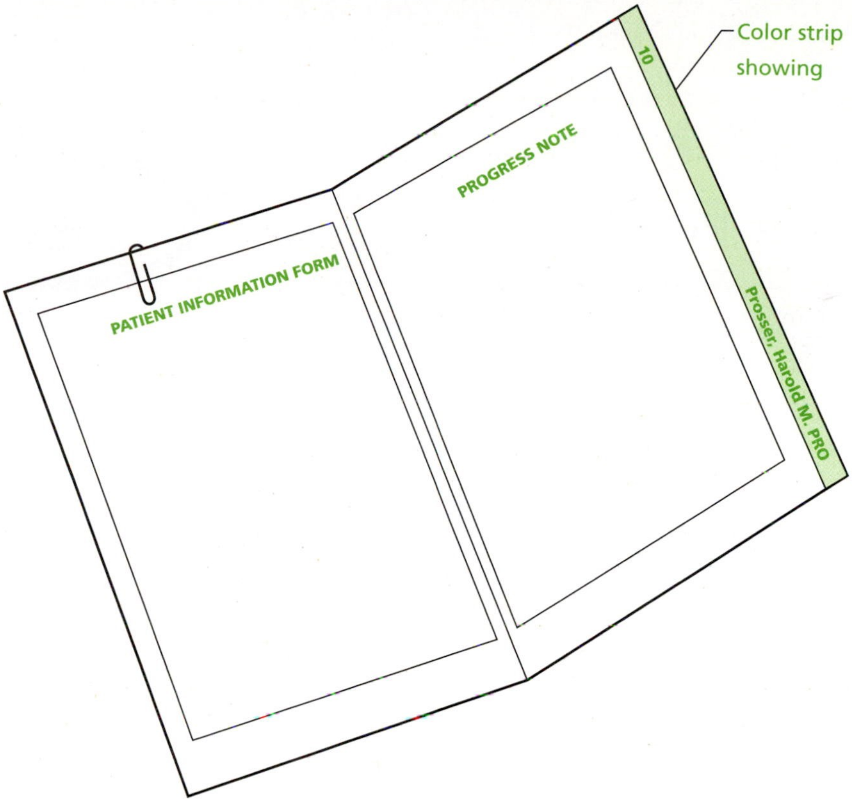

Source: Delmar/Cengage Learning

basic data entry, updating, and entering patient information into the computer as patients check in. *Before beginning this exercise, log in to MOSS and begin at the Main Menu. Be sure that Feedback Mode is turned off when completing these exercises. Information about logging in to MOSS and using Feedback Mode is found in Appendix C.*

INSTRUCTIONS

A. **Mr. Prosser checks in first.** He is a patient of Dr. Mendenhall's and is returning for his one-month follow-up visit for a gastrointestinal problem. Mr. Prosser has updated his Patient Information Form today. Using his completed Patient Information Form, update his information in the computer using the following steps.

1. From the Main Menu screen of MOSS, click on Patient Registration.

2. Type "Prosser" in the Search Criteria field and click the Search button (see Figure 5-2). (You can also use the arrow key and scroll bar to scroll down to find the name "Prosser" in the list of patient names.)

3. Since Mr. Prosser is an established patient of Dr. Mendenhall, he is already in the system. Single click on his name in the patient list and click on the Select button, since you will be updating his information. (You would choose Add if you were adding a new patient into the system.)

4. Double-check his demographic information (address, phone number, social security number, date of

FIGURE 5-2
Using the search screen in MOSS

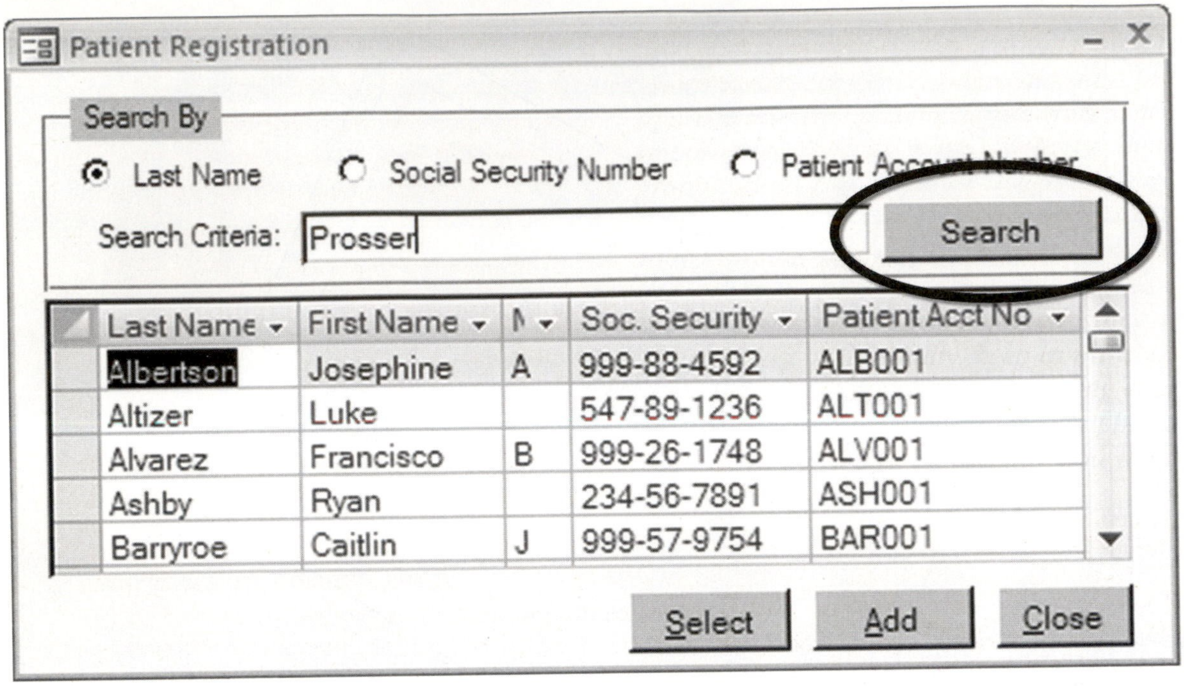

Source: Delmar/Cengage Learning

birth, etc.) shown on the Patient Information screen by comparing it to his Patient Information Form. (For Field 21 in the program, Mr. Prosser is the Responsible Party, meaning that he is responsible for paying the bill; he carries the insurance, which is Century SeniorGap, as noted on his Patient Information Form.) If all information is correct, click on tab for Spouse/Parent/Other, since Mr. Prosser is married and has also listed a next of kin.

5. On the Spouse/Parent/Other tab, add Mr. Prosser's spousal information, including name, date of birth, and social security number. Select the radio button next to Female (the default for this is Male). Check your work with Figure 5-3 and click Save. Click through the prompts, confirming you have saved the information.

6. While on the Spouse/Parent/Other tab, click the Address button. Since Mrs. Prosser's address is the same as Mr. Prosser's, click the button Copy Pt Addr. When you do, the address populates automatically (see Figure 5-4). Click Close when you are finished with the address window. Always click Save before proceeding to the next window.

7. Next, click on the Primary Insurance tab to update Mr. Prosser's insurance information. Mr. Prosser is the policyholder, and Century SeniorGap is his insurance. Be sure to enter his ID# (Field 8) from the Patient Information Form. If his name is not populated in Fields 3 and 4, enter it now. Dr. Mendenhall accepts assignment and is a participating physician with Century SeniorGap, so the Yes boxes in Fields 13 and 15 should be selected. Mr. Prosser's signature is on file, so you may select the Yes box in Field 14. Check your work with Figure 5-5 and click Save.

FIGURE 5-3

Check your work for Step 5

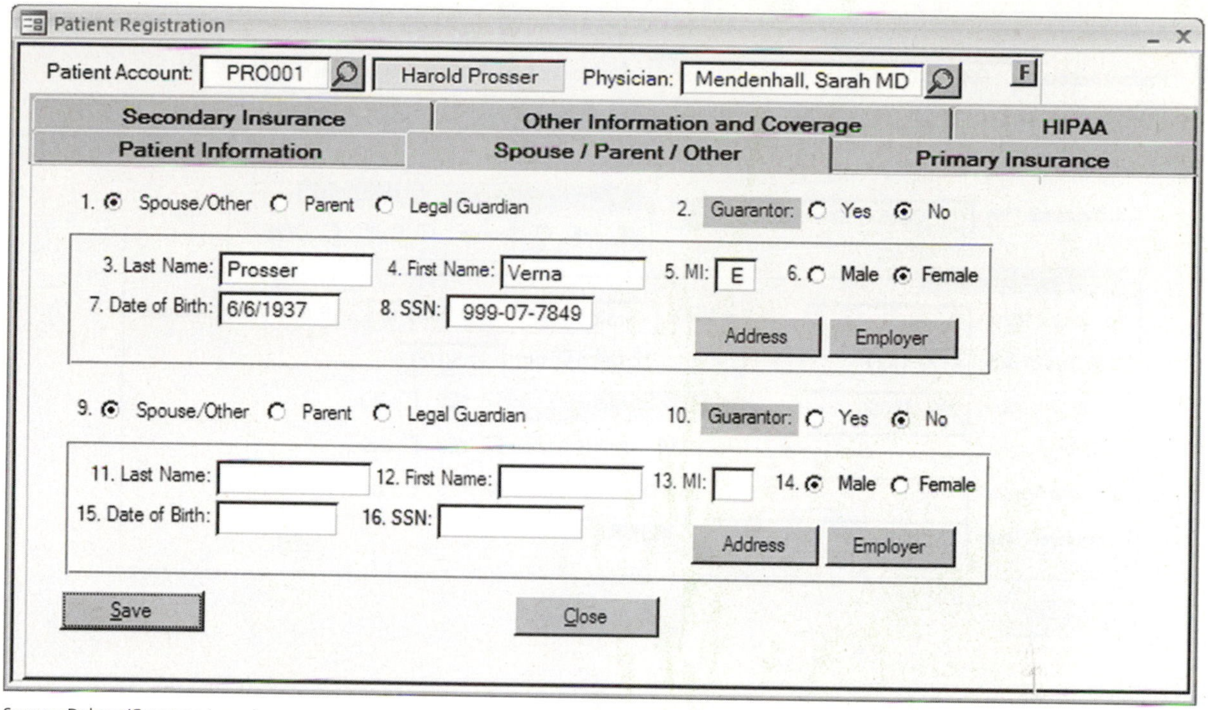

Source: Delmar/Cengage Learning

FIGURE 5-4

Check your work for Step 6

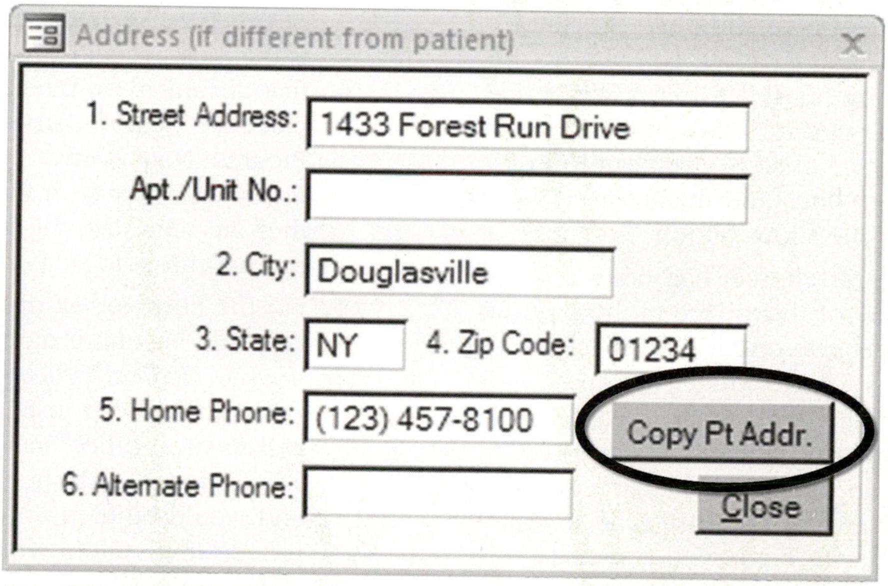

Source: Delmar/Cengage Learning

8. Finally, it is important to ensure that Mr. Prosser has received a copy of the HIPAA (Health Insurance Portability and Accountability Act) Privacy Notice.

Click on the HIPAA tab. On that screen, click on the Privacy Notice button. You will see the Privacy Notice for Douglasville Medicine Associates. (This should be printed

FIGURE 5-5
Check your work for Step 7

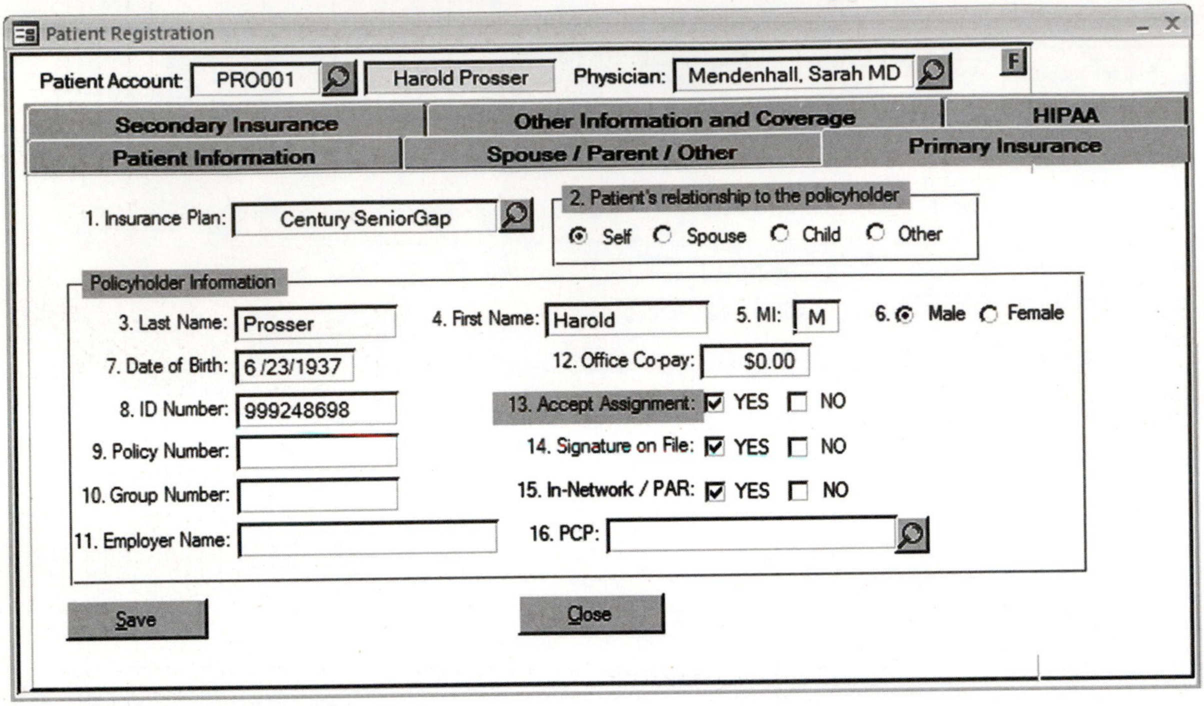

Source: Delmar/Cengage Learning

out for each patient if the field next to "HIPAA form given to patient/guardian box" indicates No. Since this is a simulation, you will not be printing out this form; however, in a real medical office, a HIPAA Privacy Notice is given out to every patient once and documented.) Click the Close button.

9. Since Mr. Prosser had not received a copy of this notice in the past, he will receive one today. Check the boxes for Yes in Fields 1 and 2, indicating that he received the form and that the form was signed by him. In the date fields, enter today's date, October 8, 2010. Check your work with Figure 5-6 and click Save. Click through the prompts. Click Close until you have returned to the Main Menu screen.

10. You have now finished data entry for Mr. Prosser. File his Patient Information Forms, new on top of old, on the left side of his chart.

Now find his Progress Note and H&P, and file them on the right side of his chart. Since his Progress Note is the most recent document, place that document on the top, and place the H&P underneath the Progress Note. (Always file the most recent documents on the top so that they are seen first; this is known as reverse chronological order.)

11. For the purposes of this simulation only, file his entire medical record in your *Medical Office Practice* package, keeping in mind that in a real medical office, medical records would never leave the premises and would be filed in an established filing system with the highest confidentiality.

B. **Mr. Raymond Nolte comes to the front desk to check in next.** He is being seen for a severe case of sunburn from his recent trip to the Caribbean. Since he is a new patient, you will need to add his information

FIGURE 5-6
Check your work for Step 9

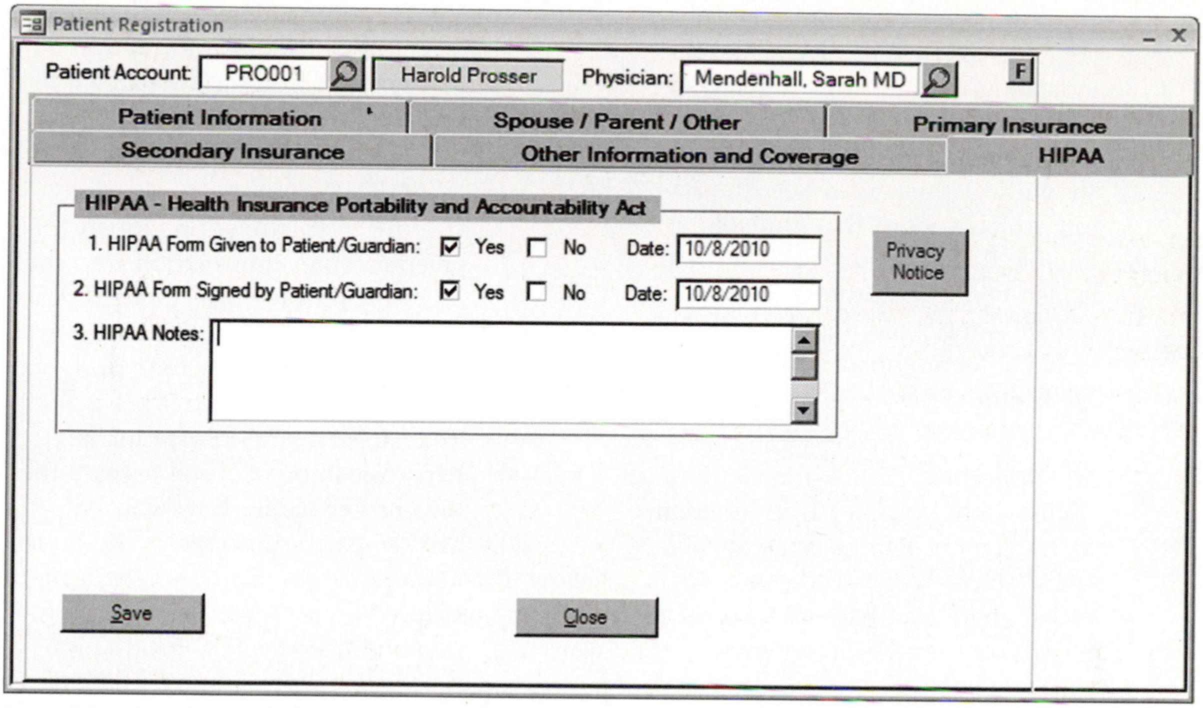

Source: Delmar/Cengage Learning

into MOSS. Mr. Nolte has already completed his Patient Information Form. Additionally, he has received, read, and signed the HIPAA Privacy Notice.

1. From the Main Menu, click Patient Registration. Type "Nolte" in the search box. *(Note: Even though Mr. Nolte is a new patient to the practice, it is important to always begin by typing the name into the computer system first. In this particular case, Mr. Nolte called to make his appointment to see Dr. Mendenhall, and some information was taken over the phone and entered into the system; therefore, his name is already entered into the system. Additionally, if Mr. Nolte had been a patient of the practice years ago, it would be important to ensure that you did not add him without double-checking that he was not already in the system.)* Highlight Mr. Nolte's name in the patient list and click the Select button.

2. Proceed through each screen (Patient Information, Spouse/ Parent/Other, Primary Insurance, and HIPAA) as you did in the previous case study, making sure to save your data with each screen as you go along. Some information may already be entered; double-check this information for accuracy. When you have finished, click Close until you return to the Main Menu screen.

3. Since Mr. Nolte is a new patient today, you will need to verify his insurance eligibility through the online eligibility feature in MOSS. From the Main Menu, click Online Eligibility. Type "Nolte" in the search box (or scroll down to choose Raymond Nolte from the patient list) and click Search. Highlight Mr. Nolte in the patient list, and click Select.

4. Review the information for accuracy, and then click the Send to Payer

button at the bottom right corner of your screen. This will begin the online process of verification. When verified, you will receive a message indicating that transmission is complete (see Figure 5-7). Click "View" to see the transmission report, shown in Figure 5-8. (Note the status, which verifies that Mr. Nolte is Eligible through Signal HMO. There is also verification that the policyholder is the patient and the provider is Dr. Mendenhall, whom he will be seeing today.)

5. When you are finished entering Mr. Nolte's data, click the Close button until you return to the Main Menu screen. File his Patient Information Form on the left side of his chart. File his entire medical record in your *Medical Office Practice* package.

C. **Theresa Lingard checks in next.** She is also a new patient to Dr. Mendenhall. However, most of her information was retrieved over the phone prior to her appointment and entered into the computer. You will need to verify that this information is correct by comparing it with her Patient Information Form. She comes in today with flu-like symptoms. After being given the HIPAA Privacy Notice, she reads and signs the form.

1. Use the instructions previously given to enter information into the MOSS system for Mrs. Lingard. Use caution when entering data into the Patient Information screen and the Primary Insurance screen. Mrs. Lingard is the Responsible Party, meaning she will receive the bills in her name; however, Mrs. Lingard's husband is the guarantor since the insurance is in his name. You will need to enter information and/or verify information on the following screens: Patient Information, Spouse/Parent/Other—including spouses address and employer, Primary Insurance, and HIPAA. Be sure to note that

FIGURE 5-7
Online eligibility status screen

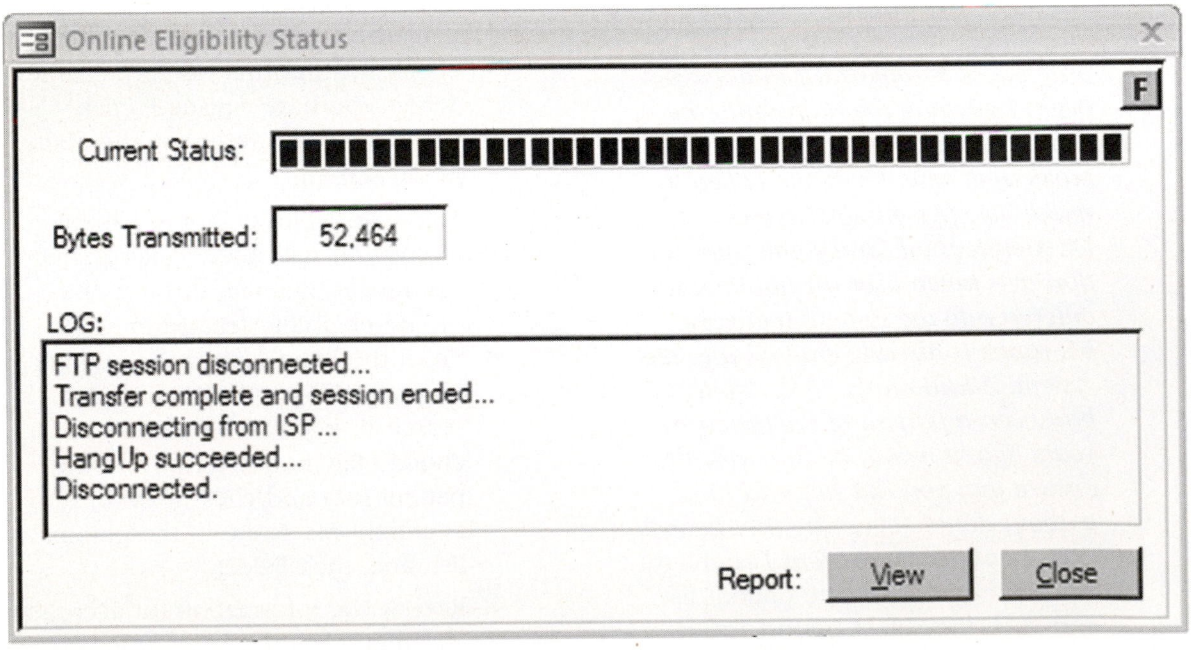

ONLINE ELIGIBILITY TRANSMISSION REPORT

Date: 2/5/2010

User ID: Student1

Insurance Provider: SIGNAL HMO

Policyholder: Nolte, Raymond

Status: ELIGIBLE

Patient Name: Nolte, Raymond

Date of Birth: 6/10/1971

Gender: Male

Account No

NOL001

Provider Name: Mendenhall, Sarah

Office CoPayment: $10.00

Office Deductible: $0.00

Source: Delmar/Cengage Learning

the patient's signature is on file at the Primary Insurance screen. Since Theresa's husband, Robin, is employed, you may click on the Employer button at the Spouse/Parent/Other screen to verify that this information has been filled in (hint: be sure the ID and Group Numbers are updated). Be sure to save your work on each screen. Return to the Main Menu when finished.

2. Since Theresa Lingard is a new patient today, you will also need to verify her insurance eligibility. Using the instructions given for Mr. Nolte's online eligibility

verification, complete the process for Mrs. Lingard. When verified, you will receive a message indicating that transmission is complete. Click View to see the transmission report. (Note the status, which verifies that Mrs. Lingard is Eligible through FlexiHealth PPO In-Network. There is also verification that the policyholder is her husband, Robin, and that her provider is Dr. Mendenhall, whom she will be seeing today.)

3. After you have completed data entry for Mrs. Lingard, file her Patient Information Form in her chart on the left-hand side. File the

verification of insurance underneath her Patient Information Form. File her entire medical record in your *Medical Office Practice* package.

D. Enter the remaining patients' (Julia Richard, Francisco Alvarez, and John Wittmer) details in MOSS, making sure to update the HIPAA tab and run online eligibility reports. File all the hard copy forms properly in each patient's chart. Arrange all your patient charts in alphabetical order in your *Medical Office Practice* package.

Correcting/Editing Patient Information in MOSS: Once data are saved, you can edit it by going back into Patient Registration, selecting the patient's name, choosing the correct tab (such as Primary Insurance, for example), editing the data you need to change, and clicking on Save.

JOB 6
Administrative Functions—Scheduling Patient Appointments

MATERIALS AND SUPPLIES

- Medical Office Simulation Software (MOSS)

TIME ALLOTMENT

1.5 hours

OCTOBER 11, 2010

Today Mrs. Fleet has assigned you to the front desk to work with Mei Ling Chun, RMA. Mei Ling will be assisting you today as you learn computerized patient scheduling. This will be accomplished as patients reschedule for follow-up appointments after seeing the physician, as well as through telephone appointment requests. Your goal in appointment scheduling is to satisfy the patients' requests while adhering to your employers' wishes.

As you know, Douglasville Medicine Associates utilizes a medical office software program known as MOSS, and there are ways to input patient data specific to our practice. For example, all new patients are to be scheduled for 45-minute time slots. Therefore, when scheduling them in the computer, it is imperative that you block out three time slots, since each time slot represents 15 minutes. Established patients are scheduled for 15-minute time slots when they are being seen for follow-up appointments; however, if they are being seen for a physical examination, they should be scheduled for 30 minutes. This means that you must block out two time slots.

Before beginning this exercise, log in to MOSS and begin at the Main Menu. Be sure that Feedback Mode is turned off when completing these exercises. Information about logging in to MOSS and using Feedback Mode is found in Appendix C.

INSTRUCTIONS

1. From the Main Menu, click on Appointment Scheduling. Using the calendar in the upper right-hand corner of the Practice Schedule window, navigate to today's date, October 11, 2010 (use the M−/M+ and Y−/Y+ buttons, or type in today's date in the Go To field).

2. The first patient to arrive at the desk is Francisco Alvarez. He is a patient of Dr. Mendenhall, and he is being seen today for complications related to his diabetes. Dr. Mendenhall has requested that he return in one month for follow-up. Four weeks from today is November 8; however, you are able to schedule Mr. Alvarez any time during

that week. We will first look at Monday, November 8. Use the M+ key to advance to November on the Practice Schedule, and then click on November 8. You will note that Dr. Mendenhall's schedule is open, both in the morning and in the afternoon. However, you understand that Mr. Alvarez usually needs a fasting blood sugar drawn and therefore suggest a morning appointment; Mr. Alvarez agrees and is available anytime in the early morning. You will schedule Mr. Alvarez for a 9:00 a.m. appointment. Since Mr. Alvarez is an established patient, he will only need a 15-minute time appointment.

a. Single click on the 9:00 a.m. time slot on Dr. Mendenhall's schedule and then click on View/Create

Appointment at the bottom of the appointment screen (Figure 6-1).

b. A search screen appears. Enter "Alvarez" and click Search. Highlight Mr. Alvarez's name in the patient list and click Add (Figure 6-2), since you are adding a new appointment.

c. Now, the Patient Appointment Form appears. In Field 2 (physician), click on the magnifying glass and select Dr. Mendenhall (you can either scroll down and click Select or search for her name and click Select). In Field 5, keep the duration at 15 minutes. In Field 6 (reason), use the drop-down menu to select Office Visit (V2). Check your work with Figure 6-3 and click Save Appointment. Click OK

FIGURE 6-1

Single click in the available appointment slot, and then click View/Create appointment

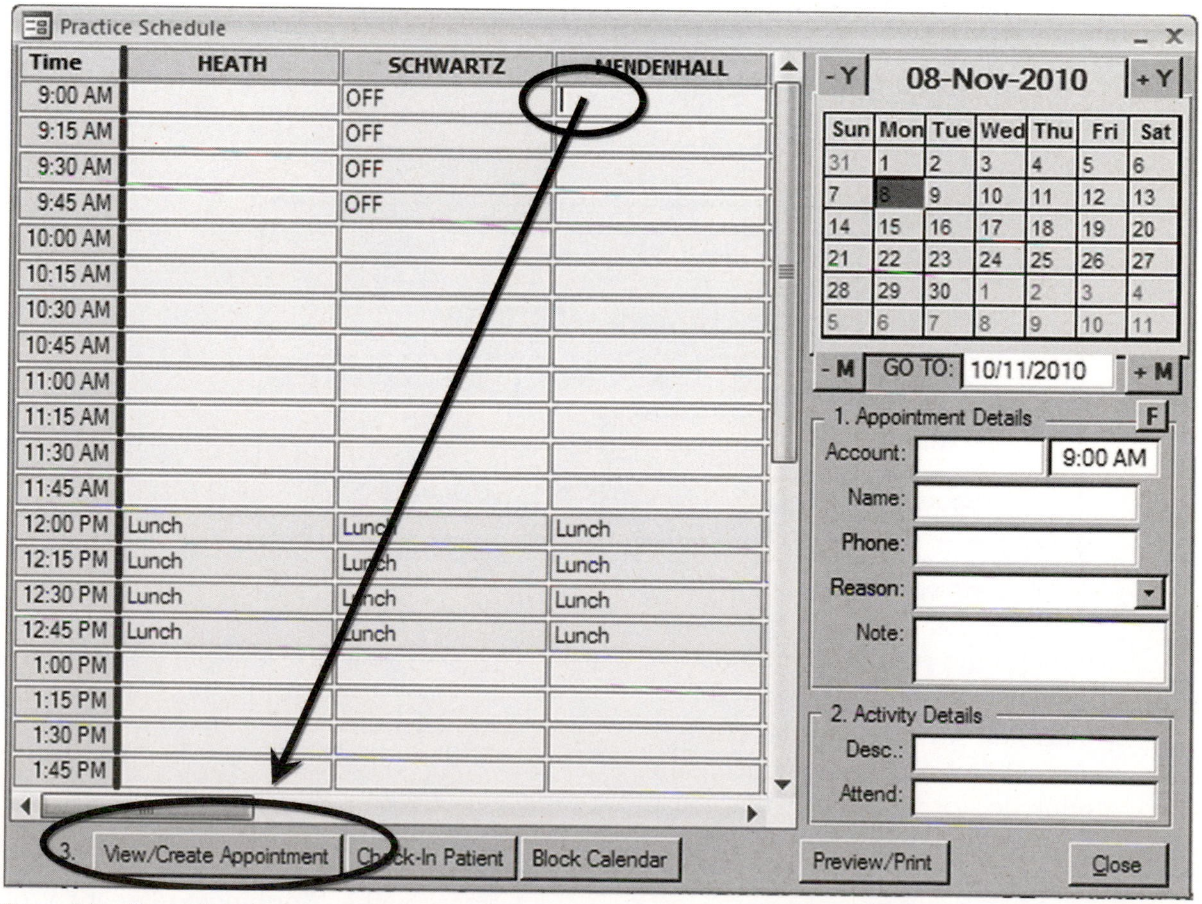

Source: Delmar/Cengage Learning

FIGURE 6-2

Select the patient's name and click Add, to create a new appointment

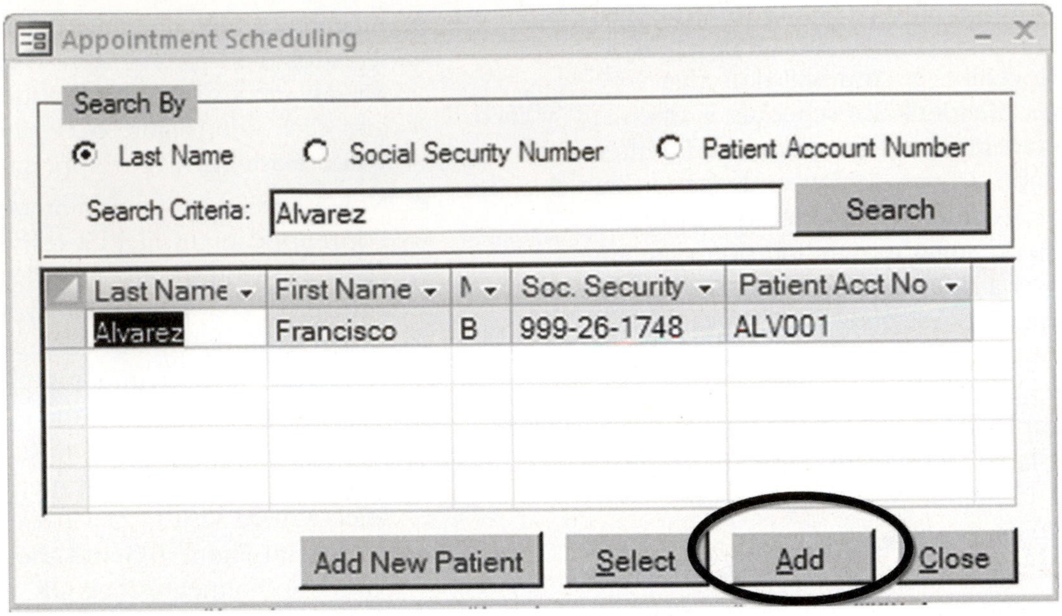

Source: Delmar/Cengage Learning

FIGURE 6-3

Check your work for Step 2C

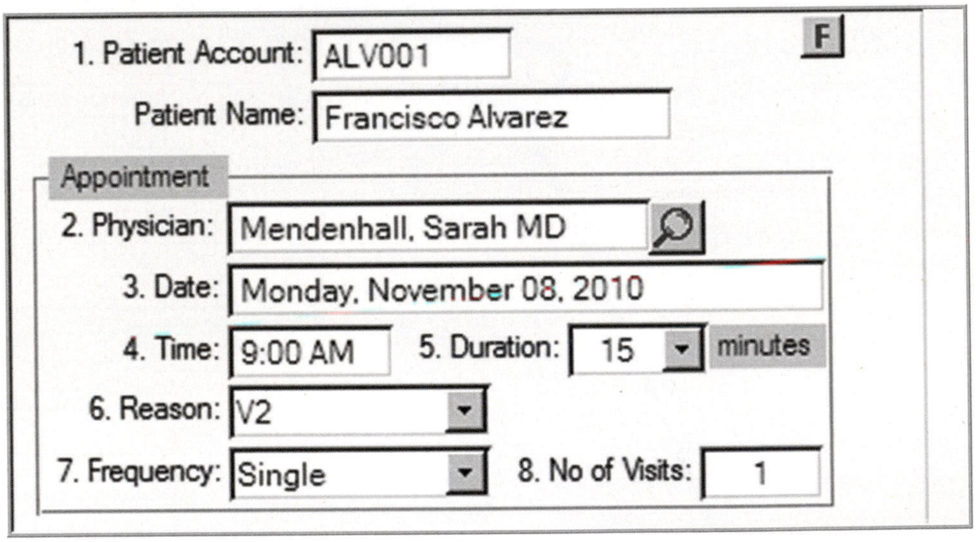

Source: Delmar/Cengage Learning

through the prompt, indicating the appointment has been posted.

d. Since Mr. Alvarez is in the office, you will print an appointment slip reminder for him. To do this, click Print at the bottom of the Patient Appointment Form (Figure 6-4).

e. As this is a simulation, file the appointment slip in your Completed Work folder. Click Close to return to the Practice Schedule. You should now see that Mr. Alvarez is scheduled for 9:00 a.m. on Dr. Mendenhall's schedule.

3. Next you receive a telephone call from Cynthia Worthington, a patient of Dr. Heath. She is complaining of sinus

FIGURE 6-4

An appointment slip can be generated by clicking the print button

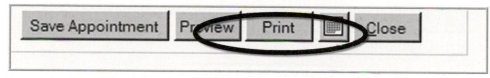

Source: Delmar/Cengage Learning

congestion, pressure, and pain that has been ongoing for a week or so. However, she is requesting an appointment close to lunch since she must use her lunch break to see the doctor. After consulting with Mei Ling, RMA, you schedule Ms. Worthington for an appointment tomorrow, Tuesday, October 12, 2010. Click on October 12, 2010, on the appointment calendar. Note that Dr. Heath goes to lunch at noon, so the closest available appointment would be 11:45 a.m. Ms. Worthington would prefer 11:30 so that she has time to get back to her office; therefore, you will need to schedule a 15-minute appointment for her at 11:30 a.m.

a. Begin by single clicking in the 11:30 time slot on October 12 in Dr. Heath's schedule and clicking the View/ Create Appointment button. Search for Ms. Worthington in the patient list, highlight her name, and click Add.

b. Complete the Patient Appointment Form with the appropriate information. When finished, compare your screen with Figure 6-5 and click Save Appointment. Click OK through the prompt, indicating the appointment has been posted.

c. Click on Close to return to the Practice Schedule. Ms. Worthington should now appear on Dr. Heath's schedule at 11:30 a.m. on October 12.

4. Elaine Ybarra comes to the desk after her appointment with Dr. Schwartz today. She needs to schedule a follow-up appointment for one month. She is being seen by Dr. Schwartz for depression. Ms. Ybarra is requesting a morning appointment.

a. Navigate to Friday, November 12, 2010, to view Dr. Schwartz' availability. Note that Dr. Schwartz does not begin seeing patients until 10:00 a.m. and then takes lunch from 12 to 1. After discussing this with Mrs. Ybarra, she determines that a 10:30 appointment will be the best option for her, and since she is an established patient, she will only require 15 minutes. Single click in the 10:30 slot and click View/Create Appointment. Search for Ms. Ybarra in the patient list.

b. When Mrs. Ybarra's name appears, you notice that her first name is spelled incorrectly. When you ask her to spell her first name, she states it is spelled "E-L-A-I-N-E." You will need to make this correction in the computer before proceeding.

c. Close the search screen and minimize the Practice Schedule to go back to the Main Menu. From there, click on Patient Registration. Search for "Ybarra" in the patient list, highlight her name, and click Select. In Field 2, make the appropriate change to her first name, making sure that it is spelled correctly. Click Save. Click OK through the confirming prompt, and then click Close.

d. Maximize the Practice Calendar and proceed in making Ms. Ybarra's appointment. When all information is correct, click Save Appointment. Then, print an appointment slip for the patient to take home. When you are finished, Ms. Ybarra should now appear on the Practice Schedule, scheduled for 10:30 a.m. on November 12, 2010.

FIGURE 6-5
Check your work for Step 3b

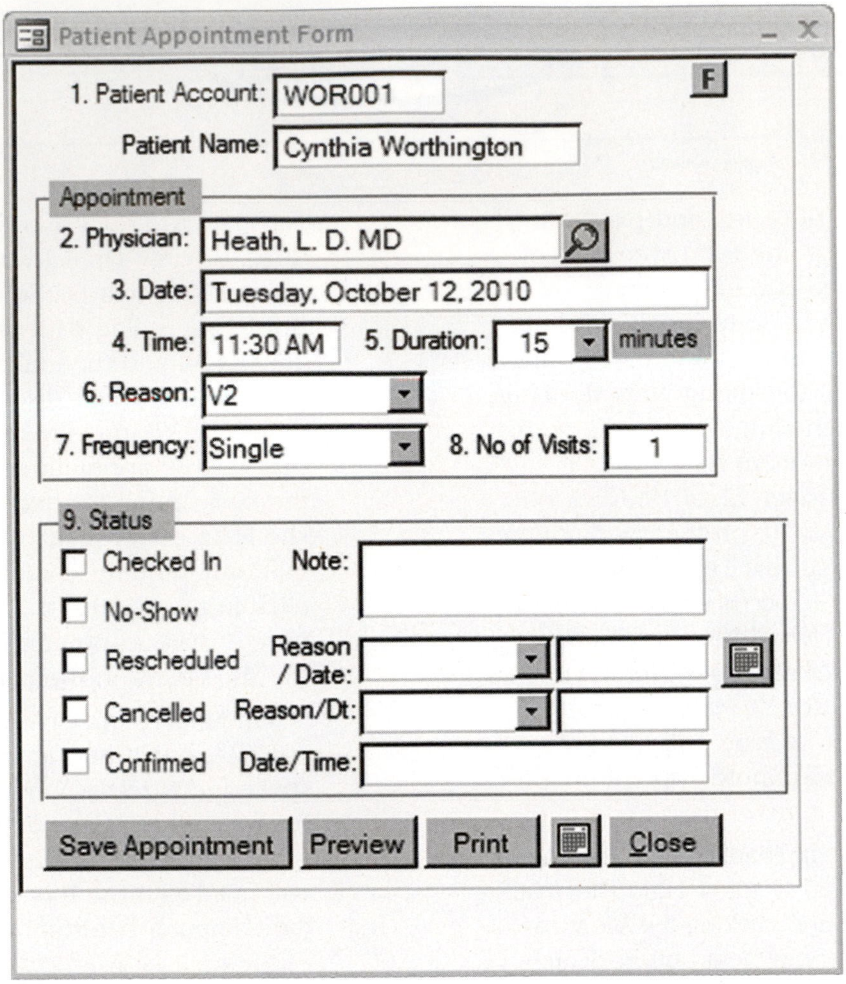

```
┌─────────────────────────────────────────────────────┐
│ ▣ Patient Appointment Form                    _  X   │
│ ┌─────────────────────────────────────────────────┐ │
│ │                                            ┌───┐ │ │
│ │    1. Patient Account: │WOR001        │    │ F │ │ │
│ │                                            └───┘ │ │
│ │       Patient Name: │Cynthia Worthington      │  │ │
│ │ ┌─Appointment────────────────────────────────┐  │ │
│ │ │  2. Physician: │Heath, L. D. MD      │ ┌─┐  │  │ │
│ │ │                                        │⌕│  │  │ │
│ │ │                                        └─┘  │  │ │
│ │ │     3. Date: │Tuesday, October 12, 2010  │  │  │ │
│ │ │                                             │  │ │
│ │ │   4. Time: │11:30 AM│ 5. Duration: │ 15 │▼│ minutes │
│ │ │                                             │  │ │
│ │ │  6. Reason: │V2           │▼│               │  │ │
│ │ │                                             │  │ │
│ │ │ 7. Frequency: │Single      │▼│ 8. No of Visits: │ 1 │ │
│ │ └─────────────────────────────────────────────┘  │ │
│ │ ┌─9. Status──────────────────────────────────┐  │ │
│ │ │  ☐ Checked In    Note: │              │     │  │ │
│ │ │  ☐ No-Show              │              │     │  │ │
│ │ │  ☐ Rescheduled  Reason │      │▼│ │    │ ▣   │  │ │
│ │ │                 / Date:                     │  │ │
│ │ │  ☐ Cancelled  Reason/Dt:│      │▼│ │     │   │  │ │
│ │ │  ☐ Confirmed  Date/Time:│              │    │  │ │
│ │ └─────────────────────────────────────────────┘  │ │
│ │ ┌──────────────┬─────────┬───────┬───┬────────┐  │ │
│ │ │Save Appointment│ Preview │ Print │ ▣ │ Close  │  │ │
│ │ └──────────────┴─────────┴───────┴───┴────────┘  │ │
│ └─────────────────────────────────────────────────┘ │
└─────────────────────────────────────────────────────┘
```

Source: Delmar/Cengage Learning

5. Christopher Snider calls in to the office next, requesting an appointment with Dr. Heath. He is a new patient to the practice. He just moved to the area and would like to schedule an appointment for his yearly physical.

  a. Since Mr. Snider is a new patient to the practice, you will have to enter him into MOSS before you can schedule an appointment. Therefore, you will need to get some information from him over the telephone. Minimize the Practice Schedule and return to the Main Menu. Click Patient Registration. Search for "Snider" in the patient list, noting the spelling of his last name. *It is always important that you confirm the spelling of a patient's first and last name upon entering names into the computer for the first time. Do not assume the patients spell their names in specific ways. If spelled incorrectly, there is a "trickle-down" effect that takes place in the medical office, as charts are created, bills are generated, and letters are transcribed—all erroneously.* Mr. Snider is a new patient, and clicking on Search will confirm that he is not in the system already.

  b. You will need to add him by clicking on "Add" at the bottom of the screen. On the Patient Information screen, insert the following information in the appropriate fields:

- Last name, first name, middle initial (Fields 1–3): Snider, Christopher A.
- Social security number (Field 4): 999315364
- Gender, marital status, date of birth (Fields 5–7): Male, Married, October 20, 1972
- Address (Fields 8–11): 1853 Felker Road, Douglasville, NY 01234
- Home phone (Field 12): (123) 457-6215
- Employment status (Field 14): Employed

c. Click Save. Click OK through the confirming prompt.

d. Click on the Primary Insurance tab, and complete the following fields:

- Insurance plan (Field 1): FlexiHealth PPO In-Network
- In Field 2, select the radio button next to Self. When you do, fields 3–7 automatically populate based on what you entered on the previous screen.
- ID Number (Field 8): DBX4570
- The co-pay for FlexiHealth is $20 (Field 12)
- Dr. Heath does accept assignment (Field 13) and is a participating provider with FlexiHealth (Field 15)
- Since the patient is new to the practice, his signature is not on file (Field 14). You will have to change this when Mr. Snider comes in for his appointment.

e. Click Save. Click OK through the confirming prompt. You can collect the rest of Mr. Snider's information when he comes in for his appointment. Click Close until you return to the Main Menu. You are now ready to schedule his appointment.

f. Maximize the Practice Schedule. Mr. Snider would like an appointment in about five weeks (around the week of November 15), as he will be on a business trip until that time. He is requesting a Wednesday in the afternoon. Navigate to Wednesday, November 17, 2010, on Dr. Heath's schedule. You will note that Dr. Heath has rounds at Retirement Inn in the afternoon. After conveying this to the patient, Mr. Snider decides that a Friday morning appointment that week would also be a possibility. Click on Friday, November 19, 2010, and schedule Mr. Snider for a new patient appointment (three time slots) anytime that is available for this duration on Friday morning with Dr. Heath. (On the Patient Appointment Form, make sure the duration [Field 5] is 45 minutes and the reason [Field 6] is new patient visit.) When you are finished, click Save Appointment, and then Close to return to the Practice Schedule. You tell Mr. Snider that he will need to come 15 minutes early and bring his insurance cards with him.

6. After seeing Dr. Mendenhall today for complications related to hypertension, John Wittmer comes to the desk needing a follow-up appointment in one week, around the same time of day (in the morning, around 11:00 a.m.). Using the steps learned previously, schedule Mr. Wittmer and print out an appointment reminder slip for him. File the printed appointment slip in your Completed Work folder.

7. Mr. Ernesto Santana calls in for an appointment with Dr. Mendenhall. He is complaining of an extremely sore throat. He states that it hurts to swallow, and he is asking to see the doctor as soon as possible. When asked if he has any other symptoms, he states that he thinks he may have a fever and that when his wife looked in his throat, she thought she may have seen some "white patches." Schedule Mr. Santana for an appointment this afternoon at 4:00 p.m. with Dr. Mendenhall.

8. Robert Shinn's mother calls in late in the day. Robert is a patient of Dr. Heath. Mrs. Shinn explains that Robert has been having symptoms of a sore throat, cough, and tightness in his chest for more than a week now. It is now beginning to significantly affect his sleep as well as his daytime activities, and she would like him to be seen as soon as possible. Schedule Robert for an appointment with Dr. Heath tomorrow (Tuesday, October 12, 2010) at 9:00 a.m.

9. Ms. Wilma Stearn calls in to schedule her yearly physical examination with Dr. Heath. She had her last physical in November of 2009. Therefore, you will need to schedule her in November of 2010 in order for her insurance to cover it. She is requesting a Tuesday in the afternoon if possible. Schedule Ms. Stearn for an appointment the fourth Tuesday of November in the afternoon. (Remember that physical examinations require a 30-minute appointment.)

10. Paula Shektar calls in next. She is a patient of Dr. Schwartz. She states she has bronchitis. She "gets it every year at this time." She would like to be seen tomorrow, if possible. Schedule Mrs. Shektar for a 1:00 p.m. appointment tomorrow with Dr. Schwartz.

11. Richard Manaly, a patient of Dr. Schwartz, calls in complaining of peculiar skin rash all over his chest and back. He states that the rash appeared this morning and that the only other symptom is that he is feeling slightly fatigued. He is wondering if he should be seen. After consulting with Mei Ling, RMA, you explain to Mr. Manaly that he should be seen tomorrow to be evaluated. Schedule Mr. Manaly for the first available appointment tomorrow afternoon, at 1:15 p.m., with Dr. Schwartz.

12. Paula Shektar calls back to say that she forgot she had already scheduled a previous appointment that day and would like to move her appointment with Dr. Schwartz to an hour later.

   a. Double click on Mrs. Shektar's appointment on October 12, 2010, at 1:00 p.m. The Patient Appointment Form will appear.

   b. Field 9, Status, gives you several options. Check the box next to Rescheduled. Moving along the row horizontally, in the Reason/ Date field, use the drop-down menu to select Needs Different Date (R6). Check your work with Figure 6-6, and then click the rescheduling calendar icon to the right of this row.

   c. When you click on the rescheduling icon, a new Practice Schedule appears. Note the bar along the top of the schedule says "Practice Reschedule" (Figure 6-7). Be sure that you are in the Practice Reschedule calendar before proceeding.

   d. Use the scroll bar and scroll down to the 2:00 p.m. time slot with Dr. Schwartz. Double click on the 2:00 p.m. time slot. *It will appear on the Practice Reschedule calendar that nothing has happened.*

   e. Click the Close button, on the bottom right corner of the screen.

   f. Now, you are back on the Patient Appointment Form, and you should notice that the date field on the Rescheduled line has now populated (Figure 6-8).

   g. Click Save Appointment. Click OK through the confirming prompt. Click Close to return to the Practice Schedule.

   h. Note that Mrs. Shektar's appointment now appears at 2:00 p.m. on the Practice Schedule.

13. You have completed your tasks for the day. Close the Practice Schedule and return to the Main Menu screen.

FIGURE 6-6
Check your work for Step 12b. Note the rescheduling calendar icon indicated

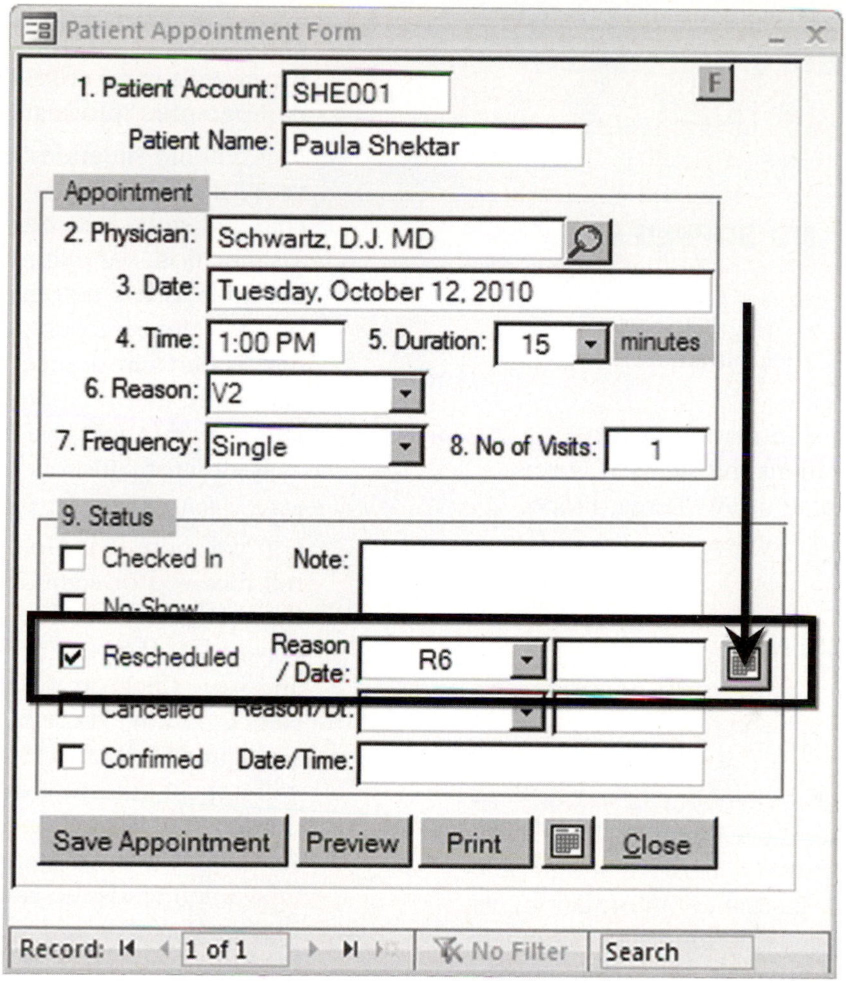

Source: Delmar/Cengage Learning

FIGURE 6-7
The practice reschedule calendar

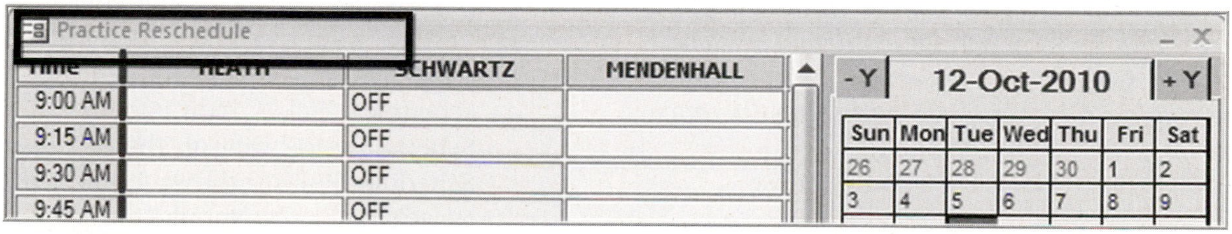

Source: Delmar/Cengage Learning

FIGURE 6-8
The reschedule date now appears on the patient appointment form

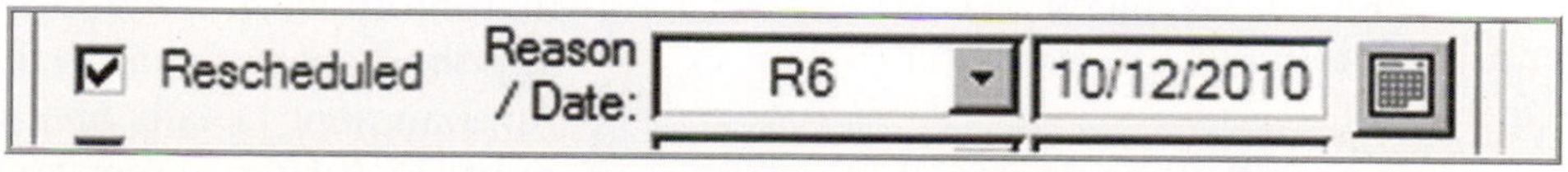

Source: Delmar/Cengage Learning

JOB 7
Administrative Functions— Patient Registration

MATERIALS AND SUPPLIES

- Medical Office Simulation Software (MOSS)
- 5 Patient Information Forms: Job 7—Patient Information Forms for Patients Furtaw, Perez, Freno, Boyd, and Brewer

TIME ALLOTMENT

45 minutes

OCTOBER 12, 2010

Today you will be checking in patients as they arrive for their appointments. Your tasks will include verifying their demographic information and insurance information, as well as checking them into the computer using MOSS. Additionally, you will ensure that all HIPAA forms have been signed. You will be working with Emily Parker, a medical assistant who has been with the practice for five years. *Before beginning this exercise, log in to MOSS and begin at the Main Menu. Be sure that Feedback Mode is turned off when completing these exercises. Information about logging in to MOSS and using Feedback Mode is found in Appendix C.*

INSTRUCTIONS

1. The first patient to check in is Robert Shinn, an adolescent male, accompanied by his mother. He has a 9:00 a.m. appointment this morning with Dr. Heath.

   a. Click on Patient Registration at the Main Menu. Type in "Shinn" and click Search. Highlight Robert Shinn's name in the patient list and click Select. This brings you to several patient registration fields where you can verify Robert's demographic information.

   b. In a real-life situation, you would verify that his address has not changed since last seen. Since this is a simulation, we will proceed as if the address has not changed. Click on the Primary Insurance tab. Verify that Robert's insurance is still Signal HMO and that it is through his father, Karl. Again, we will proceed as if all information is the same.

   c. Next, click on the HIPAA tab. Here you will note that Mrs. Shinn has not received or signed a HIPAA form. You will need to give her a copy of the HIPAA form to read and sign. Click on the Privacy Notice button. The Douglasville Medicine Associates HIPAA form will appear, and you can print this out for Mrs. Shinn. Since this is a simulation, we will assume that Mrs. Shinn reads the Notice of Privacy Practices and signs the form. Click the boxes next to Yes in Fields 1 and 2 and type today's date. Check your work with Figure 7-1 and click Save. Click through the confirming prompts, and then click Close until you are back at the Main Menu.

   d. You are now ready to check the patient in on the appointment schedule. Click Appointment Scheduling to bring up the Practice Schedule. Pull up the schedule for today's date. You should see Mr. Shinn's name in the 9:00 a.m. slot for Dr. Heath. Single click on Mr. Shinn's name on the Practice Schedule. When you do this, notice that information about Mr. Shin's appointment appears in the Appointment Details area (on the right side of the screen), as in Figure 7-2.

FIGURE 7-1

Check your work for Step 1c

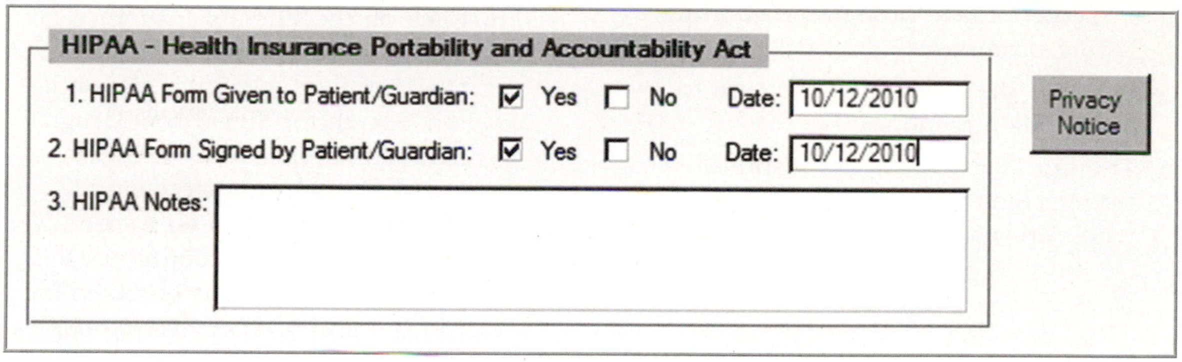

HIPAA - Health Insurance Portability and Accountability Act				
1. HIPAA Form Given to Patient/Guardian:	☑ Yes	☐ No	Date: 10/12/2010	Privacy Notice
2. HIPAA Form Signed by Patient/Guardian:	☑ Yes	☐ No	Date: 10/12/2010	
3. HIPAA Notes:				

Source: Delmar/Cengage Learning

FIGURE 7-2

Check your work for Step 1d

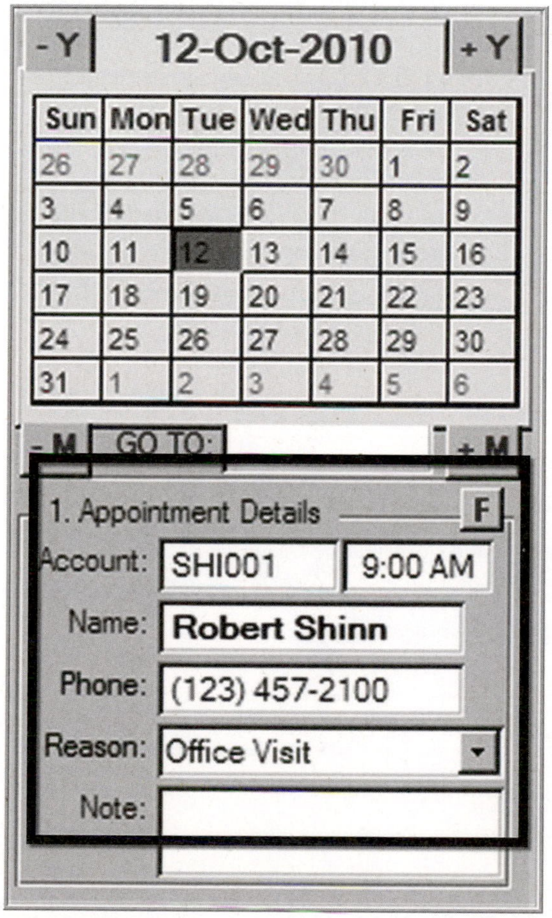

Source: Delmar/Cengage Learning

e. At the bottom of the screen, click Check-In Patient. A pop-up menu will appear, indicating "Patient Marked as Checked In!" Click OK. Close the Patient Schedule and return to the Main Menu.

f. As Robert Shinn is now checked in, file the printed Notice of Privacy Practices in your Completed Work folder. (This would have been given to the patient; however, since this is a simulation, you will file it instead.)

2. Cynthia Worthington arrives next for her 11:30 appointment with Dr. Heath.

a. From the Main Menu, click on Patient Registration. Search and select Ms. Worthington, bringing up her registration information. After verifying that all her demographic and insurance information has not changed—she states that it has not—click on the HIPAA tab. Note that Ms. Worthington needs to receive a copy of the Privacy Policy to read. She states that she did receive this on a previous visit; however, it must not have been checked off in the computer. She agrees to sign a new HIPAA form for verification. Check Yes in Fields 1 and 2 and fill in the date blocks with today's date. Click Save. Click through the confirming prompts, and then click Close until you are back at the Main Menu.

b. Open the Practice Schedule (click Appointment Scheduling from the Main Menu) and pull up today's date. Find Ms. Worthington under Dr. Heath's schedule and single click on her name. Click Check-In Patient on the bottom of the screen. Click through the confirming prompt.

c. Close the schedule and return to the Main Menu.

3. The next patient you are responsible for checking in is Richard Manaly, who appears at the desk at 1:00 p.m for his 1:15 p.m appointment with Dr. Schwartz.

a. From the Main Menu, click on Patient Registration. Search and select Mr. Manaly, bringing up his registration information. At this point, you will need to verify Mr. Manaly's demographic information. It seems that Mr. Manaly's home address and work information have not changed; however, when asked about his insurance information, he states that his insurance has changed from FlexiHealth PPO Out-of-Network to Signal HMO.

Therefore, this information will need to be updated in the computer.

b. Click on the Primary Insurance tab. Next to Field 1, Insurance Plan, click on the magnifying glass button. Search for Signal HMO, highlight it, and click Select. As Mr. Manaly's insurance has changed, you will need to see his insurance card in order to get the current ID and group numbers for Fields 7 and 9. After making copies of his card, type 99998621 in Field 8 (ID number) and WF3103 in Field 10 (Group number). There is now a $10.00 co-payment; enter this in Field 12. Since Dr. Schwartz is a participating provider with Signal HMO and is considered an "in-network" physician, make sure Yes is checked in Fields 13 and 15. Check your work with Figure 7-3 and click Save. Click through the confirming prompt.

FIGURE 7-3
Check your work for Step 3b

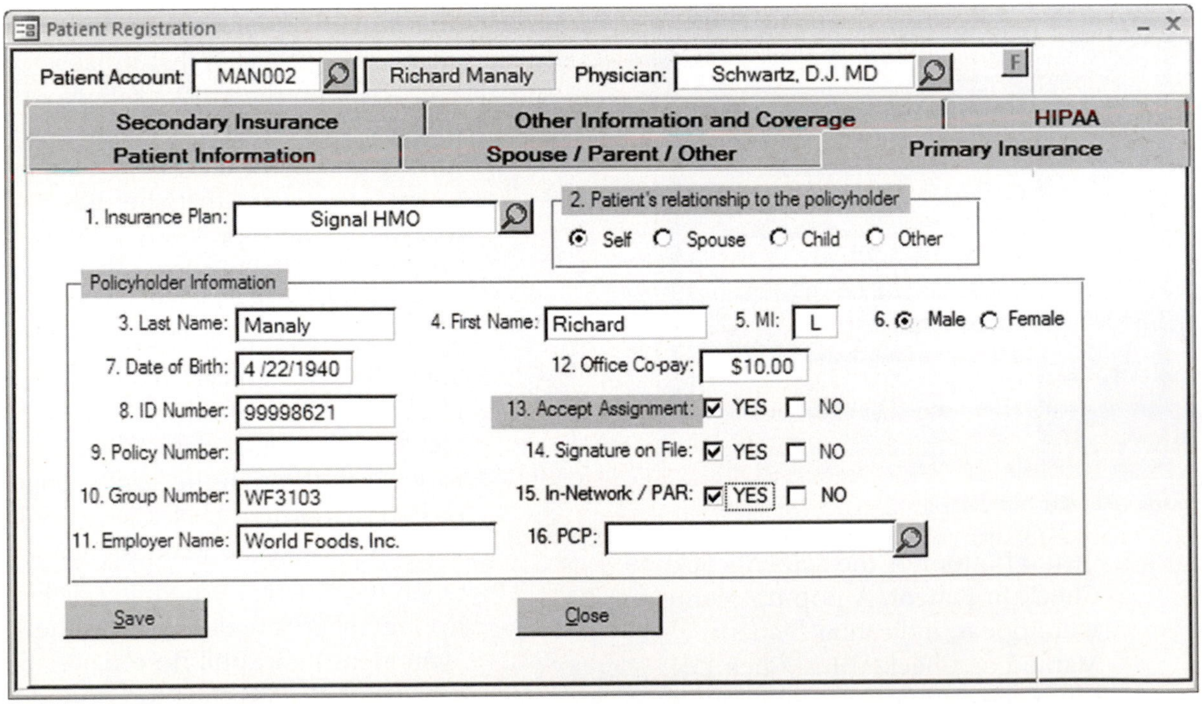

Source: Delmar/Cengage Learning

c. Now Click on the Secondary Insurance tab. Note that Mr. Manaly also has Medicare, and Dr. Schwartz does not participate in Medicare, so you will need to verify that Fields 14 and 16 are checked No. Click Save.

d. Click on the HIPAA tab. Mr. Manaly needs to receive and sign a copy of the Notice of Privacy Practices for Douglasville Medicine Associates. (Although you will not print out a copy of the privacy act for Mr. Manaly now, in a real-life situation, you would ensure that he received a copy and signed the HIPAA form.) Check Yes in Fields 1 and 2 and fill in the date blocks with today's date. Click Save. Click through the confirming prompts, and then click Close until you are back at the Main Menu.

e. Click on Appointment Scheduling and pull up today's date. Find Mr. Manaly's name on the schedule and indicate that he is checked in. Close the schedule and return to the Main Menu.

4. It is now 2:30 p.m., and Paula Shektar seems to be a No-Show for her 2:00 p.m. appointment with Dr. Schwartz. Emily Parker, another medical assistant in the office, tells you that Mrs. Shektar has failed to show for her appointment three times in a row this month. She would like you to document her missed appointment.

a. From the Main Menu, click on Appointment Scheduling and pull up today's date. Find "Shektar" under Dr. Schwartz' schedule and double-click on her name. The Patient Appointment Form will appear.

b. In Field 9 (Status), note that this is already a rescheduled appointment. Click the box next to No-Show (when you do this, the box next to Rescheduled is automatically

unpopulated, although the date field remains). In the Note section, type "Third missed appt in a row." Check your work with Figure 7-4, and then click Save Appointment. Click through the confirming prompt, and then click Close until you return to the Main Menu.

5. It is 2:45 p.m., and you receive a telephone call from Edward Gormann, an established patient of Dr. Schwartz. He is asking if he can come in today to see the doctor. Mr. Gormann is complaining of a productive cough, chest tightness, fever, and malaise for a week now. He is feeling awful and has missed work for a few days. He states he can be there in 5 minutes.

a. After consulting with Emily Parker, the medical assistant, and Dr. Schwartz, you schedule Mr. Gormann for a 3:00 p.m. appointment with Dr. Schwartz.

b. When Mr. Gormann arrives at the office, utilize the Patient Registration function of MOSS to verify Mr. Gormann's demographic information (for the purpose of this simulation, no information has changed) and to ensure that he has read and signed the HIPAA form.

c. However, you notice on the Patient Information screen that Dr. Heath is listed as Mr. Gormann's physician. Click on the magnifying glass next to Physician, search for Dr. Schwartz, and click Select. Click Save, and then OK through the confirming prompt.

d. Check Mr. Gormann in on the Practice Schedule.

6. Now that you have some basic experience with the computerized medical software, Emily gives you five patient information forms to enter into the computer from today. She has already verified the insurance and checked the

FIGURE 7-4
Check your work for Step 4b

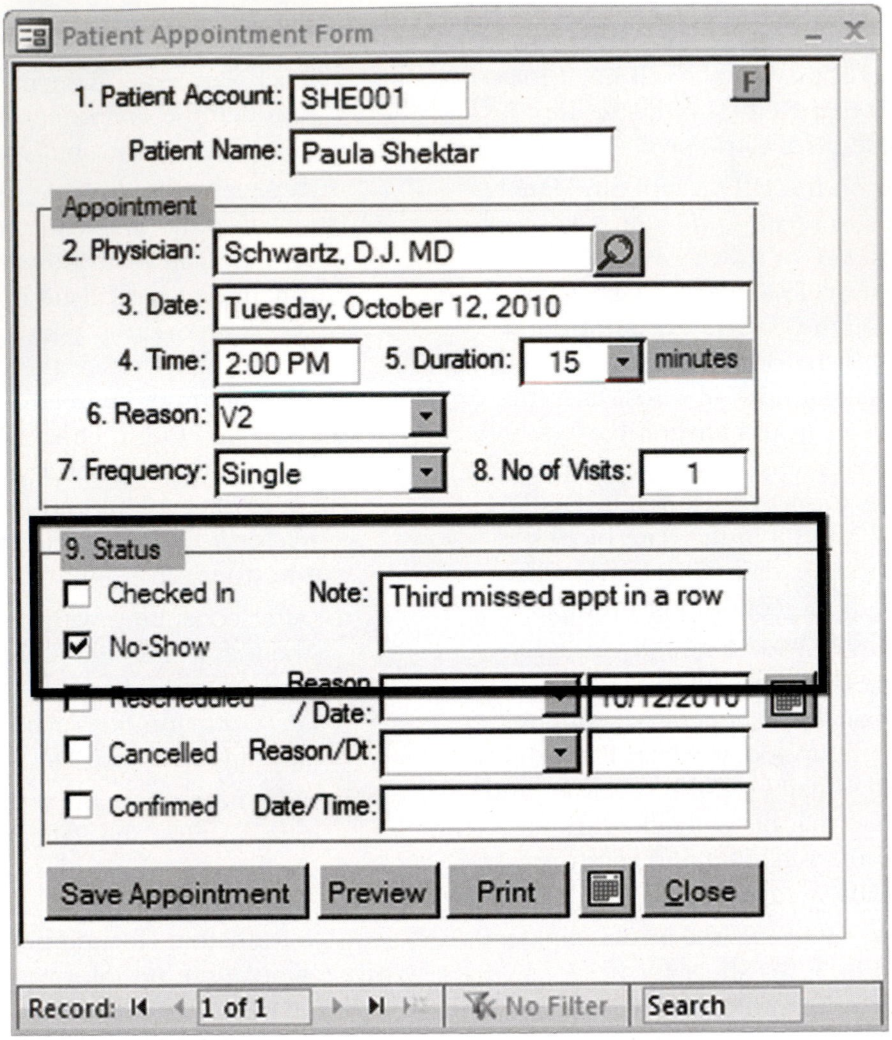

Source: Delmar/Cengage Learning

patients in but was unable to enter all the information into the computer system since she was also answering telephones and checking patients out. All patients are being seen by Dr. Mendenhall.

a. At the Main Menu, click Patient Registration and complete all applicable tabs for the following patients:

- Thomas Furtaw (enter his insurance co-payment as $20.00)

- Raul Perez (enter his insurance co-payment as $15.00)

- Elmer Freno (enter his insurance co-payment as $20.00)

- Karen Boyd (enter her insurance co-payment as 20.00)

- Edward Brewer (has no insurance; select Self-Pay in the insurance list)

b. Be sure that you change the Physician to Dr. Mendenhall for all patients (see Figure 7-5).

c. When you have completed the exercise, close out of MOSS and file the patient information forms in your Supplies folder.

FIGURE 7-5

Be sure Dr. Mendenhall is selected in the patient registration screen

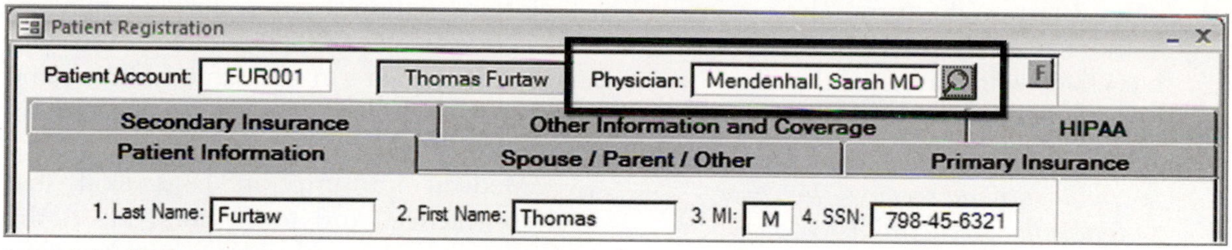

Patient Registration						— X
Patient Account: FUR001		Thomas Furtaw	Physician: Mendenhall, Sarah MD 🔍		F	
Secondary Insurance		Other Information and Coverage			HIPAA	
Patient Information		Spouse / Parent / Other			Primary Insurance	
1. Last Name: Furtaw	2. First Name: Thomas		3. MI: M	4. SSN: 798-45-6321		

Source: Delmar/Cengage Learning

JOB 8
Legal Implications—Request for Release of Medical Information

MATERIALS AND SUPPLIES

- Form: Job 8—Authorization to Release Medical Information

TIME ALLOTMENT

20 minutes

OCTOBER 13, 2010

Miriam Pinnerwell, a patient of Dr. Heath, is here today requesting that her records be transferred to a new family practice office in Florida. She explains that she is moving there within the next six weeks to live with her daughter and grandchildren.

INSTRUCTIONS

(As this is a simulation, this Job can be effectively done with a partner or classmate. However, if you do not have a partner, you may read Step 1 but proceed to Step 2.) Prior to beginning Step 1, familiarize yourself with the Authorization to Release Medical Information form.

1. Explain to Ms. Pinnerwell (your partner) that she will need to complete a Release of Information form, which authorizes Douglasville Medicine Associates to release information to her new provider.

2. Assist her in completing the form, using the information provided below:

   Provider Name: Gulf View Associates

   Provider Address: 3500 Tamiami Trail South, Sarasota, FL 34239-5280

   Phone Number: (941) 555-3980

   Fax Number: (941) 555-3900

   Records Authorized to be Released: Check "Other" and write in "Entire Chart." Since Ms. Pinnerwell is moving to a new permanent address, she is requesting that her entire medical record be copied and sent.

   Information to Be Used for the Purposes of: Continuity of Care

   Method of Release: US Mail

3. Have Ms. Pinnerwell (your partner/classmate) read the final paragraph of the release form and then ask if she has any further questions. Explain that you will be making a copy of the release for her records *(simulation only)*. If there are no further questions, Ms. Pinnerwell (your partner/classmate) should sign and date the release form.

4. As the witness, you, the student medical assistant, will now sign and date the release form. (If this was a real-life scenario, you would copy this form,

and Ms. Pinnerwell's medical record would be copied and sent to the provider listed on the form. The original authorization form would be filed in her chart, with a note of the date the chart was sent.)

**Some medical practices charge a fee for photocopying services; however, Douglasville Medicine Associates extends this courtesy to their patients at no charge.

5. File the Authorization to Release Medical Information form in your Completed Work folder.

JOB 9
Concepts of Effective Communication—
Transcription: Soap Notes

MATERIALS AND SUPPLIES

- Flash Drive
- Transcription File: Job 9A—Lee Westfail, MD (from Quali-Care Clinic)
- Transcription File: Job 9B—David L. Childs, MD (from Quali-Care Clinic)
- Form: Job 9—Quali-Care Clinic Letterhead

TIME ALLOTMENT

1 hour

OCTOBER 14, 2010

One of your responsibilities at Douglasville Medicine Associates will be performing medical transcription for the physicians here at our practice and occasionally for the physicians at Quali-Care Clinic, who submit their dictation to our transcriptionist to complete when an urgent need arises (such as when their transcriptionist is sick or when they are overloaded). We offer them the same support since we are in the same building and work closely with their physicians, making referrals as necessary.

Medical transcription is a skill that takes practice, and today Mrs. Fleet, the office manager, would like you to try your hand at some progress notes from Quali-Care Clinic. She explains that these are just "old practice SOAP notes" that she uses to train new medical assistants, so there is no pressure to be perfect this time. There will be plenty of time to hone your skills. She asks that you use all the resources available to you, as well as SOAP format, and transcribe the dictation to the best of your ability.

INSTRUCTIONS

1. Open the Transcription Folder on your flash drive to retrieve the dictation for this Job (there will be two files: Job 9A and Job 9B). Select the file type that is appropriate for your computer system.

2. You will transcribe this document in a Word file using 1-inch margins. Remember to save your work from the beginning. For the purpose of this simulation, you may want to save your documents using the last name of the patient.

3. Follow the format for SOAP notes shown in Appendix A: Reference Materials. This is the format preferred by Quali-Care Clinic.

4. A list of some of the unfamiliar words you may hear are included for you in Appendix A: Reference Materials since this is your first time transcribing. In time, and with practice, you will learn more medical terms pertinent to the specialty at hand, and transcription will become easier for you.

5. Remember to proofread your finished work. When you are ready, print out a hard copy and submit it to your instructor for review.

6. Upon return of your documents from your instructor, file both documents in your Completed Work folder.

JOB 10
Concepts of Effective Communication—Telephone Messages

MATERIALS AND SUPPLIES

- 4 Message Forms: Job 10—Message Forms for Patients Coleman, Richard, Santana, and Shektar

TIME ALLOTMENT

30 minutes

OCTOBER 15, 2010

After returning from a business meeting, Mrs. Fleet asks you to assist with taking care of telephone messages that have been piling up over the lunch hour. Douglasville Medicine Associates employs a local medical bureau to take over the phone lines during the lunch hours and after the office closes for the day, as well as over the weekends and holidays. If a message is urgent, the medical bureau operator will connect the patient with the physician on call. If the message is not of an urgent matter, a message will be taken, and the office will be notified when the medical office assistant calls in to alert the medical bureau that the office is open for the day.

Mrs. Fleet has given you four messages that were taken by the medical bureau. She would like you to handle these messages by routing them to the proper person and taking appropriate action.

Since this is only a simulation, you will not be able to actually take action on these messages; however, answering the questions below will show what you would do in each situation.

INSTRUCTIONS

1. Read each message.

2. Read the questions below pertaining to each patient. Type your complete answer to each question in a Word document and save the document to your flash drive.

3. Print out a hard copy for your instructor. Hand in or place in your Completed Work folder.

Patient: Francois Blanc

a. Is there anything missing from this message? If so, what?

b. What should you do before giving this message to Dr. Heath?

c. If you would have taken this message, what questions could you have asked Mrs. Coleman to have made the message more complete?

Patient: Julia Richard

a. What do you think when you read this message? Why?

b. What should you do before giving this message to Dr. Mendenhall?

Patient: Mr. Santana

a. Is this an important concern?

b. What things could you determine for Dr. Mendenhall before relaying the message to her?

Patient: Paula Shektar

a. Do you think this patient should be seen on the spur of the moment today?

b. Is this an ethical dilemma? Discuss.

JOB 11
Administrative Functions—Looking up a Patient Appointment, Scheduling Patient Appointments, Creating Daily Appointment Patient List, and Making New Patient Reminder Calls

MATERIALS AND SUPPLIES

■ Medical Office Simulation Software (MOSS)

TIME ALLOTMENT

60 minutes

OCTOBER 18, 2010

Today, Mrs. Fleet has assigned you to the front desk to answer the telephone calls and make appointments as needed.

Before beginning this exercise, log in to MOSS and begin at the Main Menu. Be sure that Feedback Mode is turned off when completing these exercises. Information about logging in to MOSS and using Feedback Mode is found in Appendix C.

INSTRUCTIONS

1. You receive a call from Christopher Snider, a new patient (NP) for Dr. Heath, stating that he forgot to write down the date of his new patient appointment. He is asking your assistance in finding out this information.

   a. From the Main Menu, click Appointment Scheduling.

   b. Click on View/Create Appointment (located on the bottom of the Practice Schedule).

   c. Type "Snider" in the field and click Search. (You could also use the scroll bar to locate the patient's name in the list.) Once Christopher Snider is located, click Select.

   d. A Patient Appointment Form will appear, giving you the date and time of Mr. Snider's appointment (the morning of Friday, November 19).

   e. After relaying this information to Mr. Snider, click Close.

   f. Close out of the Practice Schedule and return to the Main Menu.

2. Using MOSS, schedule appointments for the following patients tomorrow, October 19, 2010. Additionally, make any changes (indicated in parentheses next to a patient name) in Patient Registration prior to scheduling the patient appointment.

For Dr. Heath:

■ Caroline Pratt—9:00

■ Manuel Ramirez—9:30

■ Josephine Albertson—NP @ 10:00

■ David James—11:00

■ Ryan Ashby—NP @ 2:00 (Change his doctor from Dr. Murray to Dr. Heath)

■ Dinner Meeting from 4:00 onward

For Dr. Schwartz:

■ Chrissy Krouse—NP @ 1:00 (Moving; change doctor to Dr. Schwartz)

■ Eugene Sykes—2:00

■ Stanley Kramer—2:30

■ Russell Logan—NP @ 3:15 (Moved in with daughter and needs to change doctors; change to Dr. Schwartz)

For Dr. Mendenhall:

- Francisco Alvarez—9:00
- Julia Richard—9:30
- Diane Parker—10:30
- John Wittmer—11:00
- Tina Rizzo—NP @ 11:15 (Was scheduled originally as a NP to Dr. Heath but prefers a female doctor; change physician to Dr. Mendenhall.)
- Quality assurance meeting from 1:00 onward

3. Later in the afternoon, Mrs. Fleet explains that a list of patients to be seen the next day is printed out for the doctors. Today, this will be your responsibility.

   a. From the Main Menu, click Appointment Scheduling (if not already open). As today is Monday, October 18, you will be printing out the schedule for Tuesday, October 19. Navigate to Tuesday, October 19, 2010, on the Practice Schedule.

   b. Click the Preview/Print button at the bottom right of the Practice Schedule screen. (When the document is created, you may need to maximize it and then use Zoom in order to properly view the schedule prior to printing.)

   c. Use the Print icon at the top left of your tool bar (see Figure 11-1) to print the physicians' schedule. Compare to Figure 11-2. You will use this schedule, and the MOSS software, to perform the next phase of this job.

   d. Click the X on the top right corner of the physician schedule preview to return to the Practice Schedule. Click Close to return to the Main Menu. (The Main Menu may need to be maximized on your screen.)

4. Finally, Mrs. Fleet would like you to make reminder calls to the new patients who will be seen by each of the physicians tomorrow. These are done out of courtesy to the patients. Additionally, reminder calls decrease the number of "no-shows" and allow

FIGURE 11-1

The print icon is located at the top left of the screen

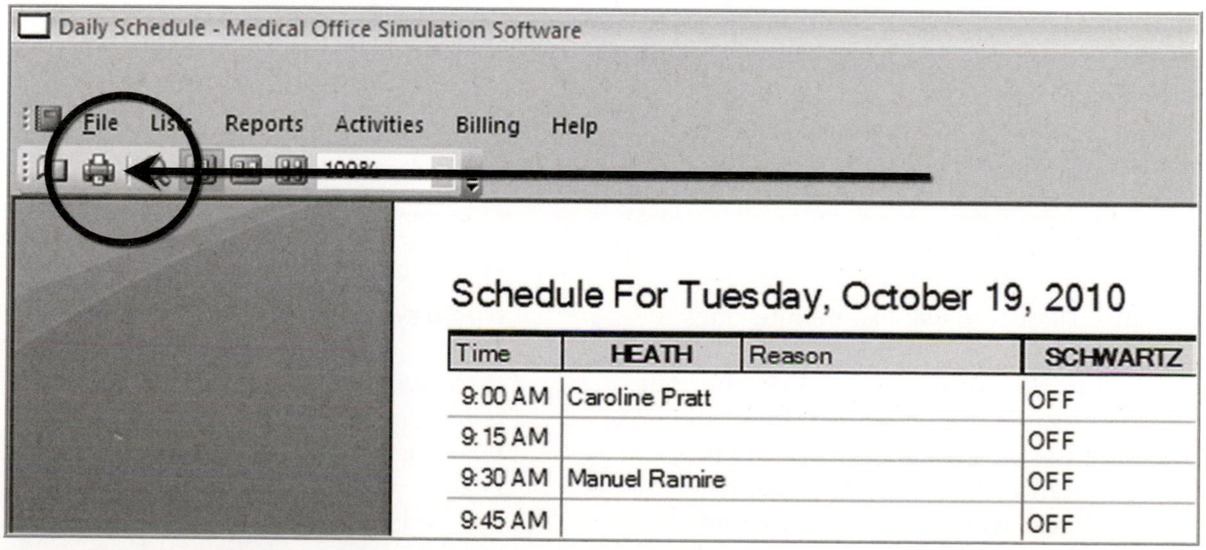

| Daily Schedule - Medical Office Simulation Software |
| File   List   Reports   Activities   Billing   Help |

Schedule For Tuesday, October 19, 2010

Time	HEATH	Reason	SCHWARTZ
9:00 AM	Caroline Pratt		OFF
9:15 AM			OFF
9:30 AM	Manuel Ramire		OFF
9:45 AM			OFF

Source: Delmar/Cengage Learning

FIGURE 11-2
The practice schedule for October 19, 2010

Schedule For Tuesday, October 19, 2010

Student No: Student1

Time	HEATH	Reason	SCHWARTZ	Reason	MENDENHALL	Reason
9:00 AM	Caroline Pratt		OFF		Francisco Alvar	
9:15 AM			OFF			
9:30 AM	Manuel Ramire		OFF		Julia Richard	
9:45 AM			OFF			
10:00 AM	Josephine Alber		Rounds @ Com			
10:15 AM	Josephine Alber		Rounds @ Com			
10:30 AM	Josephine Alber		Rounds @ Com		Diane Parker	
10:45 AM			Rounds @ Com			
11:00 AM	David James		Rounds @ Com		John Wittmer	
11:15 AM			Rounds @ Com		Tina Rizzo	
11:30 AM			Rounds @ Com		Tina Rizzo	
11:45 AM			Rounds @ Com		Tina Rizzo	
12:00 PM	Lunch		Lunch		Lunch	
12:15 PM	Lunch		Lunch		Lunch	
12:30 PM	Lunch		Lunch		Lunch	
12:45 PM	Lunch		Lunch		Lunch	
1:00 PM			Chrissy Krouse		QA Meeting @	
1:15 PM			Chrissy Krouse		QA Meeting @	
1:30 PM			Chrissy Krouse		QA Meeting @	
1:45 PM					QA Meeting @	
2:00 PM	Ryan Ashby		Eugene Sykes		QA Meeting @	
2:15 PM	Ryan Ashby				QA Meeting @	
2:30 PM	Ryan Ashby		Stanley Kramer		QA Meeting @	
2:45 PM					QA Meeting @	
3:00 PM					QA Meeting @	
3:15 PM			Russell Logan		QA Meeting @	
3:30 PM			Russell Logan		QA Meeting @	
3:45 PM			Russell Logan		QA Meeting @	
4:00 PM	Dinner Meeting				QA Meeting @	
4:15 PM	Dinner Meeting				QA Meeting @	
4:30 PM	Dinner Meeting				QA Meeting @	
4:45 PM	Dinner Meeting				QA Meeting @	
5:00 PM	Dinner Meeting		OFF		OFF	
5:15 PM	Dinner Meeting		OFF		OFF	
5:30 PM	Dinner Meeting		OFF		OFF	
5:45 PM	Dinner Meeting		OFF		OFF	

Source: Delmar/Cengage Learning

the patients to ask last-minute questions, such as directions—if they are still unclear. At the same time, the staff can remind the patients to bring the necessary documents (i.e., insurance cards and lab results, if appropriate), and to arrive early to their appointment to complete any necessary documentation. *This step should be done with a partner, in simulation, if possible. You, as the student medical office assistant, will make the "call" to the patient, who is your partner, to remind her of her appointment tomorrow.* Read the instructions below, and then proceed with your partner in answering the questions below and acting out this simulation.

a. Refer to the printed schedule for tomorrow. How many patients are new patients? Who is the first new patient for Dr. Heath?

b. From the Main Menu, click Appointment Scheduling and bring up the schedule for tomorrow (Tuesday, October 19, 2010), if you are not already there.

c. Single-click on the first new patient's name (Albertson). You will note that appointment details, including a telephone number for the patient, appear in Appointment Details area (Field 1) to the right of the screen, below the monthly calendar. You will use this number to "call" your patient to remind her of her appointment with Dr. Heath tomorrow at 10:00 a.m. (At this time, proceed with your partner to simulate this reminder call.)

d. When you have confirmed this appointment with your patient, double-click on Albertson's last name in the Practice Schedule. Her Patient Appointment Form appears.

e. In Field 9 (Status), click the box next to Confirmed (see Figure 11-3). In doing so, the date and time are automatically completed for you. *Note that MOSS will populate this field with the date you are performing this simulation.*

FIGURE 11-3

Selecting confirmed as the appointment status

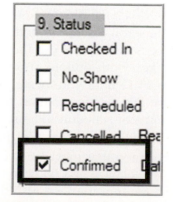

Source: Delmar/Cengage Learning

f. Click Save Appointment, and click through the confirming prompt. Close the Patient Appointment Form.

g. The next new patient is Ryan Ashby. Switch partners; now you are the patient, and your partner is making this reminder call. Confirm the appointment using MOSS.

h. Confirm all new patient appointments for Dr. Heath in MOSS, then continue with reminder calls for Drs. Schwartz and Mendenhall, taking turns with your partner.

i. When you have completed this task, file the physician schedule you printed in Step 3c for Tuesday, October 19, in your Completed Work folder.

JOB 12
Concepts of Effective Communication and Ethical Considerations—Patient Scenarios

MATERIALS AND SUPPLIES

■ Form: Job 12—Patient Scenario Sheet

TIME ALLOTMENT

30 minutes

OCTOBER 19, 2010

Yesterday, Douglasville Medicine Associates held its monthly staff meeting, which occurs on the third Monday of every month. The focus of this month's meeting was the communication process between the patient and the caregiver. Since you are currently an intern at Douglasville, you are not mandated to attend this meeting, and therefore Mrs. Fleet has asked that you spend some time with her today so that she can share with you some of the issues discussed.

Mrs. Fleet reminds you that many of these issues are difficult—most are not able to be answered with a black-and-white "cookie cutter" answer—and some even involve ethical (even legal) issues that must be addressed. She would like to examine ten different patient scenarios with you. The first five scenarios have recently occurred at Douglasville Medicine Associates. The last five scenarios have actually occurred in the past, and Mrs. Fleet is interested in your approach to these situations as a medical front office specialist.

INSTRUCTIONS

1. Read each of the scenarios on the Patient Scenario Sheet and answer the questions included with each scenario.

2. When you are finished, file your paper in the Completed Work folder.

JOB 13
Administrative Functions— Scheduling Special Procedures (Mammogram)

MATERIALS AND SUPPLIES

■ Medical Office Simulation Software (MOSS)

TIME ALLOTMENT

15–30 minutes

OCTOBER 19, 2010

It is 10:15 a.m., and Dr. Mendenhall approaches you, asking you to schedule Julia Richard for a mammogram this afternoon.

Ms. Richard was seen for a lump in her left breast, and Dr. Mendenhall would like a mammogram to be done as soon as possible. Douglasville Medicine Associates contracts with an independent diagnostic group, Wallace Diagnostics, which conducts mammograms at our facility on a monthly basis, usually the third Tuesday of the month. However, earlier this morning, we notified the technician from Wallace that no patients were scheduled for mammograms and that they would not be needed today.

Since Dr. Mendenhall approached you to handle this situation, it is now your responsibility to call Wallace Diagnostics, advise them of the current situation, schedule the patient in MOSS at the earliest convenience today, and inform the patient of her appointment time.

INSTRUCTIONS

This is a simulation exercise. Your instructor may wish to have you role-play this job with two other classmates—one being the receptionist at Wallace Diagnostics and one playing the part of Ms. Richard. If so, use the instructions below as a guideline and schedule Ms. Richard for an appropriate time slot in MOSS. When you have completed that task in MOSS, inform Ms. Richard of her appointment time today for her mammogram.

If you are completing this job independently, follow the instructions below.

1. Log into MOSS and begin at the Main Menu. Click Appointment Scheduling and navigate to today's date. (Note that this view shows the schedule for Drs. Heath, Schwartz, and Mendenhall.)

2. Use the scroll bar at the bottom of the Practice Schedule (or use the right arrow key, both options shown in Figure 13-1) until you locate the Wallace Diagnostics column of the appointment schedule (Figure 13-2).

3. After calling Wallace Diagnostics, you are informed that they can accommodate Ms. Richard at 1:00 p.m. for a 60-minute appointment; Ms. Richard is also agreeable to this time.

FIGURE 13-1

The scroll bar and arrow keys allow you to see the schedules for other physicians in the practice, as well as the schedule for Wallace Diagnostics

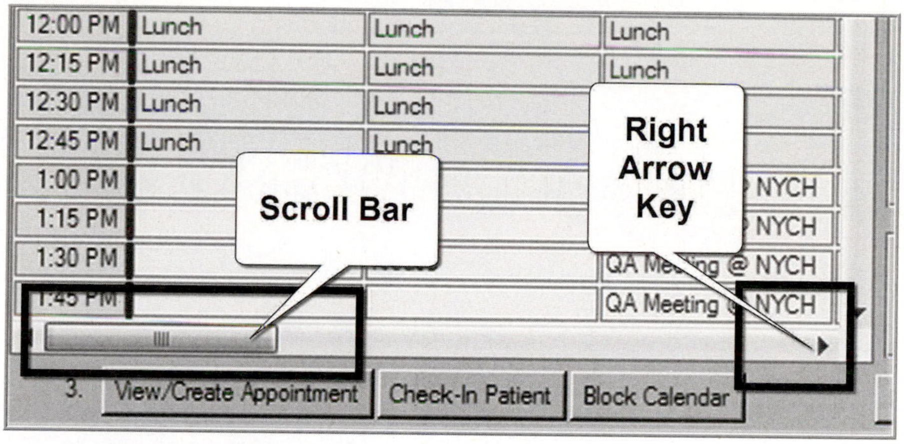

Source: Delmar/Cengage Learning

FIGURE 13-2

The Wallace Diagnostics column on the practice schedule

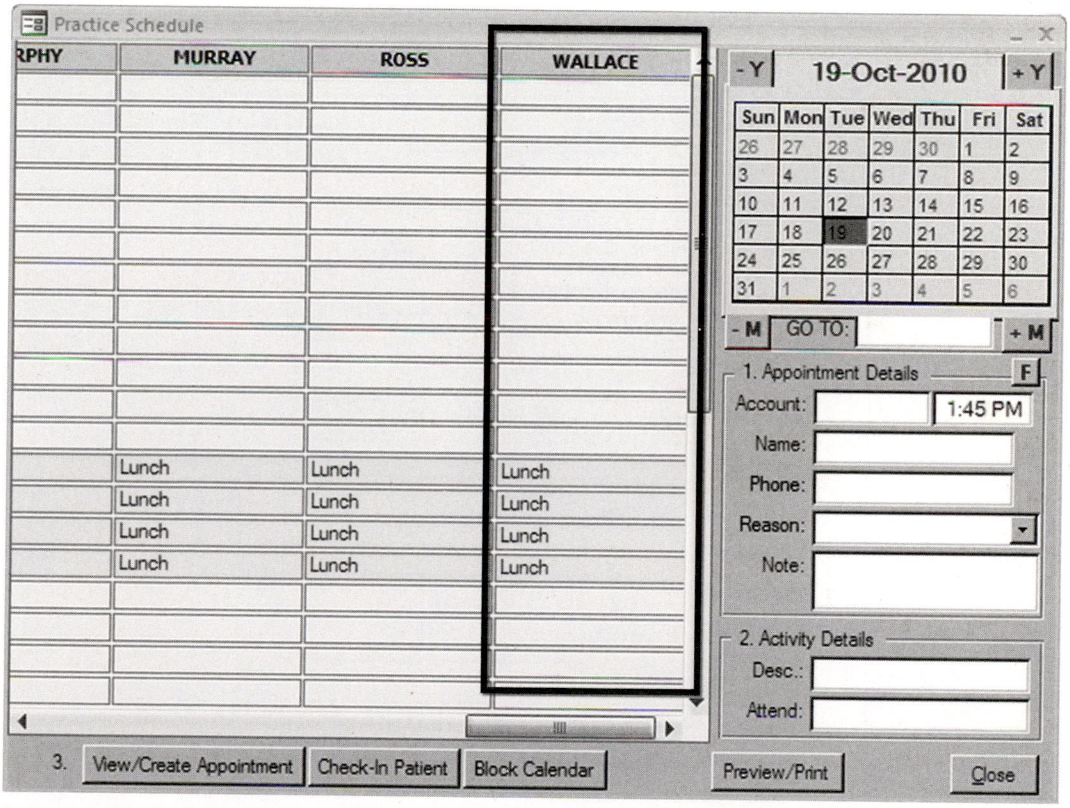

Source: Delmar/Cengage Learning

4. Single click in the 1:00 p.m. slot in the Wallace column on the Practice Schedule and click View/Create Appointment. Search for Julia Richard from the patient list and click Add, to bring up the Patient Appointment Form.

5. In Field 2 (Physician), click the magnifying glass and search for and select Greg Wallace, MD, in the physician list (Figure 13-3). (Dr. Wallace is the radiologist in charge of Wallace Diagnostics. He is also affiliated with Meadway MedSurg Clinic.)

FIGURE 13-3
Select Greg Wallace from the physician list

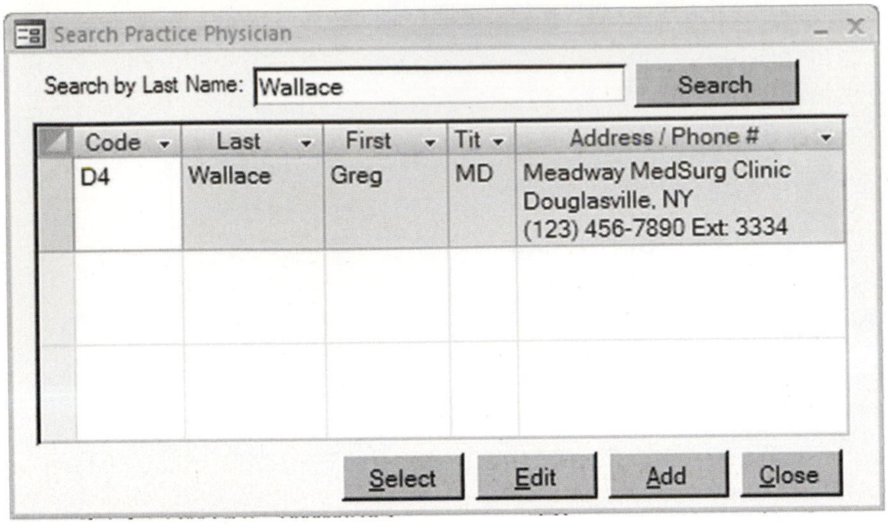

Source: Delmar/Cengage Learning

FIGURE 13-4
Check your work for Step 6

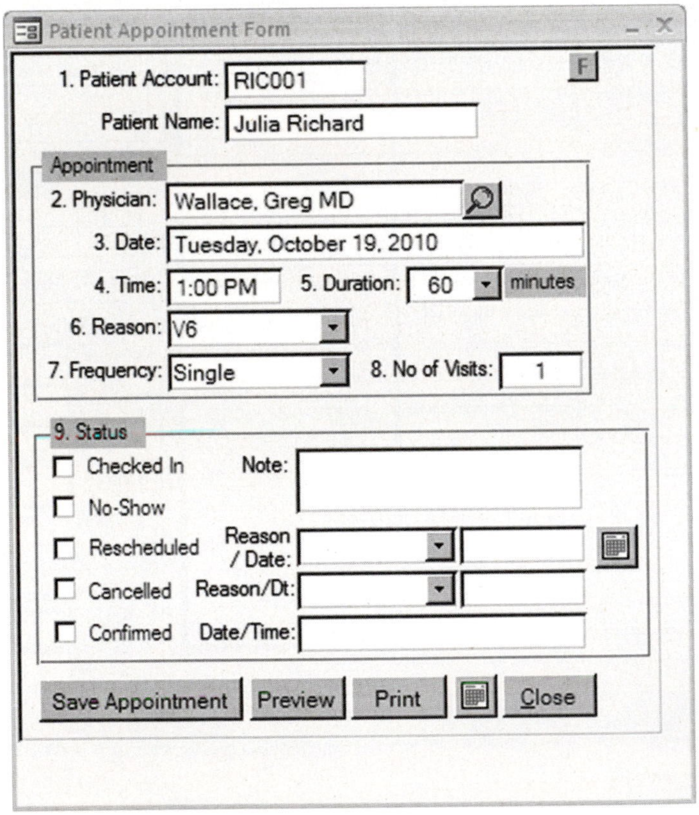

Source: Delmar/Cengage Learning

6. Continue filling out the Patient Appointment Form, selecting the correct appointment duration and reason for visit (choose Radiology, V6). Compare your screen with Figure 13-4, and then click Save Appointment. Click through the confirming prompts, and then close all windows until you return to the Main Menu.

JOB 14
Concepts of Effective Communication—Transcription: Oncology Consult

MATERIALS AND SUPPLIES

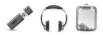

- Flash Drive
- Transcription File: Job 14— Dr. Lopez/Patient Parker
- Form: Job 14—Quali-Care Clinic Letterhead

TIME ALLOTMENT

1 hour

OCTOBER 20, 2010

Today you were asked to do substitute transcription work for Quali-Care Clinic. Dr. Lopez has completed an oncology consult on Marge Parker. You will need to review Appendix A: Reference Materials for a sample format, as well as pertinent terminology and abbreviations. It is important to note that Dr. Lopez speaks with a Hispanic accent, something you may or may not be used to. Since this is your first "real" transcription assignment, Mrs. Fleet has agreed to go over the final copy with you so that you are comfortable submitting your work.

INSTRUCTIONS

1. Open the Transcription folder on your flash drive to retrieve the dictation for this Job (there is one file: Job 14). Select the file type that is appropriate for your computer system.
2. Transcribe the dictation.

3. Save your finished work on your flash drive as Job 14.
4. Place a hard copy of the finished transcript in your Completed Work folder.

JOB 15
Concepts of Effective Communication—Making a Referral to a Specialist

MATERIALS AND SUPPLIES

- Julia Richard's medical record (in your *Medical Office Practice* package)
- Form: Job 15—Telephone Referral Information form
- Form: Job 15—Fax cover sheet
- Form: Job 15—Blank progress note
- Form: Job 15—History and Physical (Richard)
- Form: Job 15—Appointment card

TIME ALLOTMENT

30 minutes

OCTOBER 21, 2010

As you may recall, Julia Richard was seen by Dr. Mendenhall and sent for mammography after Dr. Mendenhall detected a lump in Ms. Richard's left breast. Results from mammography have confirmed a tumor of the left breast, and Dr. Mendenhall would like to refer Ms. Richard to Dr. Eric Lopez, an oncologist with Quali-Care Clinic, as soon as possible. She has dictated a brief History and Physical, which can be faxed to Dr. Lopez for his records and perusal prior to the patient's initial appointment.

INSTRUCTIONS

1. Review the procedures for making a telephone referral by reading the Telephone Referral Information form. (Since this is a simulation and you will not be able to directly call the oncologist, your instructor may have you role-play this procedure. This form guides you through the process of making a referral step by step. Make sure that you have the patient's chart in front of you—utilizing the patient information form—to convey this information to the office accepting the referral.)

2. *For the purposes of this job, Kathleen at Dr. Lopez's office schedules an appointment for Ms. Richard on Tuesday, October 26, 2010, at 2:00 p.m.*

3. Kathleen has requested that Ms. Richard's History and Physical report be faxed over to the office prior to her appointment. The fax number is (123) 456-1020. Complete the fax coversheet. *As this is a simulation, you will not be able to directly fax the form to Dr. Lopez's office. However, your instructor may demonstrate the fax procedure (or explain the procedure) to you.*

4. Document the referral on a progress note in Julia Richard's chart. Use the example on the Telephone Referral Information form as a guideline, and follow the charting instructions outlined in Appendix A: Reference Materials.

5. Complete an appointment card for Ms. Richard.

6. File the History and Physical and progress note in Julia Richard's medical record and return the record to your *Medical Office Practice* package. File the telephone referral form, appointment card, and fax coversheet in your Completed Work file.

JOB 16
Administrative Functions—Researching Drug Information

MATERIALS AND SUPPLIES

- A drug guide such as the *Physician's Desk Reference (PDR)*, most current edition
- Internet access (optional)—see Appendix A: Reference Materials for suggested Web links

TIME ALLOTMENT

60 minutes

OCTOBER 22, 2010

Jordan Connell, a patient of Dr. Heath, calls in today stating that he is currently taking Imitrex for his migraine headaches. However, Imitrex is not working for him any longer, and he has been hearing about another drug that works very well for a friend of his called Relpax. He would like to know a little more about this drug but does not have access to the Internet or to a drug reference. He is also experiencing his migraines more frequently and is interested in a medication used to help prevent migraines called Topamax. He is asking if you would be willing to research some information about these drugs today, and he will pick it up after work. He explains that having his information will help him better prepare for his upcoming appointment with Dr. Heath, as he would like to be able to discuss his treatment options further. You state that you would be happy to research these medications for him and will have it ready when he arrives after work.

INSTRUCTIONS

1. If you are using a drug guide to research this information, follow directions in steps 2 to 4. If you are using the Internet, begin with step 5.

2. Look for Relpax in the index first. Note the page number that is located across from the word "Relpax."

3. Locate the page number referenced above. You will notice that there is much information to sort through. You will need to skim through the information to find the following things:

   - Classification of drug/what is the drug used for (indications)?

   - What is the adult dosage? How many times a day is it taken?

   - Does it come in tablet or capsule form?

   - What are some of the side effects?

   - Who should NOT take Relpax (contraindications)?

   - Important patient information

4. Repeat steps 2 to 3 for "Topamax," and then go to step 6.

5. To research this information on the Internet, log onto www.Rxlist.com or www.drugs.com. Once you locate drug information for Relpax and Topamax, find the answer to all the questions listed in step 3.

6. Type a short synopsis of your findings to submit to your "patient" (instructor) or file in your Completed Work folder.

JOB 17
Administrative Functions—Creating a Travel Itinerary

MATERIALS AND SUPPLIES

- The Internet

TIME ALLOTMENT

1.5 hours

OCTOBER 25, 2010

Dr. Schwartz has indicated to you that he will be attending the American Medical Association National Convention next year in San Antonio, Texas. The dates for the convention are May 4 to 7, 2011. He would like you to make reservations for him and to create a travel itinerary that he can take with him on his trip. He will also be renting a car for sightseeing, and he would appreciate if you could get prices for him.

The convention is to be held at the Hyatt Regency San Antonio at 123 Losoya Street, San Antonio, Texas 78205. Sessions will begin at 8:00 a.m. each day of the convention and run until 5:00 p.m. except for May 7. As that is the last day, sessions will begin at 9:00 a.m. and end at 12:00 p.m.

Using the Internet to obtain lodging, flight, and car rental information, create a travel itinerary for Dr. Schwartz following the instructions below.

INSTRUCTIONS

1. View the sample travel itinerary in Figure 17-1. Note the overall format.

FIGURE 17-1
Sample travel itinerary

TRAVEL ITINERARY
FOR DJ SCHWARTZ, MD
AMA CONVENTION – MAY 4 THROUGH MAY 7, _ _ _ _

Wednesday, May 4, _ _ _ _

7:00 p.m.   Arrive at airport and check in.

8:00 p.m.   Depart on American Airlines (for example), flight #_____.
                 (If there is a connecting flight, include information here on time of departure of the next
                 flight, as well as the flight number and name of airline.)

10:00 p.m.   Arrive at _____ airport. Collect baggage and pick up rental car at the terminal. See
                 attachment A for driving directions and map to hotel. Arrive at Hyatt Regency San Antonio
                 to check in.
                 Confirmation # is _____.

Thursday, May 5, _ _ _ _

        7:30 a.m.   Continental breakfast

        8:00 a.m.   Sessions begin. (Lunch is provided.)

        5:00 p.m.   Sessions end.
                         (Include suggestions here on places to dine and/or sites of interest to visit
                         this evening. Include maps from the hotel to the destination, if Dr. Schwartz
                         will be driving, and reference them as attachments here.)

Source: Delmar/Cengage Learning

2. Read the instructions for creating a travel itinerary in Appendix A: Reference Materials.

3. Log on to the Internet. Using the sites listed in the instructions for creating a travel itinerary (in Appendix A), locate flight information first. Keep in mind that there is a difference in time between Douglasville, New York, and San Antonio, Texas. Therefore, flight times will be increased on the return flight home. See Figure 17-2 for a time zone map.

4. Next, locate hotel information. Pay particular attention to check in/check out time, room information (nonsmoking/smoking, number and size of beds), facilities (restaurant on the premises, fitness center, etc.), and parking information (cost per night). It may be helpful to print out this information for later use in composing the actual itinerary.

5. Locate car rental information and print out.

6. As Dr. Schwartz is interested in doing some sightseeing during his free time, locate some information on places of interest in the surrounding San Antonio area. Include restaurant and dining information.

7. Following the format of the sample itinerary provided, type a travel itinerary, save it, and print it out. You may want to attach some of the supplemental information on the hotel, car rental, and places of interest/dining information with the travel itinerary so Dr. Schwartz can review it during his flight.

8. File your finished work in your Completed Work folder.

FIGURE 17-2
Time zone map

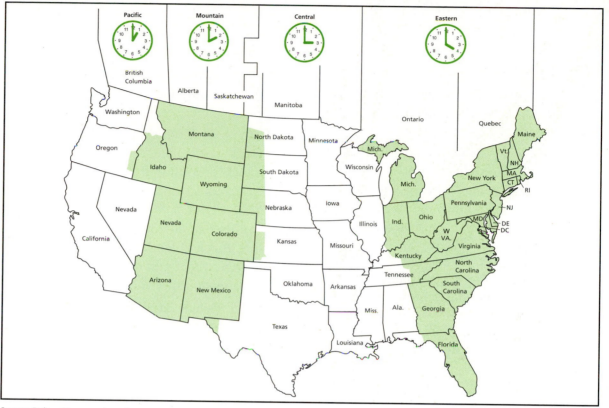

Source: Delmar/Cengage Learning

JOB 18
Administrative Functions—Blocking the Physicians' Schedule

MATERIALS AND SUPPLIES

- Medical Office Simulation Software (MOSS)

TIME ALLOTMENT

30 minutes

OCTOBER 25, 2010

Since Dr. Schwartz will be attending the American Medical Association National Convention next year in San Antonio, Texas, you will need to block his schedule in the computer so that no patients are scheduled for him during this time. You may recall that you already have some practice with schedule blocking from completing Job 3. Therefore, Mrs. Fleet has entrusted you with this task. Using instructions given below, block Dr. Schwartz' schedule from May 4, 2011, to May 6, 2011. (You will not need to block off the schedule for May 7th since May 7th is a Saturday and Dr. Schwartz does not have Saturday hours.)

Mrs. Fleet has informed you that even though Dr. Schwartz does not usually start seeing patients until 10 a.m., you should block out his schedule beginning at 9 a.m. in the morning. This avoids all confusion in the appointment schedule in the future once scheduling begins for the new year.

INSTRUCTIONS

1. Log into MOSS and click Appointment Scheduling from the Main Menu. Navigate to May 4, 2011.

2. Click Block Calendar, and click Yes through the confirming prompt.

3. As the physicians' lunch hours are already blocked into the permanent schedule, Mrs. Fleet has suggested that you block off the morning hours for all three days first and then proceed to the afternoon hours. Complete the Block Calendar screen for the mornings of May 4 to 6. (Remember: You will need to figure out the duration of time in *minutes* for the morning for Field 5.) Check your work with Figure 18-1, and click Save. Click through the confirming prompt, and click Close to return to the Practice Schedule.

Correcting Mistakes in Block Scheduling: If you make a mistake in blocking off the schedule and you have already saved your work, follow the steps below to correct it:

- Click on Appointment Scheduling in the Main Menu (if you are not already there).

- Single click on any time slot within your "error" time. (For example, if you blocked off time past 5:00 p.m., and you should have only blocked off time UNTIL 5:00 p.m., click anywhere within that time frame and then click on "Block Calendar.") This should bring up that particular blocking information that you wish to edit.

- Click Delete Break. This will delete the current information from the calendar and allow you to insert the correct information into the system.

- Be sure to click on "Save" when you are through entering the correct information and double check your work in the calendar when you are finished.

FIGURE 18-1
Check your work for Step 3

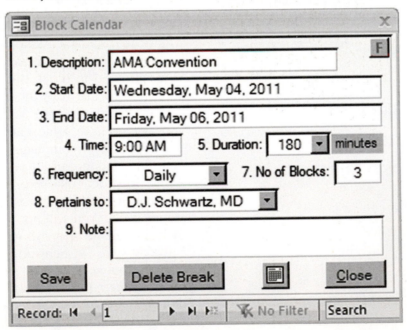

Source: Delmar/Cengage Learning

FIGURE 18-2
The practice schedule for May 4, 2011

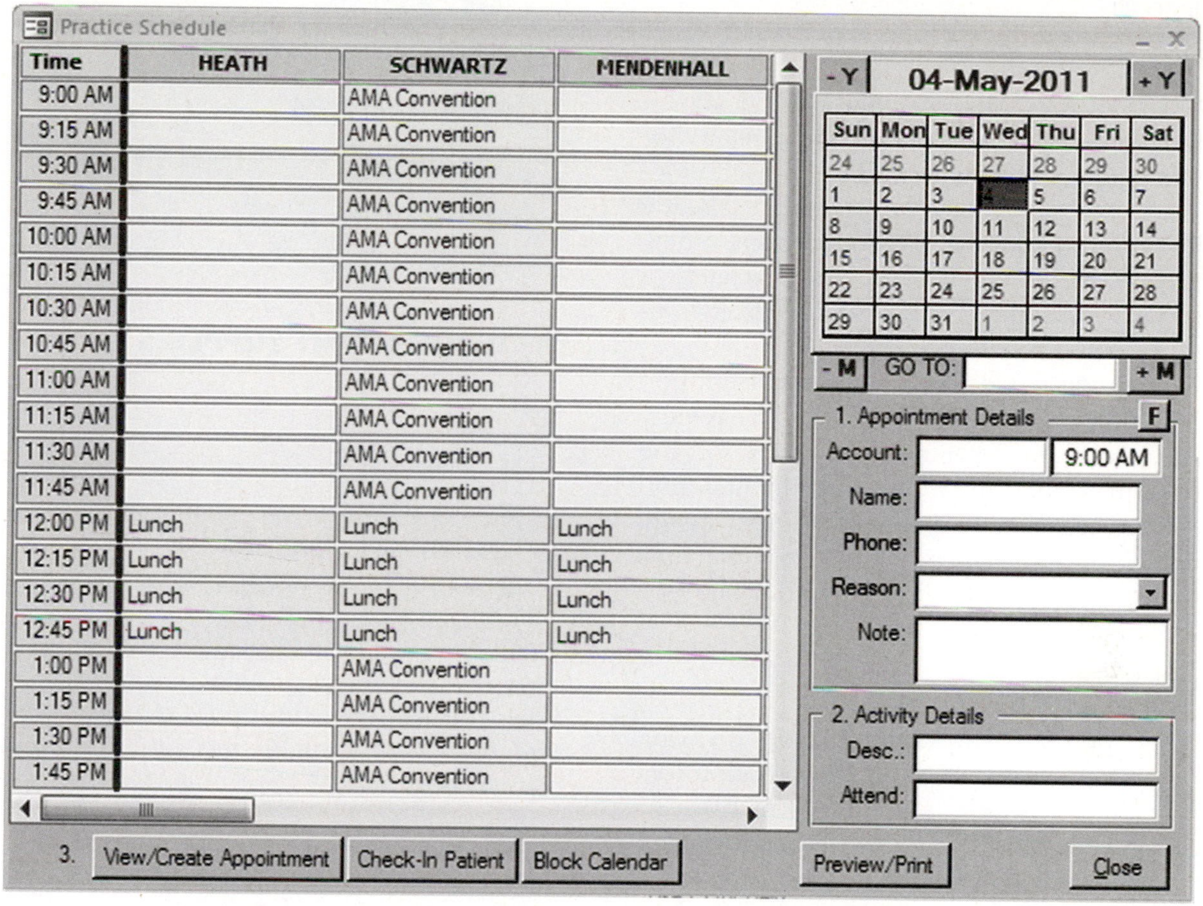

Time	HEATH	SCHWARTZ	MENDENHALL
9:00 AM		AMA Convention	
9:15 AM		AMA Convention	
9:30 AM		AMA Convention	
9:45 AM		AMA Convention	
10:00 AM		AMA Convention	
10:15 AM		AMA Convention	
10:30 AM		AMA Convention	
10:45 AM		AMA Convention	
11:00 AM		AMA Convention	
11:15 AM		AMA Convention	
11:30 AM		AMA Convention	
11:45 AM		AMA Convention	
12:00 PM	Lunch	Lunch	Lunch
12:15 PM	Lunch	Lunch	Lunch
12:30 PM	Lunch	Lunch	Lunch
12:45 PM	Lunch	Lunch	Lunch
1:00 PM		AMA Convention	
1:15 PM		AMA Convention	
1:30 PM		AMA Convention	
1:45 PM		AMA Convention	

Practice Schedule

04-May-2011

Sun	Mon	Tue	Wed	Thu	Fri	Sat
24	25	26	27	28	29	30
1	2	3	4	5	6	7
8	9	10	11	12	13	14
15	16	17	18	19	20	21
22	23	24	25	26	27	28
29	30	31	1	2	3	4

GO TO:

1. Appointment Details

Account: 9:00 AM
Name:
Phone:
Reason:
Note:

2. Activity Details

Desc.:
Attend:

3. View/Create Appointment | Check-In Patient | Block Calendar

Preview/Print | Close

Source: Delmar/Cengage Learning

4. Next, block off his afternoon schedule for all three days. After you have finished blocking Dr. Schwartz' schedule for all three days, compare your Practice Schedule screen for May 4, 2011, with Figure 18-2.

5. Close out of MOSS. You have completed your assignment for the day.

JOB 19
Concepts of Effective Communication— Transcription: Oncology Consult

MATERIALS AND SUPPLIES

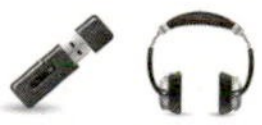

- Flash drive
- Transcription File: Job 19— Dr. McCracken

TIME ALLOTMENT

1 hour

OCTOBER 26, 2010

This morning, Mrs. Fleet has asked you to transcribe another oncology consult for Quali-Care Clinic. One of their transcriptionists is out sick today, and they are already behind in their work. Dr. McCracken, a new physician to Quali-Care, has dictated a report on Sterling Peak and needs it transcribed as soon as possible.

As with your previous transcription assignment, you will need to review Appendix A: Reference Materials for the sample format, as well as pertinent terminology and abbreviations. Once again, Mrs. Fleet has agreed to go over the final copy with you when you have finished.

INSTRUCTIONS

1. Open the Transcription folder on your flash drive to retrieve the dictation for this Job (there is one file: Job 19). Select the file type that is appropriate for your computer system.

2. Transcribe the dictation. Save your finished work on your flash drive as Job 19.

3. Place the finished transcript in your Completed Work folder or hand in to your instructor.

JOB 20
Concepts of Effective Communication— Completing Finished Copy from Rough Draft

MATERIALS AND SUPPLIES

- Flash drive
- Form *on flash drive*: Job 20—Procedure-Vasectomy
- Form *in Job Training Manual*: Job 20—Rough Draft Procedure-Vasectomy

Note: You will be using BOTH the electronic and hard copy form in this Job. The hard copy form in the Job Training Manual contains proofreaders' marks to indicate how you should correct the electronic file.

TIME ALLOTMENT

30 minutes

OCTOBER 27, 2010

Several days ago, Dr. Mendenhall dictated an informational vasectomy consent form. The resulting transcript has been edited and is now ready for you to prepare in final form. The words "PROCEDURE: VASECTOMY" are to be used as a heading. In the future, Dr. Mendenhall wishes to provide a copy for each patient who requests a vasectomy.

INSTRUCTIONS

1. Open your flash drive and find the file for Job 20: Procedure-Vasectomy.

2. Find the form for Job 20 in this Job Training Manual (Rough Draft, Procedure-Vasectomy). The hard copy provides the proofreaders' marks and edit notations.

3. Prepare the electronic document, proofread, and correct all errors noted on the Rough Draft form. Appendix A: Reference Materials contains a page with Proofreaders' Marks to help you complete this job.

4. Save your finished work on your flash drive as Job 20.

5. Print a copy of the finished document and place it in your Completed Work folder.

fallen into one of the drawers under the examination table (evidently left open). When you reached in to check the supply of paper drapes kept in that drawer, you were exposed to the needle.

Mrs. Fleet informs you to immediately wash your hands thoroughly with soap and water, following proper Occupational Safety and Health Administration (OSHA) exposure protocol. Additionally, she retrieves an Occupational Exposure Incident Form and asks you to complete it as soon as possible.

INSTRUCTIONS

1. Complete Page One of the report.

2. Place the report in your Completed Work folder.

JOB 21
Safety and Emergency Practices/Legal Implications—Preparing Occupational Exposure Incident Report

MATERIALS AND SUPPLIES

- Form: Job 21—Occupational Exposure Incident Report

TIME ALLOTMENT

15 minutes

OCTOBER 28, 2010

This morning, Mrs. Fleet asked you to assist her in doing the monthly inventory of the clinical areas in preparation for ordering supplies. While completing this task in one of the examination rooms, you accidentally pricked your finger on a needle, which had

JOB 22
Administrative Functions—Ordering Office Supplies and Preparing a Purchase Order

MATERIALS AND SUPPLIES

- Form: Job 22—Purchase order
- Internet access

TIME ALLOTMENT

1 hour

OCTOBER 28, 2010

At Douglasville Medicine Associates, an inventory is taken on a monthly basis of all medical office supplies to determine which supplies need to be replenished. Douglasville Medicine Associates has been using a local medical office supplier for reorders; however, today Mrs. Fleet has asked you to do some research on the Internet to find the "best" prices for the supplies that need to be ordered. She would prefer to order all the supplies online from the same company.

The following items need to be purchased:

- three aural (tympanic) thermometers
- ten boxes each of small, medium, and large Latex-free, powder-free gloves
- ten boxes of Dynarex alcohol prep pads
- ten boxes of Tegaderm Foam Adhesive Dressing (4-inch square pad)
- five boxes of Monoject tuberculin safety syringes (1 mL 25-gauge × 5/8" needle)
- ten reusable tie-back patient examination gowns (one size fits all)
- one Accu-Chek Aviva glucometer
- four Accu-Chek Aviva test strips
- one Accu-Chek Aviva 2-level control solution
- one Accu-Chek Softclix lancet device
- one Accu-Chek Softclix lancets

After determining which medical supply company to use, you are to complete a purchase order for the requisition.

INSTRUCTIONS

1. Using an Internet search engine (such as Google or Yahoo), search for a medical supply company that offers the above-listed products. Then, search a second site to determine which company has the "best" price. (Be sure to look at shipping and handling charges in your comparison.) If you have time, a third site can be reviewed.

2. Once you have determined which medical supplier to use, write down the name, address, and phone number

of the company, as well as the pricing information. You will need this to complete the purchase order.

3. Open your flash drive and download the form for Job 22—Purchase Order. Use your flash drive to save your work.

4. Prepare the purchase order, save it, and print it out.

5. Place the paper copy in your Completed Work folder.

JOB 23
Administrative Functions—Manual Appointment Scheduling

MATERIALS AND SUPPLIES

- Folded Appointment Schedule from your *Medical Office Practice* package (for the week of November 1–5 and 8–12)
- Physicians' schedule from Job 2 (use as a reference)
- Form: Job 23—Appointment Cards

TIME ALLOTMENT

45 minutes

OCTOBER 29, 2010

When you arrive at Douglasville Medicine Associates today, you are greeted by Mrs. Fleet, who informs you that the computers have "crashed" and that she will need you to assist Emily, one of the medical assistants, in scheduling appointment requests in the appointment book. Since Douglasville has converted to computerized appointment scheduling, the appointment book will first need to be properly blocked out according to the current physician schedule. Second, appointments which have already been scheduled will need to be written in the book. Finally, all appointment requests will have to be scheduled manually and then posted in the computer when it becomes accessible.

As the computers crashed early this morning just after the office opened, there has been little time for the manual appointment schedule to be completed. Emily has managed to block next week's appointment schedule off accordingly for each physician, and with the help of Mei Ling (who manually pulled encounter forms to determine dates and times), she was able to fill in the names of patients who have already been scheduled for next week and the week of November 8. Additionally, some patients from today need to be scheduled for rechecks in the next week or two.

Emily has asked you to block the appointment schedule for the week of November 8 through November 12, using the physician practice schedule from Job 2 and the previous week's appointment book sheet as a guide. Once that is completed, you will assist her for the rest of the morning in scheduling patient appointments manually in the appointment book.

INSTRUCTIONS

Use a pencil to complete this assignment!

1. Using the appointment schedule from the week of November 1st as a guide, and referencing the physicians' work schedules from Job 2, block the appointment schedule for the week of November 8th. Blocking the schedule means placing an X through, or drawing a line through, times when physicians are unavailable to see patients (i.e., before the office opens, after the office closes, lunchtime, physician rounds, etc.). You must be careful to block the correct physician's schedule with the correct times; otherwise, the physician may not be

available when the patient arrives for his or her appointment. When you have finished with the above task, schedule the following patients in the order they are listed. *Remember to schedule patients for the correct time allotments: New patients 45 minutes, physical examinations 30 minutes, established patients/rechecks 15 minutes.* **Additionally, fill out an appointment card for each patient who actually makes their appointment in the office. (If this were a real situation, you would give the completed appointment card to the patient to take home instead of printing out a reminder sheet since the computer system is down.) **There are extra appointment cards provided in case you make an error.**

A. Christopher Vioni, a patient of Dr. Schwartz, calls to request an appointment for a medication check the week of November 8th. He is available later in the morning (as close to lunchtime as possible) on Tuesdays and Wednesdays.

B. While scheduling Mr. Vioni, you discover that Dr. Schwartz has three patients who were scheduled during the time of his morning rounds at Community General. These patients were scheduled in error and must be rescheduled as soon as possible. Reschedule these patients for Wednesday, November 10th, in the morning.

C. Edward Pinny, a patient of Dr. Mendenhall, stops by during his lunch hour to make an appointment for his annual physical examination. He is requesting either a Tuesday or a Friday morning the week of November 8th.

D. Beverly Phipps, an established patient, calls asking for an appointment with Dr. Heath ASAP as she is going out of the country and needs the proper immunizations.

She would like the earliest appointment possible. However, she has not been seen by Dr. Heath for over a year, and it is the policy of the practice to schedule patients for a 30-minute examination if they have not been seen within a year's time.

E. Maria Gomez was in today to see Dr. Schwartz for a blood pressure check and will need an appointment for a recheck in two weeks.

F. Yvonne Peterson sees Dr. Heath for chronic osteoarthritis. This morning she calls stating that the pain in her knee is increasing. She would like to see him as soon as possible Monday afternoon.

G. Aubrey, a receptionist from Dr. Torres' office (located in Sarasota Florida), calls to refer a patient and her husband who are moving into the Douglasville Area next week. She would like to set up two new patient appointments with one of the physicians the week of November 8th, possibly Thursday or Friday afternoon. The patients' names are Roy and Kay Baker. Their telephone number here in Douglasville will be (123) 457-8809. Aubrey states that Kay will need a late afternoon appointment since her husband works until 3:30 p.m.

H. Eva Valez calls asking if she can change her appointment with Dr. Schwartz from Thursday, November 11, at 4:00 p.m., to Thursday, November 11, at 2:00 p.m. She is going out of town and would like to leave earlier.

I. Rod Spencer, an elderly gentleman, comes to the appointment desk after seeing Dr. Heath. He needs a recheck in one week. He tells you that this time (close to lunchtime) was very inconvenient since he relies on his neighbor to bring him to his appointments, and his neighbor volunteers at the Senior Center

on Friday afternoons. He is requesting an appointment in the morning as early as possible but not before 10:00 a.m. because he is having difficulty "getting around" these days, and it takes him a while to get ready. Mr. Spencer prefers if the appointment be some time between 10:00 and 10:45.

J. A new patient, Gladys Baker, calls in asking to schedule an appointment with Dr. Mendenhall. She tells you she works second shift at Community General as a surgical technician; therefore, she will need a morning appointment. Mrs. Baker also tells you that she babysits her granddaughter on Mondays, Wednesdays, and Fridays.

2. After you have completed scheduling patients A–J, file the appointment schedule and the appointment cards in your Completed Work folder.

JOB 24
Basic Practice Finances—Posting Entries on a Day Sheet

MATERIALS AND SUPPLIES

- Appointment Schedule for October 29, 2010 (Figure 24-1)
- 8 Encounter Forms: Job 24— Encounter Forms for the following patients: Wittmer, Furtaw, Perez, Guest, Freno, Santana, Boyd, and Brewer
- CPT (Current Procedural Terminology) code list and fee schedule (in Appendix A: Reference Materials)

- Folded Day Sheet from your *Medical Office Practice* package
- Deposit Slips (example , Figure 24-3)
- Form: Deposit Slip (blank)
- Calculator
- Pencil and eraser

TIME ALLOTMENT

60 minutes

OCTOBER 29, 2010

This morning you were asked by Mrs. Fleet to assist Emily in scheduling appointments manually since the office computer system was down. This afternoon, Mrs. Fleet would like you to gain some basic knowledge in the financial aspect of a medical practice by learning how to "post" debits and credits on a day sheet. She explains that this is usually done on the computer; however, since the computer system is still unavailable, this procedure will have to be done manually. Mrs. Fleet will be helping you as you complete this process.

Mrs. Fleet explains that "posting" simply means to make an entry on the day sheet (or in the computer) of debits (charges) and credits (payments). This must be done accurately each time a patient comes in for services. Mrs. Fleet has completed this morning's entries, and she will be assisting you with posting the entries for the remainder of the day.

INSTRUCTIONS

1. Unfold the day sheet and examine the contents. You will be working from left to right as you post entries. Begin by looking at Line 1 at the top of the day sheet; the patient is Aimee Bradley. Mrs. Fleet has posted this entry, noting the date as October 29 (10–29). (It is important to note that ALL the entries on this day sheet will be 10–29 since each sheet must represent the SAME day.) Next is the description of services. Ms. Bradley had an office visit (OV). She was charged $140 (**Column A**) and made a payment of $140 (**Column B**). Since the patient had no previous balance on her account (**Column E**), her current balance as of today is $0 (**Column D**).

Looking to the RIGHT side of your day sheet, you will see a receipt number for Ms. Bradley of 21925. The receipt number is generated by the computer when the encounter form is printed out for the patient at the time of check-in. However, since the computer system is down, this number has been written on the day sheet as a reference number for each encounter form and is specific to each patient. Additionally, receipt numbers are sequential, so the next patient's receipt number is 21926, and so on.

Continuing on to the next column, Ms. Bradley saw Dr. Heath today (see appointment schedule, Figure 24-1); therefore, the charge of $140 is posted under Dr. Heath's column (**Column 1**). Nothing is posted in Dr. Schwartz's or Dr. Mendenhall's columns (**2 and 3**) since she was not seen by either of those physicians today. Ms. Bradley's payment of $140 is posted on her account under Services—Paid (**Column 4**). Nothing is posted under Services—Charge (**Column 5**) since Ms. Bradley paid in full. The *paid on account* column (**6**) is used to post a payment that is received on account (ROA) without services being rendered; for example, a patient mails a payment to the office for services rendered on a previous date, and you post the payment the day you receive it in the mail. (The patient does not actually come in that day to see the physician.) The next three columns are important when making the daily deposit and include *description*, *cash* (**Column 7**), and *checks* (**Column 8**). As you will note, nothing is posted in these three columns for Ms. Bradley because she paid $140 with a credit card (specifically, Master Card). This is posted in **Column 9**. The last column, *Memo*, indicates the type of credit card used to make the payment. However, when a patient makes a payment by check, you must write the patient's last name in the *description* column and post the payment amount under *check*. If the patient makes a

FIGURE 24-1
Manual appointment schedule for October 29, 2010

	Heath	Schwartz	Mendenhall
8:00			
:15			OFF
:30			
:45			
9:00	Bradley, A		
:15	↓ (PE)		
:30			
:45	Camille, E.		
10:00		Leighton, L.	
:15	Herbert, N.		
:30	Suggs, R.	Gordon, E.	
:45			
11:00		Lagasse, E.	
:15	Yamagata, N.		
:30	Jefferson, A.	Pinkston, A.	
:45		↓ (PE)	
12:00			
:15			
:30			
:45			
1:00		Wittmer, J	
:15			
:30	Furtaw, T.		
:45			
2:00	Perez, R.	Guest, D.	
:15		(NP)	
:30		↓	
:45			
3:00	Freno, E.	Boyd, K.	
:15			
:30	Santana, E.		
:45			
4:00			
:15	Brewer, E.		
:30			
:45			
5:00			
:15			
:30			
:45			
6:00			

Source: Delmar/Cengage Learning

payment with cash, the payment amount is posted under *cash*, and nothing is written under *description*.

At the time of checkout, the patient is given a copy of the encounter form and, if the patient paid by debit or credit card, a receipt of the transaction. (This is not possible in simulation, but be aware that the patient should always get a copy of their financial transactions.)

2. Now that you have some understanding of the day sheet, it is your turn to try to post entries on the next patient. You will begin on the next available open line on the day sheet. Mrs. Fleet hands you John Wittmer's encounter form. Write "Wittmer, John" in the *Name* column on the left side of the day sheet.

   a. Write today's date in the date column of the day sheet.

   b. Mr. Wittmer was here for an office visit (OV). (Note that "Office" is checked as the Place of Service on his encounter form.

   c. Next you must determine today's charge by adding up the fees for Mr. Wittmer's procedures in the top portion of his encounter form (anything circled in Sections A through H). In order to do this, you will need to reference the CPT code list, which includes a fee schedule for each procedure. The first code circled is 99214 (a detailed examination for an established patient). The CPT code list is referenced in order of **number (0–9)**. Therefore, begin by looking in the codes starting with the number **9**. You will find that the charge for 99214 is $180. There is also a Medicare Allowable charge; however, Mr. Wittmer does not have Medicare, and therefore you will use the $180 charge. The second procedure listed for Mr. Wittmer is EKG w/interpretation (93000). The charge for this code is $131. There are no other procedures circled. (There are NO charges for diagnosis codes.) The total for Mr. Wittmer for today is $311. Write this number in **Column A** (Charge).

   d. Mr. Wittmer has no co-payment and therefore makes no payment for today. Place a zero in **Column B** (Payments).

e. There is no note on his encounter form that indicates he has a previous balance on his account (this would be written above "Date of Service" on the top right of the form). Place a zero in **Column E** (Previous Balance).

f. Since Mr. Wittmer's charge for today was $311, and he made no payments and had no previous balance, his current balance is still $311 (**Column D**).

g. Mr. Wittmer's receipt number can be found at the top right of his encounter form. (Once again, these numbers are sequential; therefore, his receipt number should be 21937; double check this number and write it in the *receipt number* column.)

h. Mr. Wittmer saw Dr. Schwartz today; therefore, the total amount for services rendered ($311) must be written in Dr. Schwartz's Column (**2**).

i. No payment was made for today, so a zero is noted in **Column 4**.

j. The entire balance for today's visit ($311) will be charged to his account (**Column 5**).

k. The remainder of the day sheet for Mr. Wittmer will remain blank since he did not make a payment.

3. Your next patient is Thomas Furtaw (see encounter form), who saw Dr. Heath today for an office visit. Begin by writing this information in the appropriate columns.

a. According to his encounter form, Mr. Furtaw is an established patient who saw the doctor today for hypertension (high blood pressure). His only procedure code is 99211 (a brief office visit). You must find the correct fee for code 99211 and place the amount in the appropriate column.

b. Mr. Furtaw paid $10 in cash today and has no previous balance.

Indicate this information on his day sheet.

c. Determine Mr. Furtaw's current balance, and write this number in **Column D**.

d. Record the receipt number using the encounter form as a reference.

e. Since Mr. Furtaw saw Mr. Heath today, record the total amount of services rendered in **Column 1**.

f. Indicate Mr. Furtaw's payment of $10 in **Column 4**.

g. The remaining charge (balance) on Mr. Furtaw's account for today's services should be indicated in **Column 5**.

h. If you have not already done so, be sure to mark Mr. Furtaw's $10 cash payment in **Column 7**.

4. Mr. Raul Perez arrives at the desk to checkout after seeing Dr. Heath for an office visit. He makes a payment of $15 using his Visa debit card.

a. Complete the following columns: *Date, Description, Name,* and Columns A through E using his encounter form as a reference. (**Be sure to note Mr. Perez' previous balance.)

b. Indicate the receipt number in the appropriate column.

c. Write Mr. Perez' total charge for today in Dr. Heath's column (**1**).

d. Indicate Mr. Perez' payment in **Column 4**.

e. **Column 5** will show the difference in amount between the **charge for today's services rendered minus Mr. Perez' payment.** (**This amount will be different than the *Current Balance* on his account as Column 5 shows only TODAY'S charges to patient accounts, not ALL charges.)

f. Write Mr. Perez' payment in **Column 9**, and write "Visa" under the *Memo* column.

g. Check your work with Figure 24-2.

FIGURE 24-2

Check your work through Step 4

DAYSHEET (Daily Business Summary) SHEET NO. 24 DATE October 29, 2010

DATE	DESC.	CHARGE (A)	PAYMENTS (B)	ADJUST. (C)	CURRENT BALANCE (D)	PREVIOUS BALANCE (E)	NAME	RECEIPT NUMBER	DR. HEATH (1)	DR. SCHWARTZ (2)	DR. MENDENHALL (3)	SERVICE PAID (4)	SERVICE CHARGE (5)	PAID ON ACCOUNT (6)	DEPOSIT DESCRIPTION	CASH (7)	CHECKS (8)	CREDIT CARD (9)	MEMO
10-29	OV	140—	140—		0—	0—	Bradley, Aimee	21925	140—			140—						140—	MC
10-29	OV	85—	20—		85—	20—	Leighton, Laura	21926		85—		20—	65—			20—			
10-29	ROA		17—		0—	17—	Barrymore, Caitlin	21927				17—		17—				17—	VISA
10-29	OV	90—	45—		45—	0—	Camille, Emery	21928	90—			45—	45—		Camille		45—		
10-29	ROA (CK)		42—		0—	42—	Durand, Isabel	21929				42—		42—	Durand		42—		
10-29	OV	30—	38—		0—	8—	Gordon, Eric	21930		30—		30—		8—		38—			
10-29	OV	40—	40—		0—	0—	Herbert, Nancy	21931	40—			40—			Herbert		40—		
10-29	OV	40—	20—		49—	29—	Lagasse, Evan	21932		40—		20—	20—		Lagasse		20—		
10-29	OV	70—	15—		70—	15—	Pinkston, Anna	21933		70—		15—	55—			15—			
10-29	I (Mary)	55—	0—	15—	55—	0—	Suggs, Rachel	21934	55—				55—						
10-29	OV	70—	70—		0—	0—	Yamagata, Naomi	21935	70—			70—			Yamagata		70—		
10-29	OV	40—	40—		0—	0—	Jefferson, Andrew	21936	40—			40—				40—			
10-29	OV	311—	0—		311—	0—	Wittmer, John	21937		311—		0—	311—						
10-29	OV	65—	10—		55—	0—	Fortan, Thomas	21938	65—			10—	55—			10—			
10-29	OV	115—	15—		115—	15—	Perez, Raul	21939	115—			15—	100—					15—	VISA
TOTALS THIS PAGE →		9,473—	710—	15—	9,510—	798—		TOTALS →							TOTAL CASH/CHECKS →				
TOTALS PREVIOUS PAGE →									1	2	3	4	5	6	TOTAL DEPOSIT →	7	8	9	
MONTH-TO-DATE TOTALS →																			

PROOF OF CURRENT BALANCE THIS PAGE
$D = E + A - (B + C)$

PREVIOUS BALANCE (E)
+ CHARGES (A)
= SUBTOTAL
PAYMENTS (B)
ADJUSTMENTS (C)
– TOTAL CREDITS
= CURRENT BALANCE (D)

PROOF OF MONTH-TO-DATE CURRENT BALANCE
$D = E + A - (B + C)$

PREVIOUS BALANCE (E)
+ CHARGES (A)
= SUBTOTAL
PAYMENTS (B)
ADJUSTMENTS (C)
– TOTAL CREDITS
= MONTH-TO-DATE CURRENT BALANCE (D)

PROOF OF PAYMENTS THIS PAGE
$B = 4 + 6$

PAID SERVICE (4)
+ PAID ON ACCOUNT (6)
= PAYMENTS (B)

PROOF OF DOCTOR'S SHARE OF THIS PAGE CHARGES
$A = 1 + 2 + 3$

DOCTOR (1)
+ DOCTOR (2)
+ DOCTOR (3)
= TODAY'S CHARGES (A)

PROOF OF THIS PAGE OF SERVICE
$A = 4 + 5$

SERVICE PAID (4)
+ SERVICE CHARGED (5)
= THIS PAGE CHARGES (A)

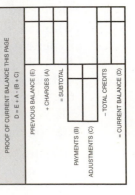

PROOF OF DEPOSIT
$B = 7 + 8 + 9$

CASH (7)
+ CHECKS (8)
= TOTAL DEPOSIT
+ CREDIT CARDS (9)
= PAYMENTS (B)

Source: Delmar/Cengage Learning

5. New patient, Denise Guest, checks out after her office visit with Dr. Schwartz. She pays her co-payment of $20 with her Visa debit card. Use Ms. Guest's encounter form and the knowledge you have gained from the above examples to complete the day sheet for this patient.

6. Your next patient is Elmer Freno. Complete the day sheet transaction for Mr. Freno, referencing the guidelines below:

   a. Remember to check for any previous balance!

   b. The amount paid today is noted on the encounter form.

   c. Check the schedule to see which physician Mr. Freno saw today.

   d. Follow patient #4's example when completing **Column 5**.

   e. Since Mr. Freno paid by check, be sure to write his last name in the *Description* column on the right side of your day sheet.

7. Now that you are feeling more comfortable with the process of posting entries on the day sheet, Mrs. Fleet has asked you to attend to the desk for the next hour. Complete the following patient entries:

   f. Ernesto Santana (usually a patient of Dr. Mendenhall, but needed to reschedule and is seeing Dr. Heath today for his three-month checkup).

   g. Karen Boyd

   h. Edward Brewer

8. When you have completed all the above transactions:

   i. Add up all of your columns individually (A through E and 1 through 9). For Columns A through E, calculate only "Totals This Page." Ex: Begin by totaling every entry in Column A and enter the total in Totals This Page.

   j. Add up Columns 7 plus 8 and write the total in the "Total

Deposit" box. (Columns 7 and 8 are cash and checks, which will need to be deposited in the bank the same day.)

   k. Next, add together the numbers in Columns A through E for "Totals This Page" and "Totals Previous Page." (Mrs. Fleet was able to get totals from yesterday's transactions from the statement that is printed out at the end of each business day.)

   l. Now it is time to "prove" the totals on your day sheet. This is a process of checks and balances. On the bottom left side of the day sheet you will see a box labeled "Proof of Current Balance This Page." Below that phrase is the formula for "proving" your totals for the **day:** $D = E + A - (B + C)$. The letters are referring to the columns you have added up. Begin by transferring the numbers you have totaled from each column under "Totals This Page" into the corresponding boxes, then follow the formula to find the current balance (D). If you have done the math correctly, the current balance (D) in the proofing box should match the "Totals This Page," Column D, which is $1775.

   m. Follow the same guidelines for the "Proof of Month-to-Date Current Balance" box; however, you will be transferring the numbers from the "Month-to-Date" totals in Columns A through E. If you have done the math correctly, the current balance in the proofing box (D) should match the "Month-to-Date Totals," Column D, which is $11,285.

   n. Continue onto the right-hand side of the day sheet to complete the next four boxes. The "Proof of Payments This Page" should add up to match the total for the day for Column B, which is $592. The "Proof of Doctor's Share of This

Page Charges" should add up to match the total for the day for Column A, which is $2133. The "Proof of This Page of Service" should add up to match the total for the day for Column A also, which is $2133. Finally, the "Proof of Deposit" should add up to match the total for the day for Column B, which is $592. If any of your total amounts are incorrect, make sure that you have entered each debit and credit correctly, *especially when the patient had a previous balance*. This seems to be a source of confusion when completing day sheets. Additionally, recalculate your columns until you are able to balance your day sheet correctly.

9. COMPLETING A DEPOSIT SLIP

   a. Deposits must be done at the end of each business day. Today you will need to complete a deposit slip by hand since the computer system is down. Mrs. Fleet has given you examples of deposit slips to review from the last time the system was down (Figure 24-3). Notice that

FIGURE 24-3
Sample deposit slips

Douglasville Medicine Associates

DEPOSIT SLIP

Record of checks for deposit

	Dollars	Cents
Cash	138. —	
Checks Fujio	45. —	
Phelan	42. —	
Serio	20.—	
Kish	40. —	
Chou	70. —	
Carchelle	67. —	
Babisz (Mo)	30. —	
Santiago (INS)	63. —	
	.	
	.	
	.	
	.	
	.	
	.	
Enter total $	515.-	

DATE February 18, - - - -

⑆606121504⑆ 162715943⑈

State Bank
3550 Commerce Blvd.
Douglasville, NY 01234

VISA		
	Chang	17. —
MC		
	Schwab	140. —
	Pennell	30. —
AE		
	Portulano	50. —
Total		237. —

Date: February 18, - - - -

Source: Delmar/Cengage Learning

there are two separate deposit slips—one for cash and checks, and one for credit cards. Using columns under "Deposit Ticket" on the day sheet, complete the deposit slip for cash and checks.

10. You have now completed Job 24. File the appointment schedule and instruction forms in your Supplies folder. File the Encounter Forms in the Encounter Forms folder. File your day sheet and deposit slips in the Completed Work folder.

JOB 25
Basic Practice Finances—Computerized Procedure Posting

MATERIALS AND SUPPLIES

- Medical Office Simulation Software (MOSS)
- Encounter Forms for the following patients from October 29, 2010: John Wittmer, Thomas Furtaw, Denise Guest, Ernesto Santana, Karen Boyd, and Edward Brewer (*these were used in Job 24 and should be in your Encounter Forms folder*)
- Form: Job 25—Patient Information Form for Denise Guest

TIME ALLOTMENT

60 minutes

NOVEMBER 1, 2010

It is Monday morning, and Mrs. Fleet welcomes you with news that the computer system has been repaired and is now functioning normally. All of the procedures and charges that were posted manually on Friday must now be posted in the computer system. Mrs. Fleet has been working on the posting process this morning, and now, with her assistance, she would like you to complete the process.

INSTRUCTIONS

1. Log into MOSS. From the Main Menu, click Procedure Posting.

2. A patient search list appears. Type "Wittmer" and click Search.

3. Highlight Mr. Wittmer's name in the patient list and click **Add**, since we are going to add procedures to his account.

4. The Procedure Posting window will appear. The top part of the window is where you will input charges, and the middle part of the screen (the Posting Detail) allows you to see charges that are posted for the visit. Using Mr. Wittmer's encounter form and the steps below, input Fields 1 to 12 for the first charge:

   a. In Field 1 (Reference Number), type "21937," Mr. Wittmer's receipt number.

   b. Leave Field 2 (Service Provider) as is. This is automatically populated based on the patient's primary physician selected in Patient Registration. *Even though Mr. Wittmer saw Dr. Schwartz today, leave this field as is.*

   c. In Field 3 (Point of Service), use the drop-down menu to choose Office.

   d. Leave Field 4 (Facility) blank. This field is only used if the patient is being seen in a facility other than the office.

   e. In Field 5 (From date), type 10/29/2010 (the date of service on the encounter form).

   f. Leave Field 6 (To date) blank and Field 7 as the default (1). These fields are only used if the service spans more than one day, such as a hospital visit. MOSS will automatically calculate Field 7 based on the To and From dates that are entered.

g. In Field 8 (CPT code), type "99214" and then press the Tab key on your keyboard. Note that when you do this, Field 10 automatically populates based on the code you have selected. The first CPT code for Mr. Wittmer's visit is 99214. Each CPT or procedure code is posted separately. *Mr. Wittmer's encounter form has two codes circled that are considered procedure codes. Procedure codes include any service the patient had during the office visit. These services incur a charge and must be posted. On Douglasville Medicine's encounter forms, procedure codes can be found in Sections A through H.* Finally, note that in MOSS you can use the magnifying glass next to Field 8 to search for CPT codes if unknown.

h. Leave Field 9 (Modifier) blank. This field is skipped since there is no modifier for this procedure. *A modifier is a code consisting of two digits that is used in conjunction with a procedure code to indicate that a procedure or service has been altered in some way, without changing the meaning of the code or the code itself.*

i. As mentioned, Field 10 is populated based on the CPT code selected. Note that the patient charges are $0, and that $180 will be billed to Mr. Wittmer's insurance.

j. Leave Field 11 (Bill To) as is. If a patient has insurance, the software automatically bills the primary insurance first. (Mr. Wittmer does not have a secondary insurance, which is indicated in Patient Registration.)

k. In Field 12 (Diagnostic Codes), we will enter the two diagnostic codes

on the encounter form. The physician has written a 1 next to angina pectoris, unspecified, indicating that it is the primary diagnosis. The primary diagnosis is the *main* reason why the patient came to see the physician. In box a, type 413.9. Again, note that you can use the magnifying glass next to the box to search for an unknown code. In Box b, enter 416.9.

Note: Angina pectoris is what the patient came in for today. In order for proper coding, billing, and subsequent reimbursement to occur, the diagnosis code must always match the procedure/service code. In other words, there always needs to be justification for a procedure/service to take place. Mr. Wittmer has an underlying heart condition (cardiopulmonary disease), which is considered his secondary diagnosis. This diagnosis code (ICD-9 or International Classification of Diseases code) must also be posted at the same time you post the procedure code (CPT code) for the office visit.

l. Leave Field 13 (Accident) as is. Mr. Wittmer's chest pain is not the result of an accident.

m. Check your screen with Figure 25-1 before proceeding.

n. When all entries are correct, click Post (at the bottom left corner of the window). When you do this, the charges are now moved into the Posting Detail area of the screen (Figure 25-2). This indicates the current charges and balance for his **first** service (99214), which is his office visit.

5. Now, we will go back to Field 1 and repeat the steps for his **second** procedure (93000). This code is for an EKG (electrocardiogram), and this was done because Mr. Wittmer was having angina pectoris, unspecified, at the time of his office visit. Since the EKG was done for that reason and not for the underlying reason or secondary

FIGURE 25-1
Check your work for Step 4

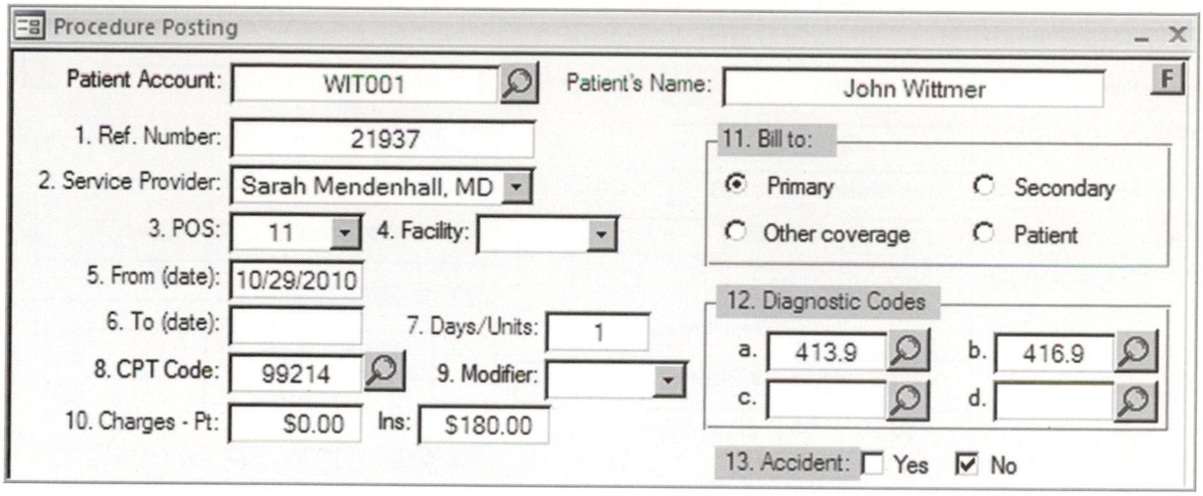

Source: Delmar/Cengage Learning

FIGURE 25-2
Check your work for Step 5

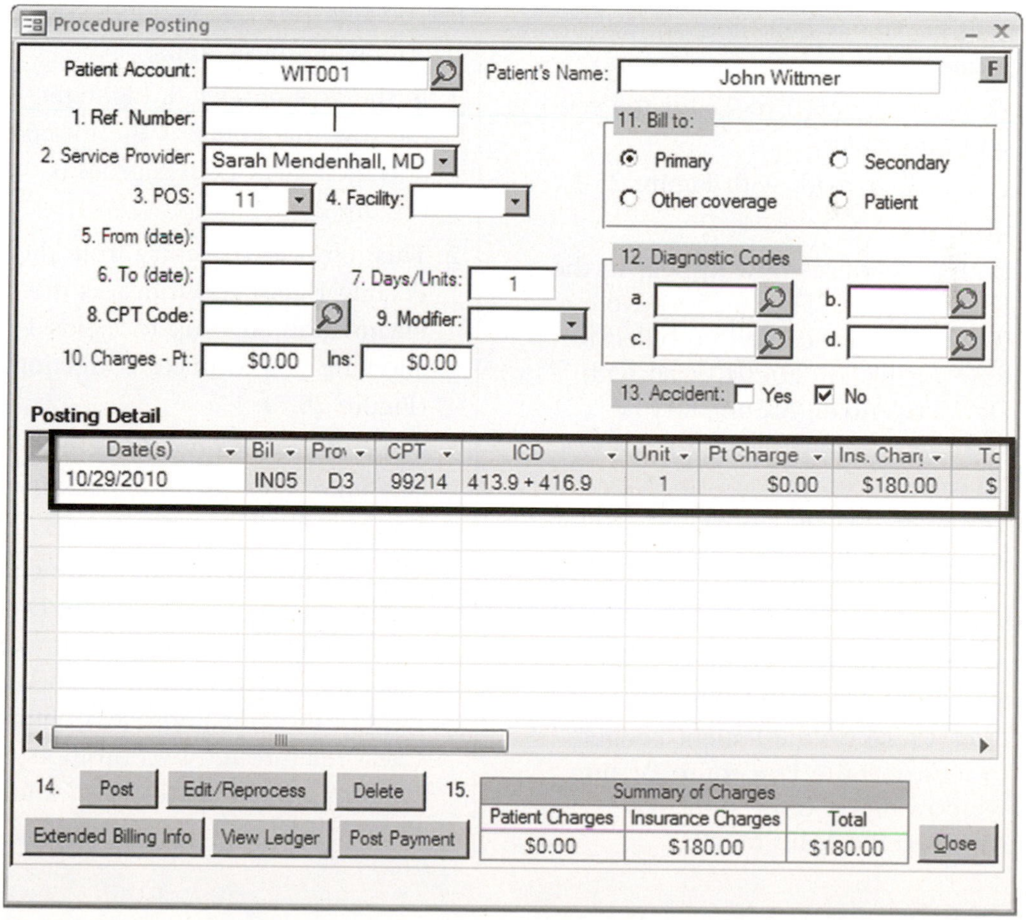

Source: Delmar/Cengage Learning

FIGURE 25-3

Check your work for Step 5b

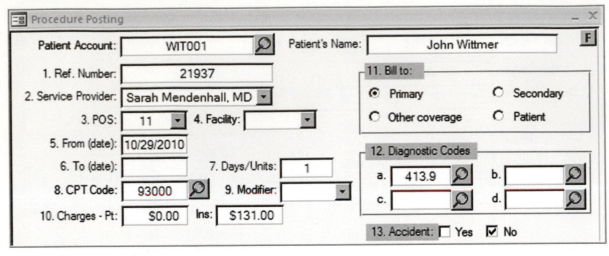

Source: Delmar/Cengage Learning

diagnosis of CAD, you will only need to post the CPT code for EKG (93000) with the ICD-9 code for angina pectoris (413.9). This is indicated on the encounter form.

a. Complete Fields 1 to 12 for the second procedure.

b. Check your work with Figure 25-3.

c. Click Post.

d. Both procedures now appear in the Posting Detail (Figure 25-4). Note that his insurance will be billed for $311 for his 10/29/2010 visit with Dr. Mendenhall. A Summary of Charges is located at the bottom of the screen.

e. You may also click on View Ledger, located at the bottom on the screen (below the Edit/Reprocess button). The ledger gives you a quick look at Mr. Wittmer's account details in a simplified way. See Figure 25-5.

f. Click Close on the Patient Ledger to return to the Procedure Posting window. Click Close until you return to the Main Menu.

Correcting Errors in MOSS: If you have made a mistake in a specific field during the posting process, you can correct it by following these steps:

1. In the Posting Detail, highlight the row that contains the mistake, and then click Edit/Reprocess (Figure 25-6).

2. This removes the entry from the Posting Detail and transfers the information back up to Fields 1 to 12, allowing you to make corrections (Figure 25-7).

3. Make the correction, and click Post. The entry now appears back in the Posting Detail, corrected.

4. You can also delete an entire charge. Again, starting in the Posting Detail area, highlight the entry to be deleted. Click the Delete button (to the right of the Edit/Reprocess button). Click Yes through two prompts, confirming that the entry should be deleted.

FIGURE 25-4
Check your work for Step 5d

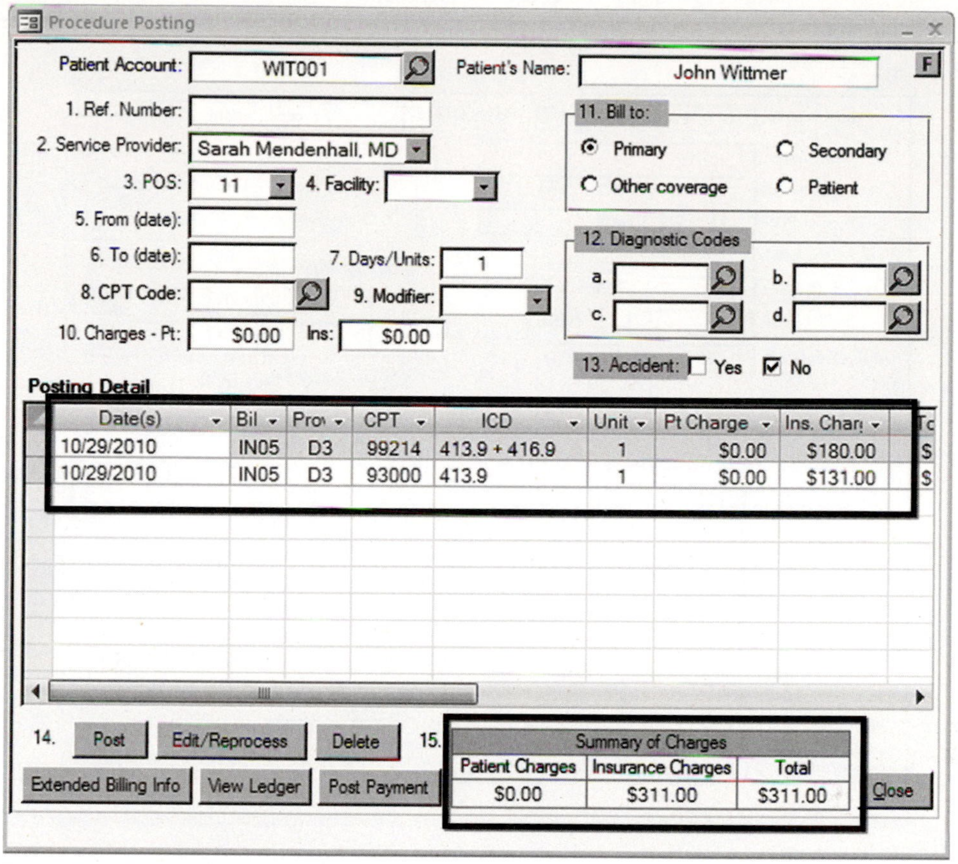
Procedure Posting

Patient Account: WIT001 Patient's Name: John Wittmer

1. Ref. Number:
2. Service Provider: Sarah Mendenhall, MD
3. POS: 11 4. Facility:
5. From (date):
6. To (date): 7. Days/Units: 1
8. CPT Code: 9. Modifier:
10. Charges - Pt: $0.00 Ins: $0.00

11. Bill to: Primary Secondary Other coverage Patient

12. Diagnostic Codes a. b. c. d.

13. Accident: Yes No

Posting Detail

Date(s)	Bil	Pro	CPT	ICD	Unit	Pt Charge	Ins. Char	Tc
10/29/2010	IN05	D3	99214	413.9 + 416.9	1	$0.00	$180.00	$
10/29/2010	IN05	D3	93000	413.9	1	$0.00	$131.00	$

14. Post Edit/Reprocess Delete

Extended Billing Info View Ledger Post Payment

15. Summary of Charges

Patient Charges	Insurance Charges	Total
$0.00	$311.00	$311.00

Close

Source: Delmar/Cengage Learning

FIGURE 25-5
The patient ledger screen

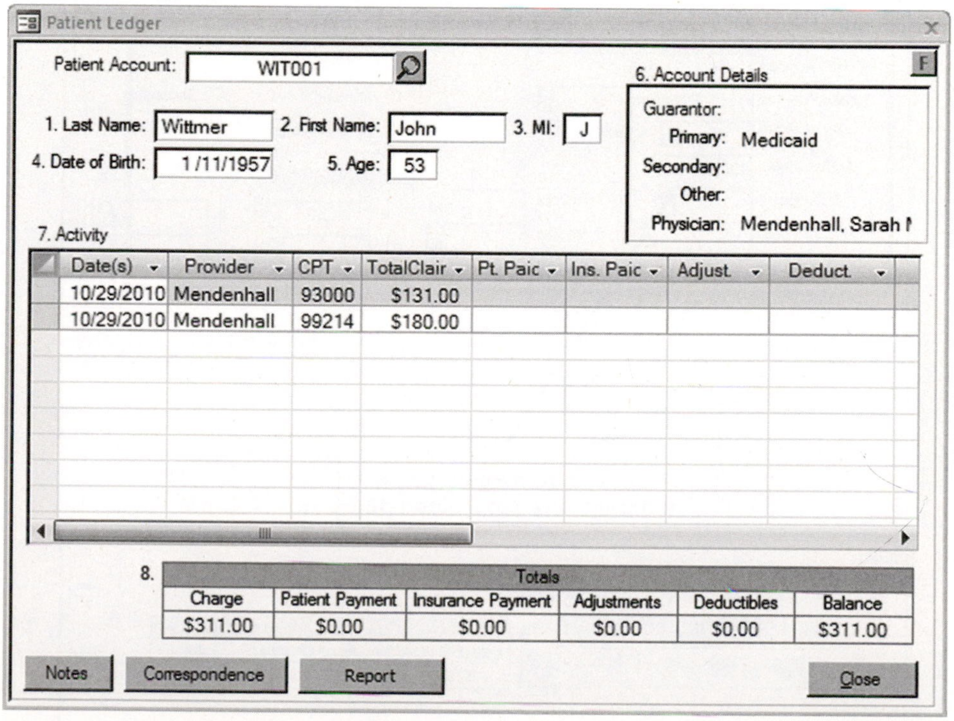
Patient Ledger

Patient Account: WIT001

1. Last Name: Wittmer 2. First Name: John 3. MI: J
4. Date of Birth: 1/11/1957 5. Age: 53

6. Account Details
Guarantor:
Primary: Medicaid
Secondary:
Other:
Physician: Mendenhall, Sarah M

7. Activity

Date(s)	Provider	CPT	TotalClair	Pt. Paic	Ins. Paic	Adjust.	Deduct.
10/29/2010	Mendenhall	93000	$131.00				
10/29/2010	Mendenhall	99214	$180.00				

8. Totals

Charge	Patient Payment	Insurance Payment	Adjustments	Deductibles	Balance
$311.00	$0.00	$0.00	$0.00	$0.00	$311.00

Notes Correspondence Report Close

Source: Delmar/Cengage Learning

FIGURE 25-6

To correct a mistake, highlight the charge in the posting detail area, and click edit/reprocess

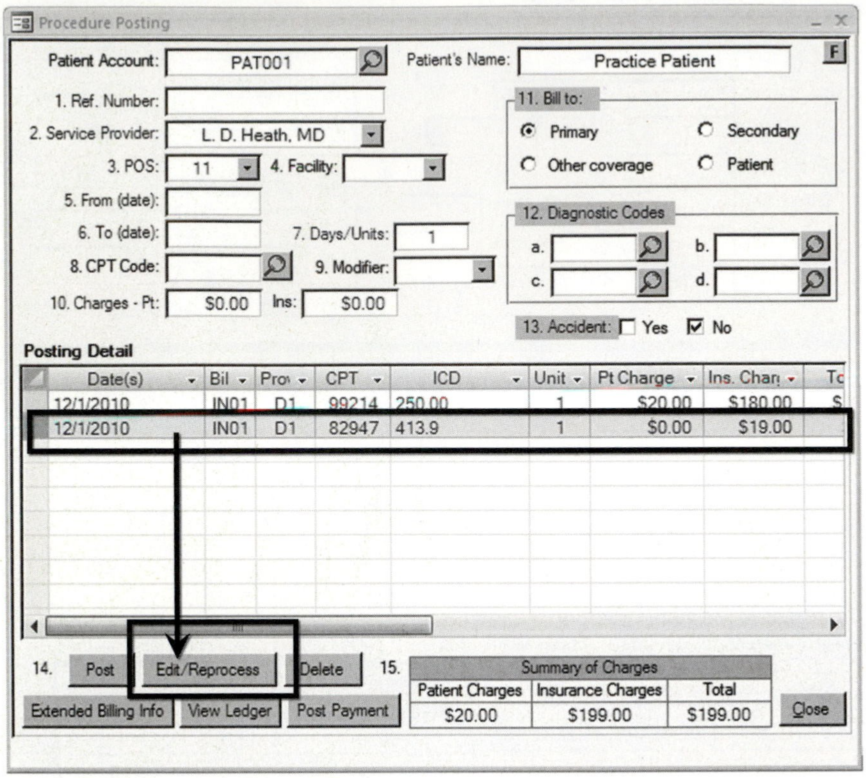

Source: Delmar/Cengage Learning

FIGURE 25-7

The entry is now transferred back to Fields 1-12, where a correction can be made

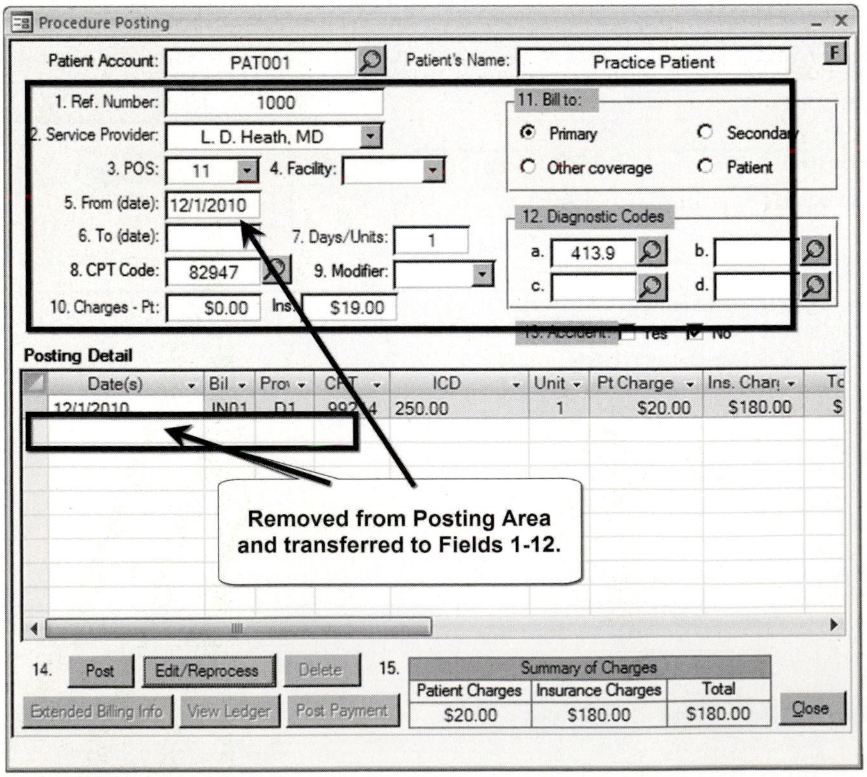

Source: Delmar/Cengage Learning

6. Next, you will post charges for patient Thomas Furtaw. Mr. Furtaw's encounter form shows one charge for his office visit (CPT code 99211).

   a. Click Procedure Posting on the Main Menu. Type "Furtaw" and click Search to find Mr. Furtaw's account. When you find him in the patient list, highlight his name and click the **Add button**, since you are adding procedures to his account (Figure 25-8).

   b. Using the guidelines learned previously, enter the charges in Fields 1 to 12. Check your screen with Figure 25-9, and click Post.

   c. When you have finished, click Close until you return to the Main Menu.

7. Denise Guest saw Dr. Schwartz as a new patient today. Due to the computer being down, her information was not put into system. Therefore, before you post procedures to her account, you will have to go to the Patient

FIGURE 25-8

Be sure to select Add when you are ready to post procedures to patient accounts

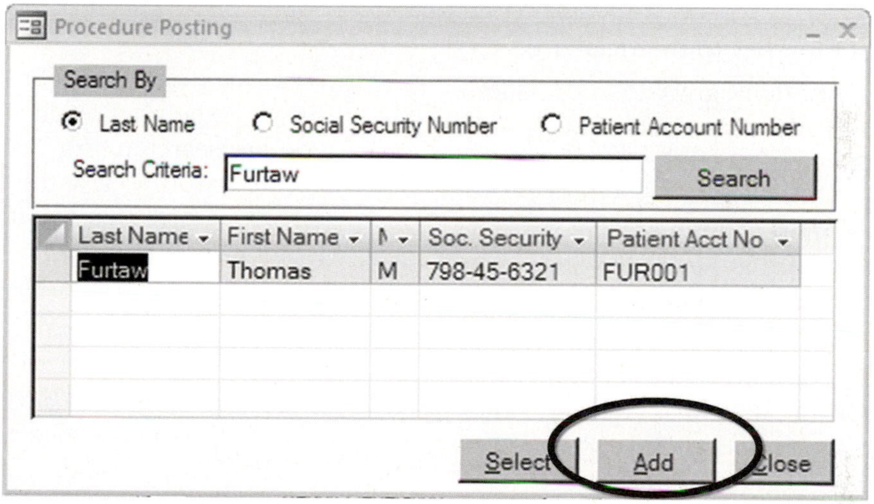

Source: Delmar/Cengage Learning

FIGURE 25-9

Check your work for Step 6b

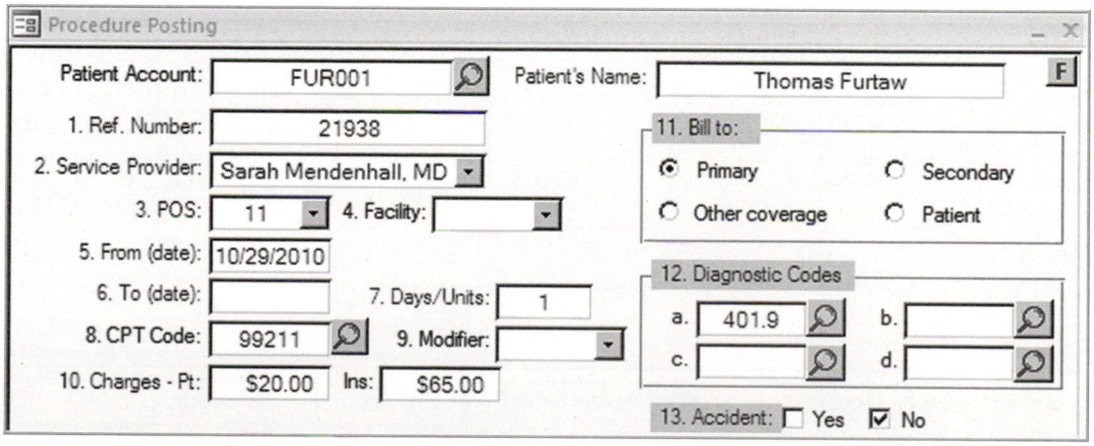

Source: Delmar/Cengage Learning

Registration area and create an account for her using the information she included on her Patient Information Form.

a. From the Main Menu, click Patient Registration, and search for "Guest." *Even though Ms. Guest is a new patient, it is good practice to always type the patient's name or social security number in to make sure that the patient does not have an account. This prevents the computer from generating two accounts for the same patient.*

b. Since Ms. Guest does not have an account with Douglasville Medicine Associates, click on Add since you are adding her to the database.

c. Enter her demographic information in the Patient Information, Primary Insurance, and HIPAA windows. Remember to save Ms. Guest's information at each screen. Make sure that her physician is Dr. Schwartz (Figure 25-10). Her insurance co-payment is $20.00.

d. When you have completed registering Ms. Guest, return to the Main Menu and click Procedure Posting. Search for and select Ms. Guest's account, and click **Add** to post her charges (refer to her encounter form):

- Post CPT 99204 with ICD-9 codes 780.79, 783.21, 311, and 599.0
- Post CPT 85031 with ICD-9 code 780.79
- Post CPT 80053 with ICD-9 code 783.21
- Post CPT 36415 with ICD-9 code 780.79 and 783.21
- Post CPT 87086 with ICD-9 code 599.0

e. Compare your Posting Detail with Figure 25-11.

f. Click Close.

8. Ernesto Santana has one procedure to be posted to his account. Remember to click **Add** after you have highlighted Mr. Santana's name on the patient account. Complete the posting process, and then compare your screen to Figure 25-12. *(Remember that Field 2, Physician, is automatically populated based on the patient's primary physician. Do not change this field.)*

9. Post two procedures for Karen Boyd. Remember to click **Add** when you are searching for Ms. Boyd's account. You review the encounter form and note that the ICD-9 code is not currently in the system, so you will need to add Ms. Boyd's ICD-9 code.

a. Complete Fields 1 to 11 on the top part of the Procedure Posting screen. When you get to Field 12, click on the magnifying glass (Figure 25-13) next to Box a.

b. An ICD-9 search box appears. Click Add.

c. Now, the list of ICD-9 codes that are currently in the system appears. Click Add.

d. When you do this, a new row appears. Click into the ICD code column and type "V72.42." Tab over to the Description column and type "Pregnancy Test, Positive

FIGURE 25-10

Be sure Dr. Schwartz is selected as the patient's physician

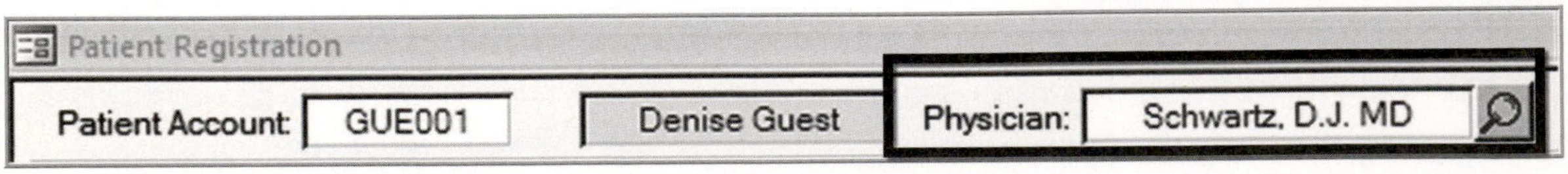

Patient Registration			
Patient Account: GUE001	Denise Guest	Physician:	Schwartz, D.J. MD

FIGURE 25-11

Check your work for Step 7

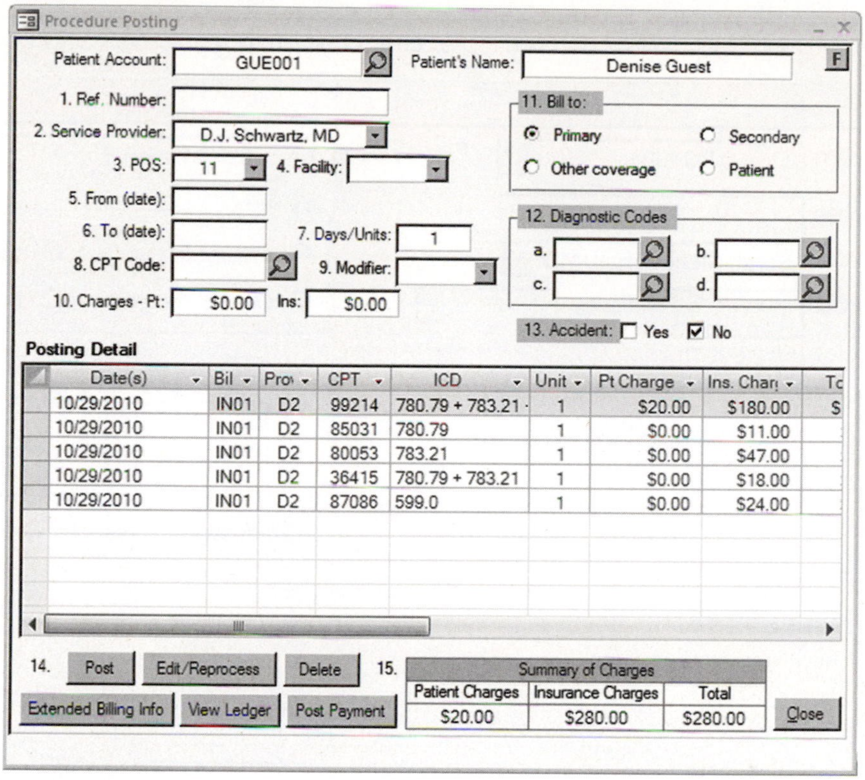

Source: Delmar/Cengage Learning

FIGURE 25-12

Check your work for Step 8

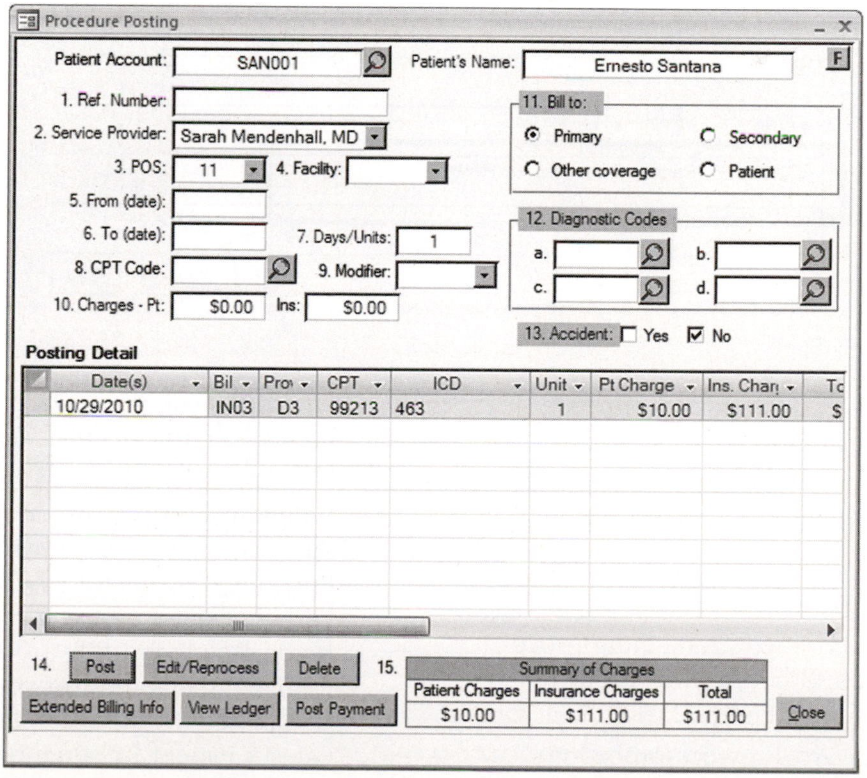

Source: Delmar/Cengage Learning

FIGURE 25-13

Clicking on the magnifying glass allows you to add ICD-9 codes, or search for ICD-9 codes already in the system

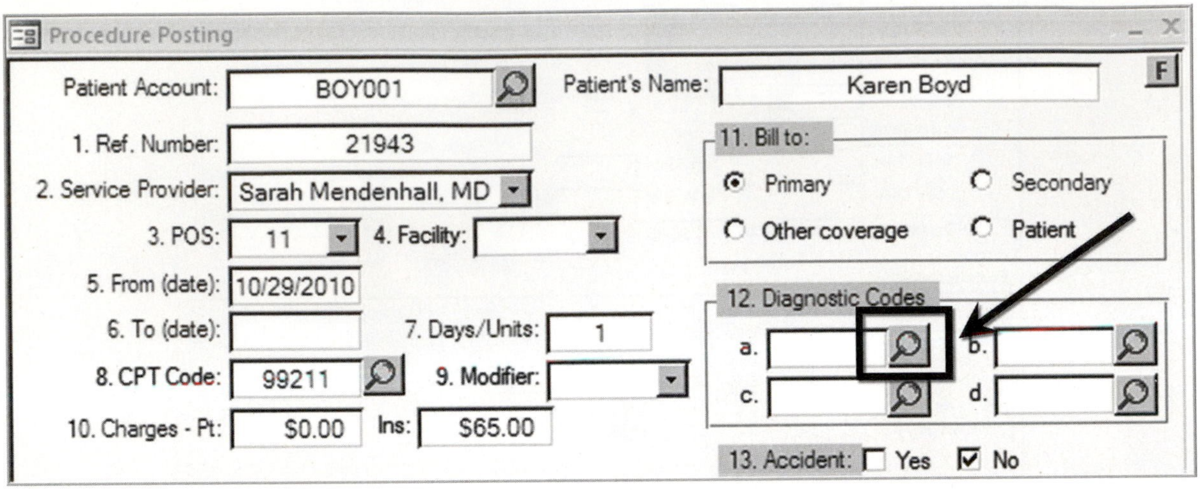

Source: Delmar/Cengage Learning

FIGURE 25-14

Check your work for Step 9d

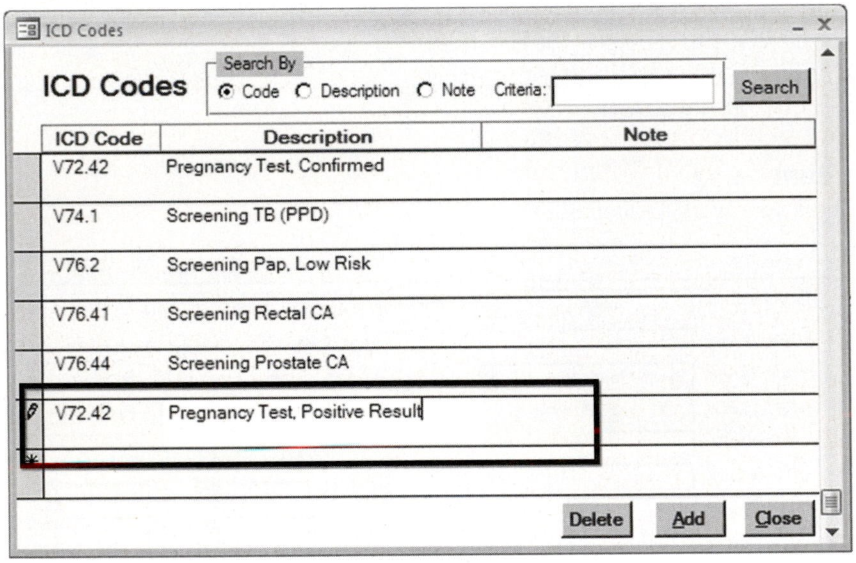

Source: Delmar/Cengage Learning

Result." Check your work with Figure 25-14.

e. When you are finished, click Close.

f. Now, back on the Procedure Posting screen, type "V72.42" in Field 12a.

g. Click Post.

h. Post Ms. Boyd's remaining procedures and check your Posting Detail with Figure 25-15.

10. Enter Edward Brewer's procedure. Check your work with Figure 25-16

and then click Post. Click Close until you return to the Main Menu screen.

11. When all postings are complete, file the following encounter forms in the Encounter Forms folder: Thomas Furtaw, Denise Guest, Ernesto Santana, Karen Boyd, and Edward Brewer. File John Wittmer's form in your Completed Work folder. Denise Guest's Patient Information Form may be filed in your Supplies folder.

FIGURE 25-15

Check your work for Step 9h

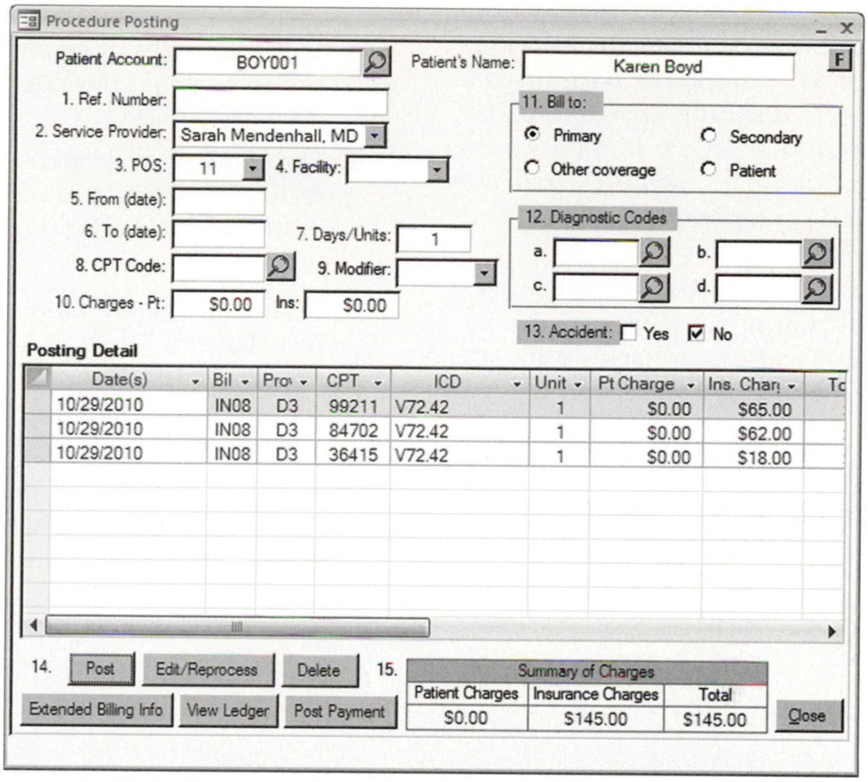

Source: Delmar/Cengage Learning

FIGURE 25-16

Check your work for Step 10

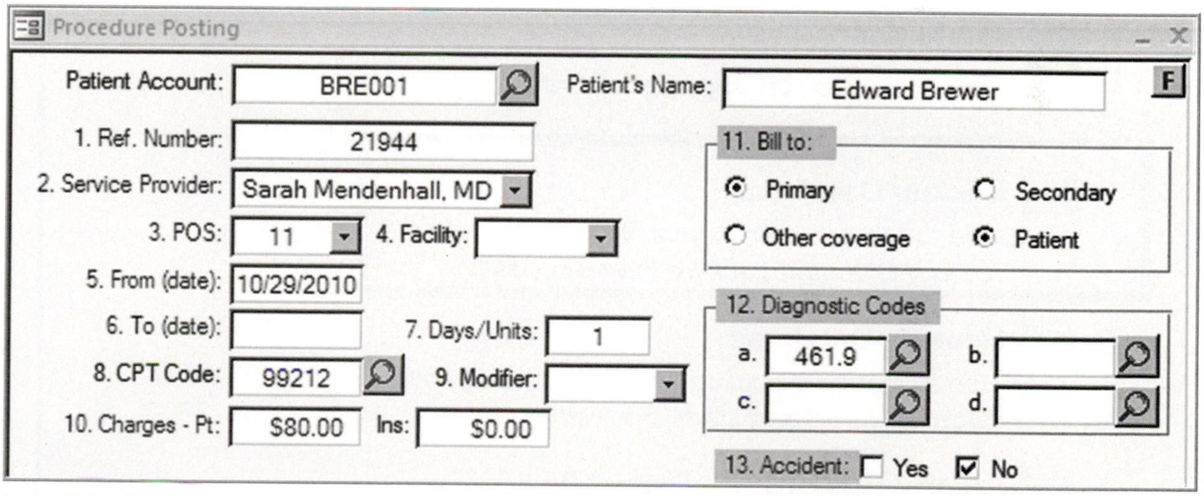

Source: Delmar/Cengage Learning

SAVING YOUR PROGRESS IN MOSS

Since MOSS is a simulation, there are certain features that have been added for training purposes. Two of these features are the Back Up and Restore functions. Backing up your MOSS database is like saving a document or other file on your computer. In the single-user version of MOSS, you can back up (save) your progress at any time by using the back up function. The restore function allows you to return to a previously saved point in the program. For instance, if you realize you have made a mistake and cannot correct it, you could restore a previous back up file and start a job over again. *If you are using MOSS 2.0 network version, you may move to the next section. The back up and restore functions are only available in the single-user version of MOSS. In the network version, the network administrator or instructor follows a different routine to back up your database.*

Now, follow these steps to create a Back Up file to save your progress through Job 25. (Steps on how to restore a back up file are found in Appendix C.)

1. Insert your *Medical Office Practice* flash drive into your computer.

2. Starting from the Main Menu screen of MOSS, click on File Maintenance.

3. In the Database Management tab, click the button next to 2. Backup Database (Figure 25-17).

4. You will receive a prompt: "Would you like to backup your current MOSS database?" Click Yes.

5. The program will open a File Save dialog box. Browse to select your flash drive as the location to save your back up file.

6. In the file name box, rename the file: "Backup Through Job 25.mde" (Figure 25-18). *It is critical to keep the file extension (.mde) at the end of the file name.*

7. Click OK through the prompt. Close the File Maintenance window and return to the Main Menu.

FIGURE 25-17
Backup up your MOSS database

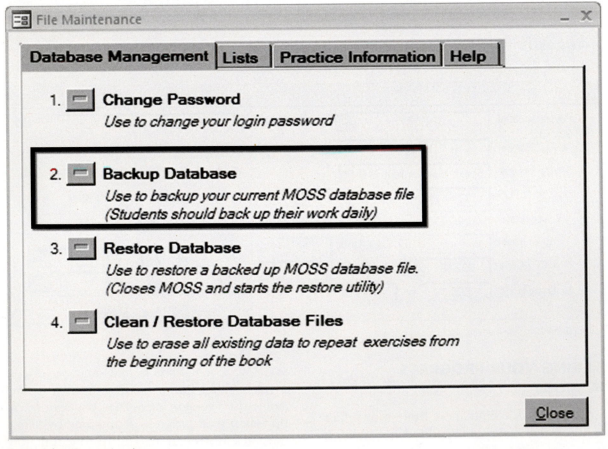

Source: Delmar/Cengage Learning

FIGURE 25-18

Naming your MOSS database, keeping the .mde file extension

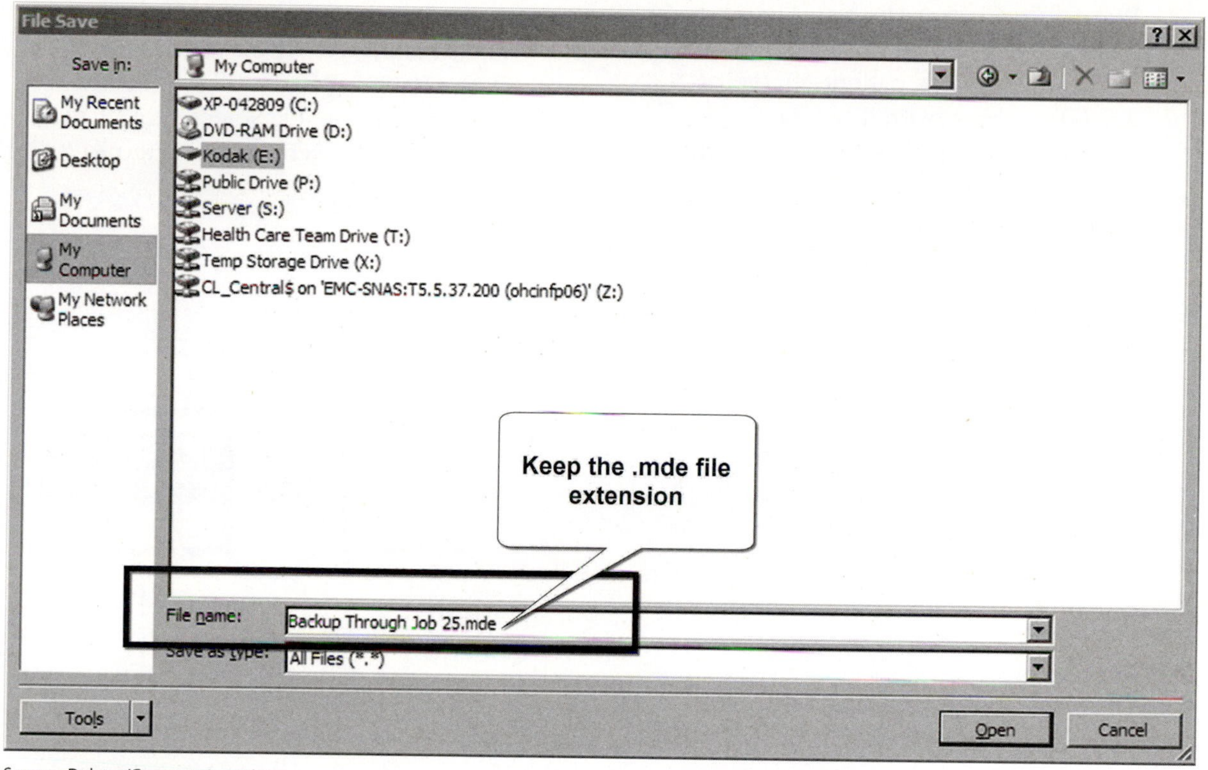

Source: Delmar/Cengage Learning

JOB 26
Basic Practice Finances—Computerized Payment Posting

MATERIALS AND SUPPLIES

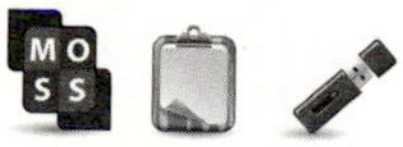

■ Medical Office Simulation Software (MOSS)

■ Encounter forms for the following patients from October 29, 2010: Thomas Furtaw, Denise Guest, Ernesto Santana, Karen Boyd, and Edward Brewer (*these were used in Jobs 24 and 25 and should be in your Encounter Forms folder*)

TIME ALLOTMENT

30 minutes

NOVEMBER 1, 2010

Now that the procedures from Friday have been posted, Mrs. Fleet would like you to learn how to post the payments received that day using the same encounter forms used to post procedures in Job 25. She explains that payments are usually posted at the same time the procedures are posted; however, since you are just learning, she would prefer you complete this in a step-by-step process before integrating both tasks.

INSTRUCTIONS

1. Log into MOSS. From the Main Menu, click Posting Payments.

2. Begin by searching for patient Thomas Furtaw in the patient list. Highlight his name in the list and click Apply Payment.

3. The Posting Payments screen should appear, which lists Mr. Furtaw's Procedure Charge History (Figure 26-1). Note that for Mr. Furtaw's charge (99211), there is a patient charge of $20.00, and his overall balance is $65.00. Reviewing his encounter form, his payment on Friday was only $10 (a partial payment).

4. In the Procedure Charge History area, click on the gray box to the left of the date (10/29/2010) to highlight the charge. Then click Select/Edit at the bottom of the screen. See Figure 26-2.

FIGURE 26-1

The procedure charge history for Thomas Furtaw

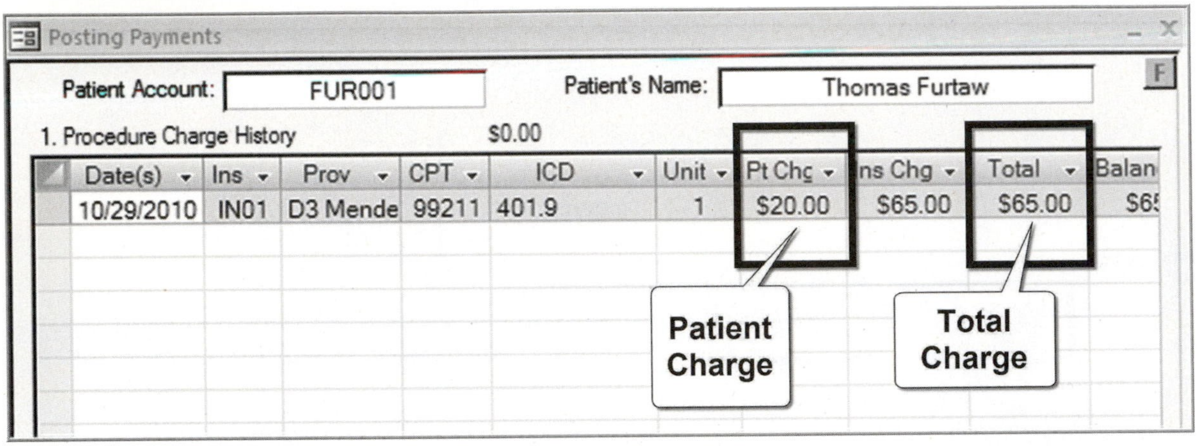

Source: Delmar/Cengage Learning

FIGURE 26-2

Highlight the 10/29/2010 charge, and click select/edit

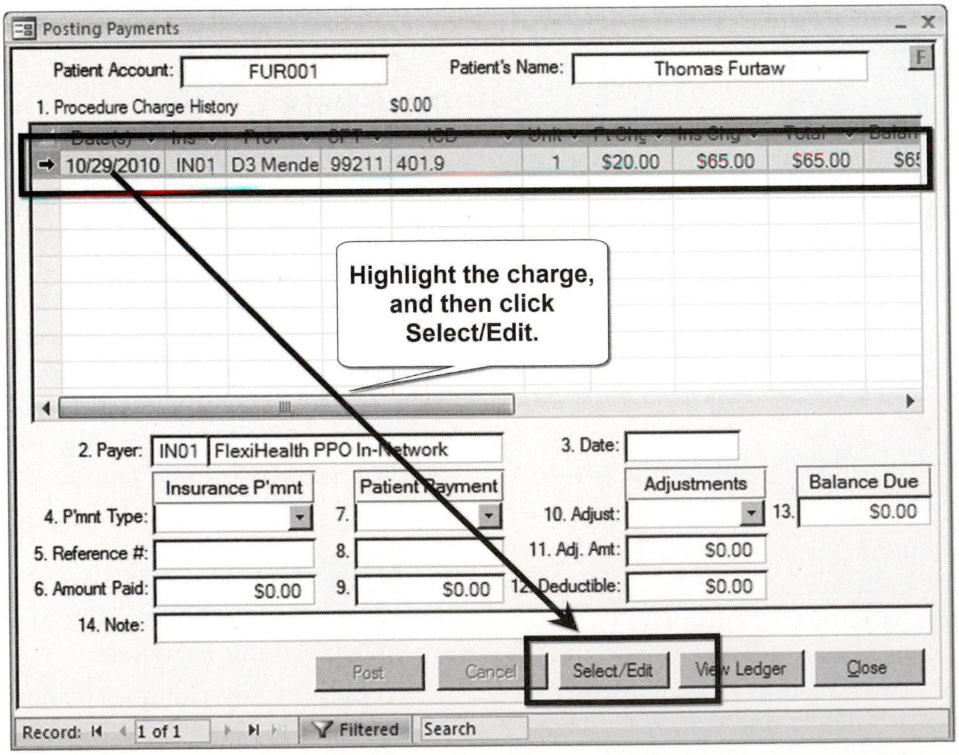

Source: Delmar/Cengage Learning

5. Note that when you do, the Balance Due field populates with $65.00 (the charges the practice is owed.) *If the Balance Due field is not populated, you have not performed Step 4 correctly. Do not proceed until the Balance Due field reads $65.00.*

6. Now that you have selected the charge against which to post the payment, fill in the following fields:

   a. Field 3 (Date): Type 10/29/2010

   b. Field 7 (Patient Payment/Payment Type): Use the drop-down menu and select PATCASH. This indicates he paid Cash.

   c. Field 8 (Patient Payment/Reference Number): Leave this blank. This is used when a patient pays by check or credit card. In the instance of a check, enter the check number here. If the patient uses a credit card, indicate the type of card (Visa, MC, etc.).

   d. Field 9 (Patient Payment/Amount Paid): Type $10.00.

   e. Leave the remaining fields as they are. (If you click out of Field 9 after the payment amount is entered, note that the Balance Due column now calculates as $55.00.) Check your screen with Figure 26-3 before proceeding.

7. Click Post. This applies the payment to the charge. Note that the Balance column in the Procedure Charge History area now reads $55.00.

8. Now click View Ledger at the bottom of the screen. In the Activity area, you can see that the $10.00 has been applied to the $65.00 charge, and his balance is $55.00 (Figure 26-4).

9. Click Close to return to the Payment Posting screen.

10. Mr. Furtaw brought in the remainder of his payment today in the form of a check (#589). This will be posted as a separate transaction of $10. Post this payment to Mr. Furtaw's account:

    a. Highlight the 10/29/2010 charge and click Select/Edit. Make sure the Balance Due field is now populated with $55.00 before proceeding.

    b. Field 3: Type 11/01/2010. (You will type over the previous date entered, 10/29/2010.)

    c. Field 7: Select PATCHECK.

    d. Field 8: Type 589.

    e. Field 9: Type $10.00.

    f. Click Post.

11. After the payment has been posted, click View Ledger. Note that the Activity area now shows two $10.00 payments. Compare your screen with Figure 26-5.

FIGURE 26-3

Check your work for Step 6

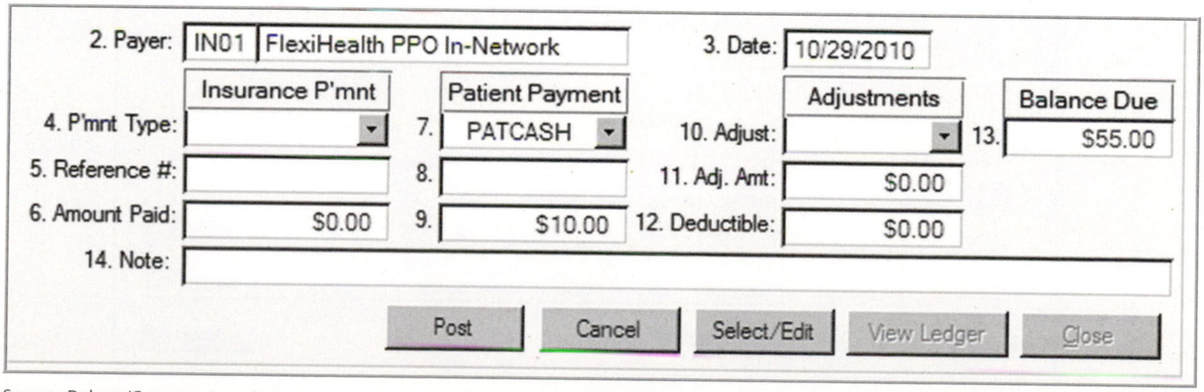

2. Payer:	IN01	FlexiHealth PPO In-Network		3. Date:	10/29/2010	
	Insurance P'mnt		**Patient Payment**	**Adjustments**		**Balance Due**
4. P'mnt Type:		7.	PATCASH	10. Adjust:	13.	$55.00
5. Reference #:		8.		11. Adj. Amt:	$0.00	
6. Amount Paid:	$0.00	9.	$10.00	12. Deductible:	$0.00	
14. Note:						

Post Cancel Select/Edit View Ledger Close

Source: Delmar/Cengage Learning

FIGURE 26-4

Patient ledger screen for Thomas Furtaw

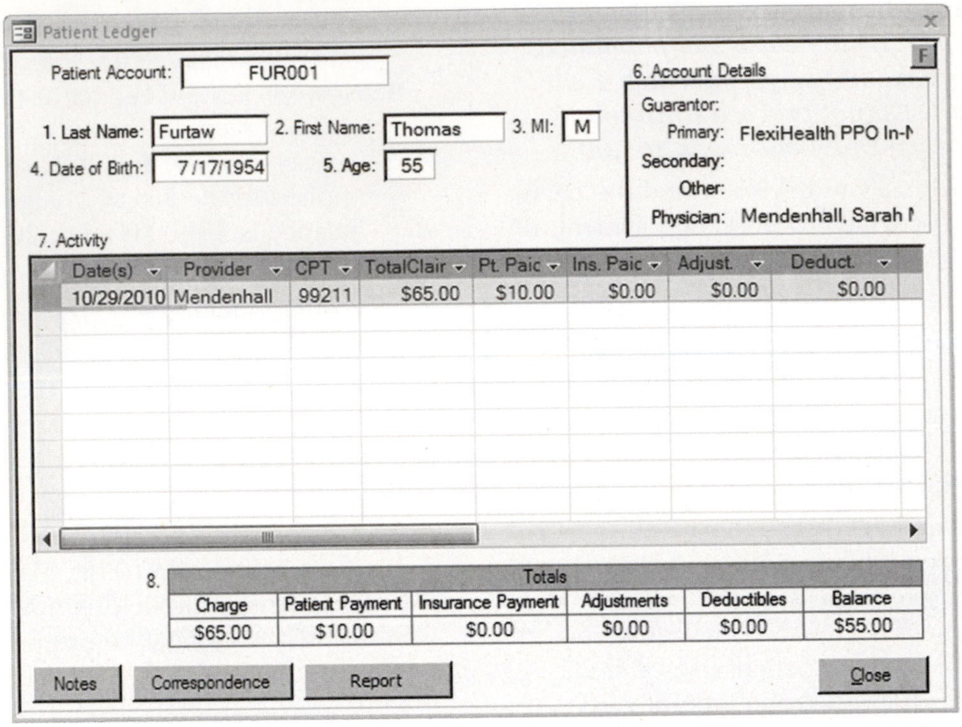

Source: Delmar/Cengage Learning

FIGURE 26-5

Patient ledger showing two payments

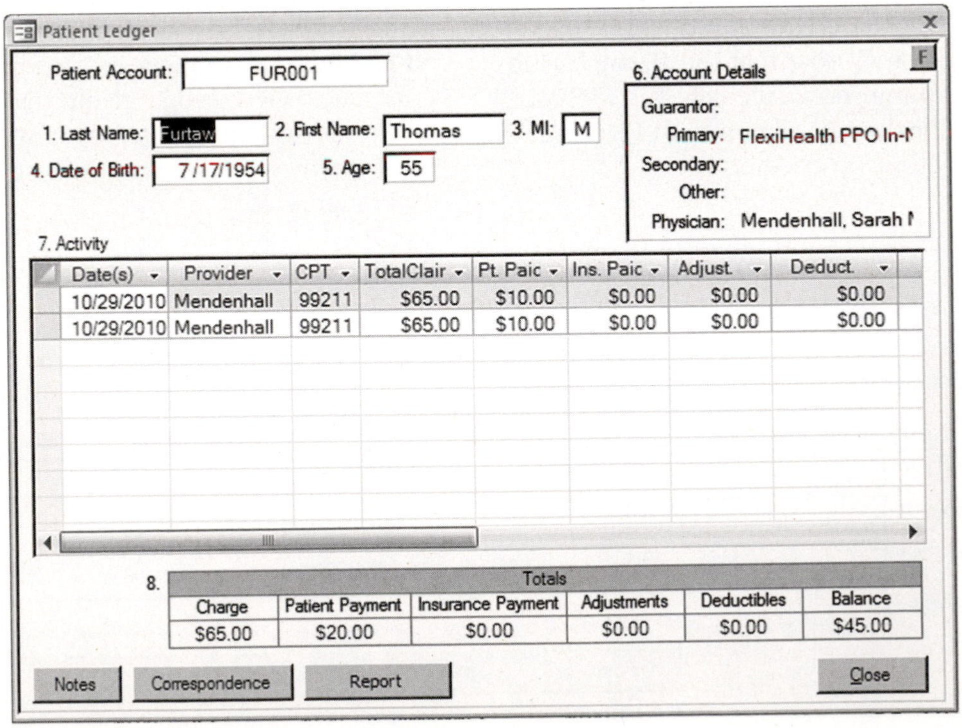

Source: Delmar/Cengage Learning

12. Click Close until you return to the Main Menu screen.
13. The next patient is Denise Guest. Ms. Guest paid with her Visa card. Her payment will be posted using the same steps used to post Mr. Furtaw's payment.
    a. From the Main Menu, click Posting Payments. Search for and select Denise Guest from the patient list. Click Apply Payment.
    b. Reviewing Ms. Guest's encounter form, she had several procedures done at her visit. However, only the office visit (99204) has a patient charge. The other charges will be billed to her insurance. In the Procedure Charge History area, highlight the 99214 charge and click Select/Edit. (Note when you do, the Balance Due field populates with $283.00.)
    c. Enter the date (Field 3) and the patient payment information (Fields 7–9). Since Ms. Guest is paying with a Visa, select OTHER in Field 7 and indicate Visa in Field 8. Compare your screen to Figure 26-6.
    d. Click Post.
    e. Click View Ledger, and view the activity area to see the payment posting.

FIGURE 26-6
Check your work for Step 13c

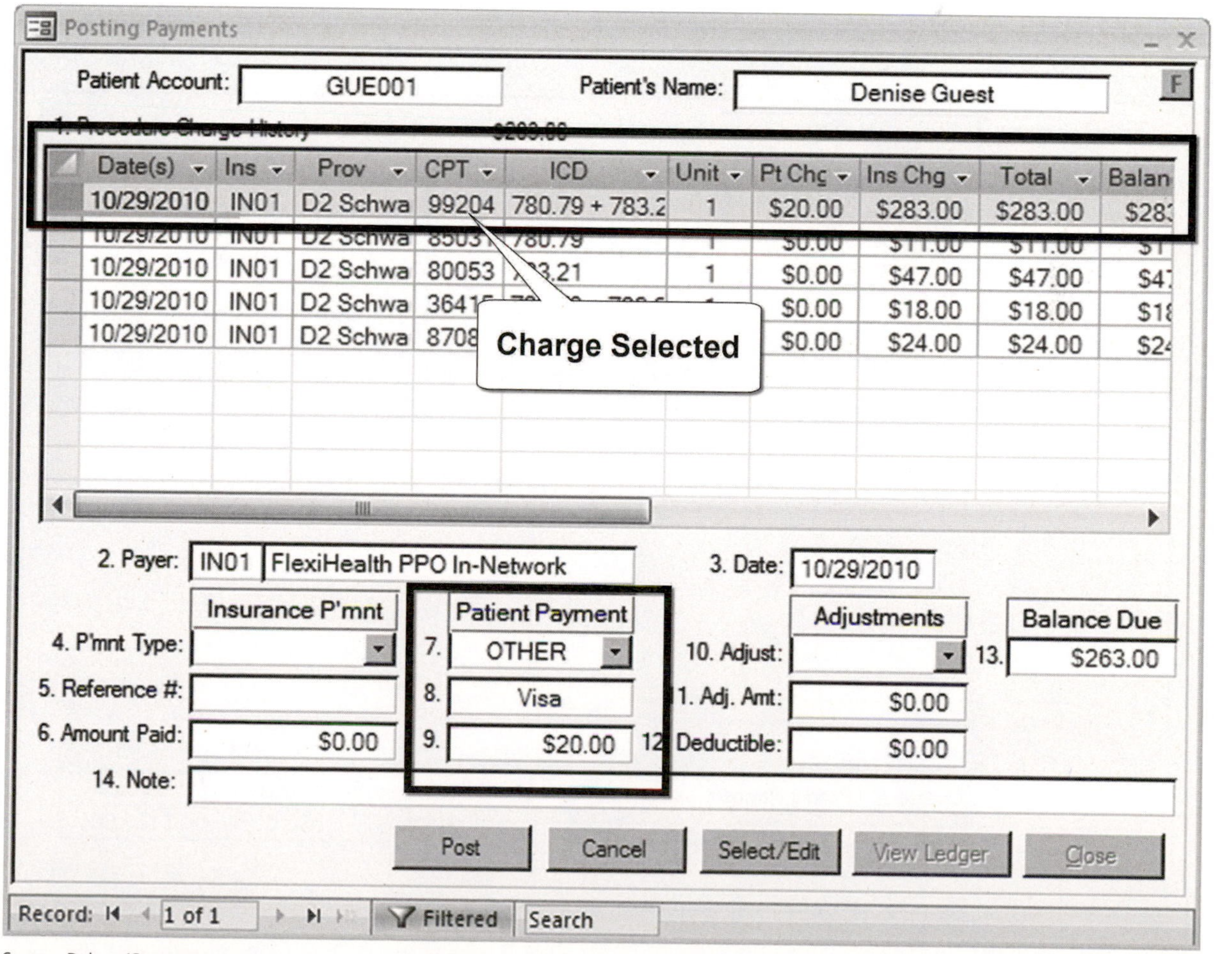

Source: Delmar/Cengage Learning

f. *At this point, you may want to create a Backup file ("Backup Through
Job 26 Step 13.mde") before posting
payments for the next patients. It is
critical to follow the same steps for
the remaining patients—most
importantly, making sure to highlight the charge line in the
Procedure Charge History, and
then clicking Select/Edit; otherwise
the payments may not be posted
correctly. MOSS does not allow
errors to be corrected after payment
posting; so if you do make an error,
restore your most recent back up file
and try the steps again.*

14. Continue to post payments for Ernesto
Santana, Karen Boyd, and Edward
Brewer. For Karen Boyd, make sure to
post her payment against the office
visit charge (99211). Compare
the Patient Ledger screens with
Figures 26-7, 26-8, and 26-9.

15. After you are finished, create a back
up file with the name "Backup
Through Job 26.mde." Return your
encounter forms to the Encounter
Forms folder.

FIGURE 26-7

Patient ledger screen for Ernesto Santana after payment has been posted

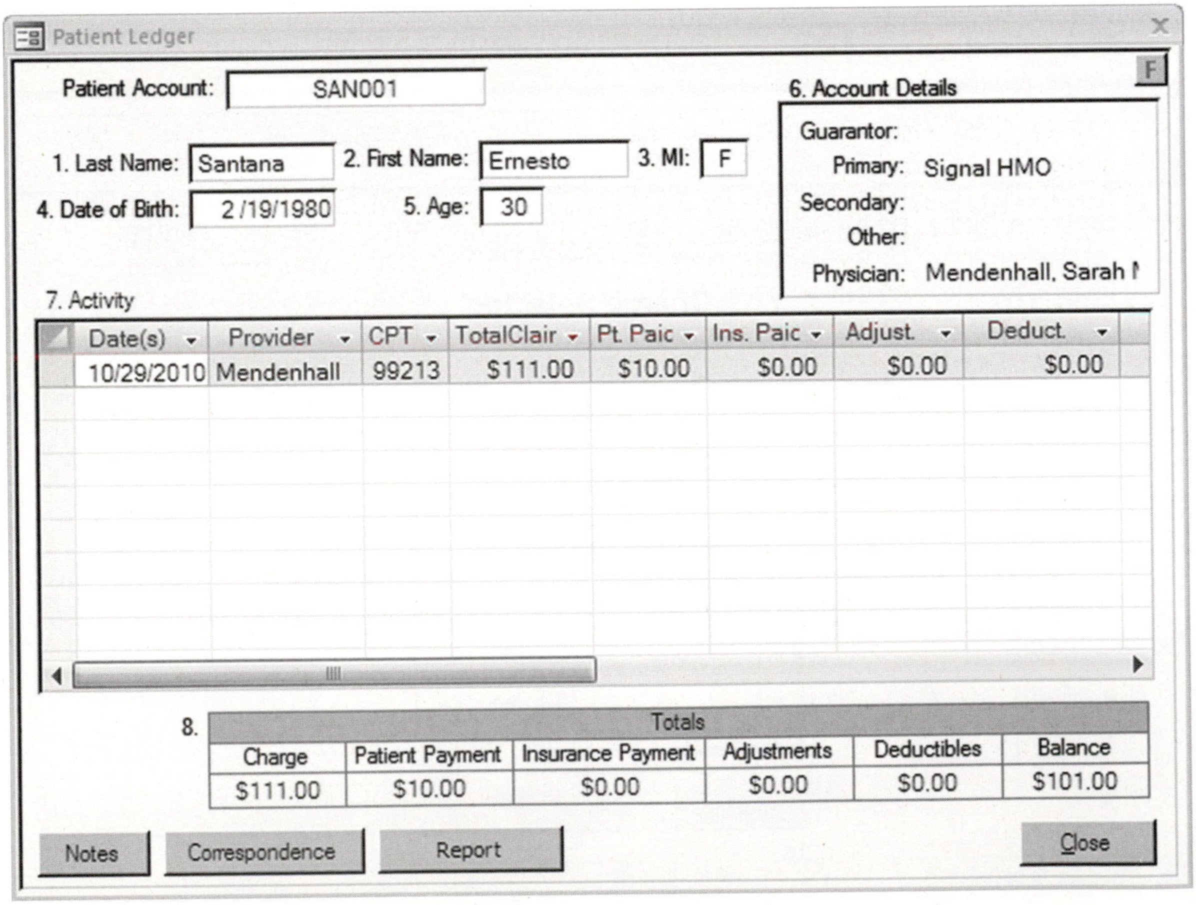

	Patient Ledger								X

Patient Account: SAN001

6. Account Details

1. Last Name: Santana	2. First Name: Ernesto	3. MI: F	Guarantor:		
			Primary: Signal HMO		
4. Date of Birth: 2/19/1980	5. Age: 30		Secondary:		
			Other:		
			Physician: Mendenhall, Sarah		

7. Activity

Date(s) ▾	Provider ▾	CPT ▾	TotalClair ▾	Pt. Paic ▾	Ins. Paic ▾	Adjust. ▾	Deduct. ▾
10/29/2010	Mendenhall	99213	$111.00	$10.00	$0.00	$0.00	$0.00

8.

	Totals					
Charge	Patient Payment	Insurance Payment	Adjustments	Deductibles	Balance
$111.00	$10.00	$0.00	$0.00	$0.00	$101.00

Notes	Correspondence	Report		Close

Source: Delmar/Cengage Learning

FIGURE 26-8

Patient ledger screen for Karen Boyd after payment has been posted

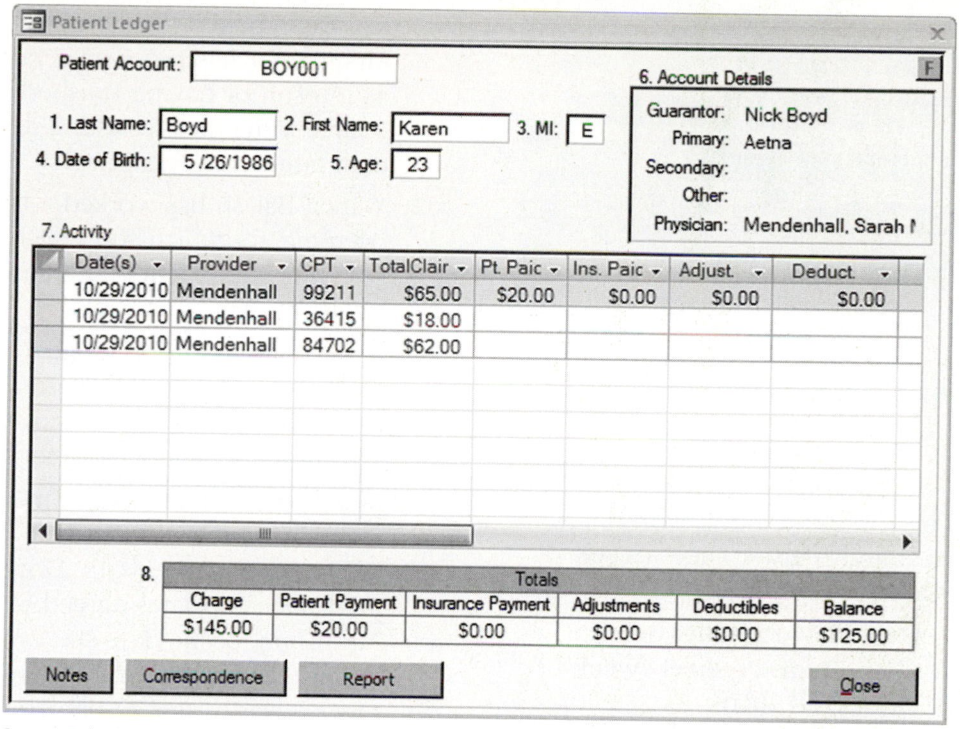

Patient Ledger									✕
Patient Account:	BOY001				6. Account Details				F

Guarantor: Nick Boyd
Primary: Aetna
Secondary:
Other:
Physician: Mendenhall, Sarah

1. Last Name: Boyd   2. First Name: Karen   3. MI: E
4. Date of Birth: 5 /26/1986   5. Age: 23

7. Activity

Date(s)	Provider	CPT	TotalClair	Pt. Paic	Ins. Paic	Adjust.	Deduct.
10/29/2010	Mendenhall	99211	$65.00	$20.00	$0.00	$0.00	$0.00
10/29/2010	Mendenhall	36415	$18.00				
10/29/2010	Mendenhall	84702	$62.00				

8.

	Totals				
Charge	Patient Payment	Insurance Payment	Adjustments	Deductibles	Balance
$145.00	$20.00	$0.00	$0.00	$0.00	$125.00

Notes   Correspondence   Report   Close

Source: Delmar/Cengage Learning

FIGURE 26-9

Patient ledger screen for Edward Brewer after payment has been posted

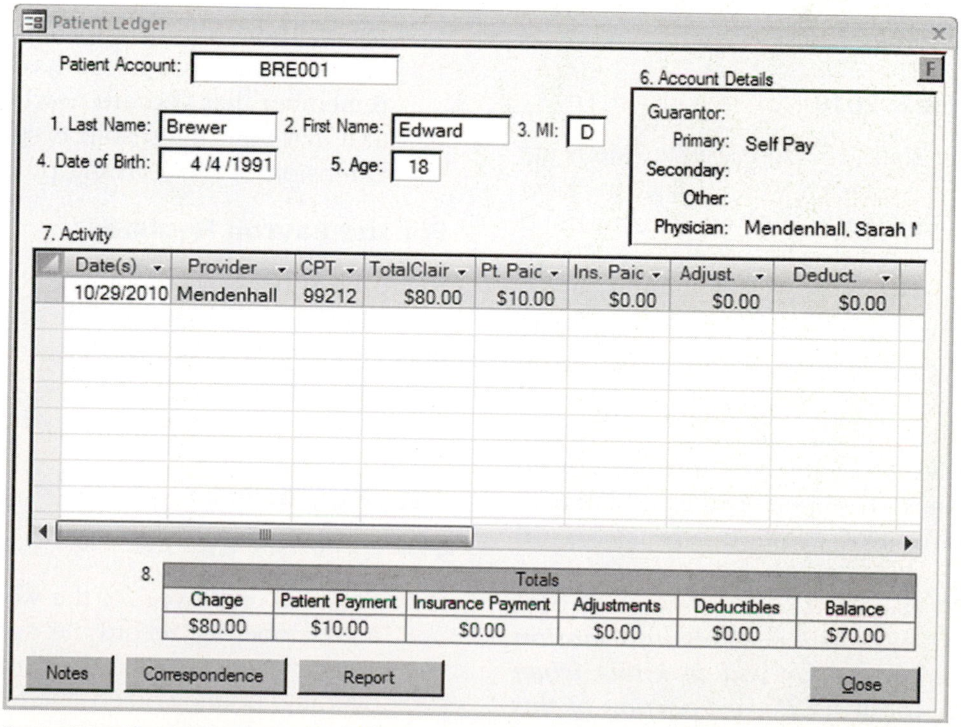

Patient Ledger									✕
Patient Account:	BRE001				6. Account Details				F

Guarantor:
Primary: Self Pay
Secondary:
Other:
Physician: Mendenhall, Sarah

1. Last Name: Brewer   2. First Name: Edward   3. MI: D
4. Date of Birth: 4 /4 /1991   5. Age: 18

7. Activity

Date(s)	Provider	CPT	TotalClair	Pt. Paic	Ins. Paic	Adjust.	Deduct.
10/29/2010	Mendenhall	99212	$80.00	$10.00	$0.00	$0.00	$0.00

8.

	Totals				
Charge	Patient Payment	Insurance Payment	Adjustments	Deductibles	Balance
$80.00	$10.00	$0.00	$0.00	$0.00	$70.00

Notes   Correspondence   Report   Close

Source: Delmar/Cengage Learning

JOB 27
Employee Payroll—Completing Work Record and Preparing and Proving Totals on Payroll Register

MATERIALS AND SUPPLIES

- Form: Job 27—Payroll work record and register sheet (week of October 22, 2010)
- Form: Job 27—Payroll work record and register sheet (week of October 29, 2010)
- Calculator
- Pencil

TIME ALLOTMENT

60 minutes

NOVEMBER 2, 2010

The office staff at Douglasville Medicine Associates is paid each Wednesday. Mrs. Fleet has given you last week's work record and asked you to complete it and the payroll register. You will need to use the previous week's records as a guide. Federal and state withholding tax schedules can be found in Appendix A: Reference Materials.

She tells you that all office staff members are full-time employees and are allowed ten **paid** sick days per year in addition to five **paid** days of vacation time and **paid** holidays.

Mrs. Fleet gives you the following payroll and tax information: *(This information will be important for you to know when completing the Work Record portion of this assignment.)*

For the Work Record

1. The time record for last week has been completed. You will notice that Mrs. Parker has received a raise in pay as a result of having finished a recent course in medical assisting at a local community college.

2. Wanda Balash has worked 4 hours overtime, for which she is to be paid time-and-a-half (1½ times her hourly rate).

3. Mr. Hasara was ill on Monday of last week. According to Mr. Hasara's records, he still has seven days of sick time left. Therefore, he will be paid for the day.

4. Mei Ling Chun attended a medical assisting conference Tuesday and Wednesday of last week. Douglasville Medicine Associates agreed to pay Mrs. Chun for the days she would be out of the office since attending the conference was related to her job. She will be paid full hourly wages for both days.

5. Emily Parker took three of her five vacation days. She will be paid for those days.

6. You worked 8 hours every day last week. Though your wages are the lowest of the group, you have to remember that you are newly hired and that your internship is still an extension of the learning process.

For the Payroll Register

There have been no employee, marital status, withholding allowance, or group insurance deduction changes since last week. Using the October 22 records as a reference guide, complete last week's payroll records.

INSTRUCTIONS
For the Work Record

1. For each employee for the week ending October 29, record the number of regular hours worked, the number of overtime hours worked, the total hours (e.g., 40 regular, overtime, and 40 total).

2. Next, compute the staff's regular earnings last week—number of regular hours worked times the hourly rate. For example, Mrs. Fleet's pay would be 40 × $20 = $800.

3. Only Wanda Balash worked overtime. Multiply her four overtime hours by her overtime rate and record it in the overtime earnings column.

4. Compute and record the total earnings for each employee.

5. For the next column, you must add last week's earnings to the total earned since January 1. For example, for Mrs. Fleet, that is her total earnings for the week of October 29, 2010, added to the $34,350 she had earned by the end of the previous week.

6. Check your work; double check your arithmetic.

For the Payroll Register

1. Enter the data you know; employee name, marital status, withholding allowances, total earnings for the week, and group insurance deduction (it is the same as last week).

2. FICA (Federal Insurance Contributions Act) tax to be withheld is to be computed as 7.65%. For Mrs. Fleet, 0.0765 × $800 = $61.20. Compute the tax for the other employees.

3. Next you need to determine the amount of federal income tax to be withheld from each employee's pay. There are two schedules (Wage Bracket Tables) in Appendix A: Reference Materials that will give you the amounts. One is for single persons; the other for married persons. For the $800 that Mrs. Fleet earned last week, with her one withholding allowance, the income tax to be withheld is $56. Determine and record the federal income tax for the rest of the employees.

4. New York does have a state income tax. As with federal income tax, there are several different tax-withholding tables in Appendix A: Reference Materials for single persons and married persons. Additionally, there is a special table for deduction and exemption allowances used for employees making more than $600 per week. This table will be used for Mrs. Fleet and Ms. Balash and can also be found in Appendix A: Reference Materials.

To compute state income tax withholdings, begin by using the state income tax table for married persons (Form T-14). Refer to the directions at the bottom in Step 1. According to the table, if an employee makes more than $600, you must use the "Exact Calculation Method" to determine the state tax to be withheld. Mrs. Fleet's total earnings for last week are $800. Therefore, refer to the Combined Deduction and Exemption Allowance Table first (Form T-12), which is Table A on the Special Tables for Deduction and Exemption Allowances of New York State. Following the left-hand column, note that Mrs. Fleet's payroll type is weekly and that she is married. With one exemption (allowance), the combined deduction and allowance for Mrs. Fleet is $163, which you should subtract from her wages according to the directions given in Table A ($800 − $163 = $637). At this point, use the Exact Calculation Method Table for Weekly Payroll (Table II-A of Form T-14), *Married*. Following the directions in Table II-A, you will note that Mrs. Fleet's net wages fall in between $385 and $1731 (line 5 of the table). Following line 5 across, subtract $385 from $637 (Mrs. Fleet's net wages) = $252. Your next step is to multiply $252 by 0.0685, which equals 17.262. The final step is to add $18.71 to $17.26. This amount ($35.97) is the exact amount of state income tax you need to withhold from Mrs. Fleet. Enter that amount in the state income tax deductions column on the payroll register.

You will need to repeat the above process for Ms. Balash; however, make sure you use the *single* Weekly Payroll table.

(You will not need to utilize the special tables for deduction and exemption allowances for the rest of the employees since they make less than $600 weekly.) You will only need to use Forms T-2 and T-3 (Method I tables) for single and married persons. Use these in the same manner as the federal income tax tables were used: find the employees' earnings in the left-hand column, then look to the right to find the tax to be withheld according to the number of allowances (deductions) they have noted on their payroll register. This is the amount of state income tax to be withheld.

5. Add and enter the total deductions for each employee.

6. Next, determine the amount of the check each employee is to receive for last week's work. For Mrs. Fleet, subtract her total deductions from her total earnings: $800 − $203.17 = $596.83. Compute and record the amount of the check for each of the other employees.

7. Total each of the columns.

8. If your computations are correct, the total earnings minus the total deductions will equal the net paid amount. If so, draw a double line below the totals.

9. Submit for review or file both payroll registers in your Completed Work folder.

JOB 28
Protective Practices—Material Safety Data Sheets (MSDS)

MATERIALS AND SUPPLIES

■ Material Safety Data Sheet (MSDS)

TIME ALLOTMENT

30 minutes

NOVEMBER 2, 2010

This morning Mrs. Fleet tells you that the supplies you ordered have come in, and she would like your assistance in stocking them, but first she would like to go over the MSDSs (Material Safety Data Sheets) with you that must be filed. She explains that MSDSs are Material Safety Data Sheets that are required by OSHA (Occupational Safety and Health Administration) as part of OSHA's mission to prevent illnesses, injuries, and deaths that are work related. MSDSs provide essential information about hazardous products that could be lifesaving in the event of an exposure incident. This information is provided by the manufacturer of the substance and must be retained by the user.

Employers must have an MSDS for every hazardous substance used in the workplace. These must be filed in such a way that they are prominently visible and available at a moment's notice should the need for reference arise, such as in an exposure incident.

Mrs. Fleet has given you an example of one of the sample MSDSs she uses for training (Figure 28-1). She points out that there are many sections containing information on various aspects of the product, from the basic identity of the product (Section I), to the health information including emergency and first aid procedures if exposure occurs (Section VII), to personal protection

FIGURE 28-1

Sample materials safety data sheet (MSDS)

MATERIAL SAFETY DATA SHEET

I – PRODUCT IDENTIFICATION

COMPANY NAME: We Wash Inc.

ADDRESS: 5035 Manchester Avenue
Freedom, Texas 79430

Tel No: (314) 621-1818
Nights: (314) 621-1399
CHEMTREC: (800) 424-9343

PRODUCT NAME: Spotfree

Product No.: 2190

Synonyms: Warewashing Detergent

II – HAZARDOUS INGREDIENTS OF MIXTURES

MATERIAL:	(CAS#)	% By Wt.	TLV	PEL
According to the OSHA Hazard Communication Standard, 29CFR 1910.1200, this product contains no hazardous ingredients.		N/A	N/A	NA

III – PHYSICAL DATA

Vapor Pressure, mm Hg: N/A
Evaporation Rate (ether=1): N/A
Solubility in H2O: Complete
Freezing Point F: N/A
Boiling Point F: N/A
Specific Gravity H2O=1 @25C: N/A

Vapor Density (Air=1) 60–90F: N/A
% Volatile by wt N/A
pH @ 1%   Solution 9.3–9.8
pH as Distributed: N/A
Appearance: Off-White granular powder
Odor: Mild Chemical Odor

IV – FIRE AND EXPLOSION

Flash Point F: N/AV

Flammable Limits: N/A

Extinguishing Media: The product is not flammable or combustible. Use media appropriate for the primary source of fire.

Special Fire Fighting Procedures: Use caution when fighting any fire involving chemicals. A self-contained breathing apparatus is essential.

Unusual Fire and Explosion Hazards: None Known

V – REACTIVITY DATA

Stability - Conditions to avoid: None Known

Incompatibility: Contact of carbonates or bicarbonates with acids can release large quantities of carbon dioxide and heat.

Hazardous Decomposition Products: In fire situations heat decomposition may result in the release of sulfur oxides.

Conditions Contributing to Hazardous Polymerization: N / A

Source: Delmar/Cengage Learning

(*continued*)

FIGURE 28-1

Sample materials safety data sheet (MSDS) (continued)

Spotfree
VI – HEALTH HAZARD DATA

EFFECTS OF OVEREXPOSURE (Medical Conditions Aggravated/Target Organ Effects,
A. ACUTE (Primary Route of Exposure)   EYES: Product granules may cause mechanical irritation to eyes.
   SKIN (Primary Route of Exposure): Prolonged repeated contact with skin may result in drying of skin.
   INGESTION: Not expected to be toxic if swallowed, however, gastrointestinal discomfort may occur.
B. SUBCHRONIC, CHRONIC, OTHER: None known.

VII – EMERGENCY AND FIRST AID PROCEDURES

EYES: In case of contact, flush thoroughly with water for 15 minutes. Get medical attention if irritation persists.
SKIN: Flush any dry Spotfree from skin with flowing water. A lways wash hands after use.
INGESTION: If swallowed, drink large quantities of water and call a physician.

VIII – SPILL OR LEAK PROCEDURES

Spill Management: S weep up material and repackage if possible.
   Spill residue may be flushed to the sewer with water.

Waste Disposal Methods: Dispose of in accordance with federal, state and local regulations.

IX – PROTECTION INFORMATION/CONTROL MEASURES

Respiratory: None needed   Eye: Safety   Glove: Not
                                                            glasses   required

Other Clothing and Equipment: None required

Ventilation: Normal

X – SPECIAL PRECAUTIONS

Precautions to be taken in Handling and Storing: Avoid contact with eyes. Avoid prolonged or repeated contact with skin.
   Wash thoroughly after handling. Keep container closed when not in use.
Additional Information: Store away from acids.

Prepared by: D. Martinez   Revision Date: 04/11/_ _

Seller makes no warranty, expressed or implied, concerning the use of this product other than indicated on the label. Buyer assumes all risk of use and/or handling of this material when such use and/or handling is contrary to label instructions.

While Seller believes that the information contained herein is accurate, such information is offered solely for its customers consideration and verification under their specific use conditions. This information is not to be deemed a warranty or representation of any kind for which Seller assumes legal responsibility.

information (Section IX). It is important to note that since products are manufactured and distributed by different companies, there will be variations in MSDS formats, including what information falls under which section. Generally, the most important information will appear first on the MSDS. This information would include such things as the chemical composition of the product and what to do if exposure occurs. Additionally, the amount and type of information available on any given MSDS may also vary according to the company or manufacturer.

OSHA regulates that each MSDS must have *at least* the following information: 1) identification of the product (as used on the label), 2) chemical and common names, 3) hazardous ingredients (includes identification of chemical and common name(s) determined to be health hazards, as well as OSHA-permissible exposure limit), 4) health information to include emergency and first aid procedures, 5) fire and explosion data, 6) safe handling and usage information, 7) spill or leak procedures, 8) personal protection information, 9) date of preparation of MSDS and last change to it, 10) demographic data (name, address, telephone number, contact person) of the manufacturer who can provide additional information about the product in an emergency.

Now that you have had time to examine the sample MSDS, Mrs. Fleet would like you to complete a short worksheet to reinforce your understanding.

INSTRUCTIONS

Using the MSDS in Figure 28-1, answer the questions below on a separate piece of paper, or type your answers, save them to your flash drive, and print out. When you are finished, file your paper in the Completed Work folder or hand in to your instructor.

1. What is this product used for?
2. Who is the supplier?
3. Is this product considered a hazardous substance or carcinogen (cancer-causing substance)?

4. When was this MSDS last revised?
5. What should you do if this substance is ingested (swallowed)? Splashes into the eyes?
6. Can you pour this substance down the drain?
7. Do you have to wear PPE (personal protective equipment) when using this product?
8. What should you do if you spill this substance?
9. Where should you store this product?
10. What number should you use to contact the company in case of an emergency?

JOB 29
Basic Practice Finances—Posting Adjustments and Collection Agency Payments and Processing Refunds

MATERIALS AND SUPPLIES

■ Medical Office Simulation Software (MOSS)

TIME ALLOTMENT

1.5 hours

NOVEMBER 2, 2010

Recently you gained some basic experience with computerized procedure and payment posting. This afternoon, Mrs. Fleet would like you to complete a tutorial on additional computerized financial transactions that may be made to a patient's account. These include transactions such as posting collection agency payments and insurance payments, as well as adjusting a patient's account balance due to a bounced check. Additionally, you will learn how to process a refund and generate common periodic financial reports. This tutorial will allow you to become more familiar with our billing software and hopefully increase your understanding of the complex financial system in place at Douglasville Medicine Associates.

Before you begin the tutorial, you will have to create two practice accounts. From the Main Menu of MOSS, click on Patient Registration and add the first patient, Jane Doe, using the information in Tables 29-1 and 29-2. (Remember to save your work after completing each screen!) Be sure Feedback Mode is Off before starting this Job.

INSTRUCTIONS

The following tutorial has been created in the form of five patient scenarios using Jane and John Doe as practice accounts, as well as a few existing patient accounts. Each scenario, with the exception of #1, builds upon itself in the billing and collection process, similar to what you may experience over time in any

medical practice, but specifically here at Douglasville. It is important that you process each step correctly, both cognitively and procedurally, so that you gain a more complete knowledge of our billing and collections system. Now is the time to ask questions. Mrs. Fleet will be available to answer any questions you may have. You may wish to create a Backup file after each patient scenario.

SCENARIO #1

1. John Doe was seen in the office as a patient of Dr. Mendenhall on October 7, 2010, for hypertension (high blood pressure). The claim was for a Level 2 office visit for an established patient. The charge for the visit was $80, which was submitted to Medicare. Mr. Doe made no payment that day since he does not have a co-payment.

   a. From the Main Menu, click on Procedure Posting. Find John Doe in the patient list and click Add, since you are adding procedures to his account.

Table 29-1
Patient Registration Information for Jane Doe

Patient Name	Jane Doe
Physician	Dr. Heath
Social Security Number	111-11-1111
Gender	Female
Marital Status	Single
Date of Birth	01/01/1969
Address	1 Keyboard Drive, Computer Way, NY 01234
Home Phone	(123) 111-1111
Employer	Minetown Video
Primary Insurance Plan	Aetna
Relationship to Policyholder	Self
ID Number	1111111
Group Number	AET111
Office Co-pay	$20.00
Accept Assignment?	Yes
Signature on File?	Yes
In-Network/PAR?	Yes

Remember to SAVE your work! When you have completed the registration process for Jane Doe, return to the Patient Registration screen to register John Doe using the information in Table 29-2.

Table 29-2
Patient Registration Information for John Doe

Patient Name	**John Doe**
Physician	Dr. Mendenhall
Social Security Number	222-22-2222
Gender	Male
Marital Status	Single
Date of Birth	02/02/1922
Address	2 Keyboard Drive, Computer Way, NY 01234
Home Phone	(123) 222-2222
Employer	Retired
Primary Insurance Plan	Medicare—Statewide Corp
Relationship to Policyholder	Self
ID Number	999222222B
Office Co-pay	0
Accept Assignment?	Yes
Signature on File?	Yes
In-Network/PAR?	Yes

Remember to SAVE your work! When you have completed the registration process for John Doe, return to the Main Menu of MOSS and begin with Scenario #1.

b. Complete the screen with the following information:
- Field 1: 22222
- Field 3: 11 (Office)
- Field 5: 10/07/2010
- Field 8: 99212
- Field 12: 401.9

c. Check you work with Figure 29-1, and then click Post.

d. Since Mr. Doe had no co-payment to make that day, click Close until you return to the Main Menu.

2. Today in the mail you receive a Medicare reimbursement check for Mr. Doe, along with an explanation of

FIGURE 29-1
Check your work for Step 1c

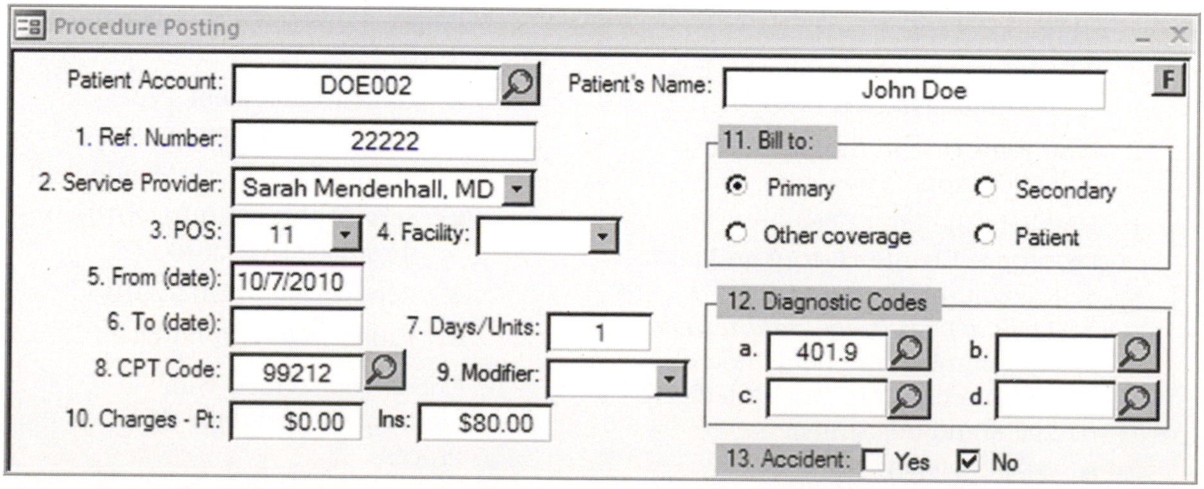
Procedure Posting
Patient Account: DOE002
Patient's Name: John Doe
1. Ref. Number: 22222
2. Service Provider: Sarah Mendenhall, MD
3. POS: 11
4. Facility:
5. From (date): 10/7/2010
6. To (date):
7. Days/Units: 1
8. CPT Code: 99212
9. Modifier:
10. Charges - Pt: $0.00 Ins: $80.00
11. Bill to: Primary (selected), Secondary, Other coverage, Patient
12. Diagnostic Codes: a. 401.9 b. c. d.
13. Accident: Yes ☐ No ☑

Source: Delmar/Cengage Learning

FIGURE 29-2

Explanation of Benefits for John Doe

Medicare Remittance Advice (MOSS Sample)									
MEDICARE CLAIMS SUBMITTED FOR Sarah O. Mendenhall 999503									
DOE, JOHN				BILLED	ALLOWED	DEDUCT	COINS	PROVPD	MC-ADJUSTMENT
HIC 999222222B				ASG Y	ICN	973332020			
ACNT	DOE002								
1007	100710	11	99212	80.00	43.77	110.00	0.00	35.02	36.23

Source: Delmar/Cengage Learning

benefits (EOB), see Figure 29-2. The EOB shows that Medicare only allows a charge of $43.77 for a Level 2 office visit. Additionally, Medicare will only pay for 80% of the allowable charge. The check, therefore, is for 80% of the *allowable charge ($43.77)*, which is $35.02. $($43.77 \times 0.8 = $35.02)$

Since the Medicare allowable is $43.77, and the original charge is $80, there will have to be an adjustment posted to Mr. Doe's account for the remainder of the amount, which is $36.23. $($80 - $43.77 = $36.23)$

However, remember that the Medicare check was only for $35.02. If the allowable charge is $43.77 and the actual check (80%) is $35.02, then there is a balance left of $8.75. $($43.77 - $35.02 = $8.75)$

This is the patient's balance. John Doe will be responsible for paying this amount.

a. You will now post the Medicare payment received today (November 2, 2010). From the Main Menu, click on Posting Payments.

b. Find John Doe in the patient list and click Apply Payment.

c. Highlight the 99212 charge in the Procedure Charge History and click Select/Edit. *(If done correctly, $80 will appear in the Balance Due field.)* Complete the fields noted below to record Mr. Doe's Medicare payment and adjustment.

■ Field 3: 11/02/2010

■ Field 4: PAYINS

■ Field 5: 98222

■ Field 6: $35.02

■ Field 10: ADJINS (use the drop-down menu to select Adjustment Insurance)

■ Field 11: $36.23

d. Check your work with Figure 29-3, and then click Post.

e. Click on View Ledger at the bottom of your screen. Compare your screen with Figure 29-4. Mr. Doe's current balance should be $8.75, which will be billed to him in his monthly statement.

f. Click Close until you return to the Main Menu.

3. Now, print out a statement for John Doe using the following steps:

a. From the Main Menu, click Patient Billing. Complete the following fields:

■ Field 1 (Statement Type): Remainder Statement

■ Field 2 (Provider): Mendenhall

■ Service Dates: 10/01/2010 through 11/02/2010

■ Report Date: 11/02/2010

■ Patient Name: John Doe

b. Check your screen with Figure 29-5, and then click Process.

FIGURE 29-3

Check your work for Step 2d

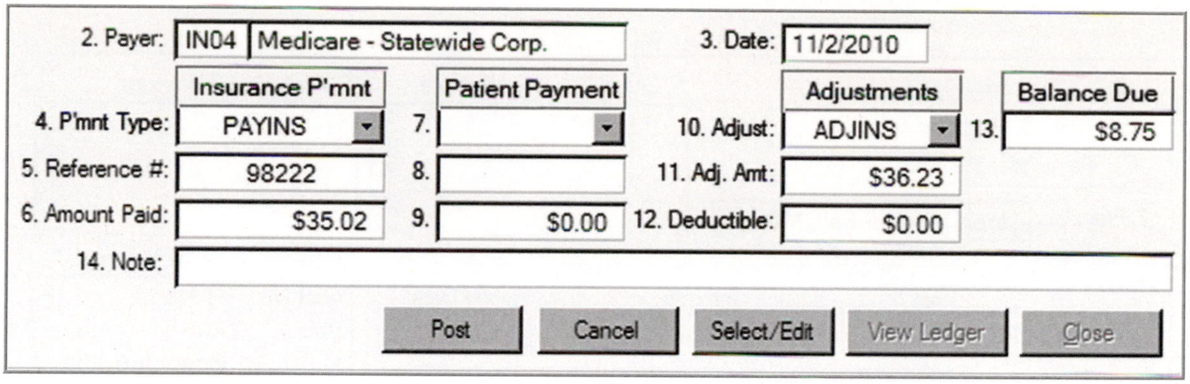

2. Payer:	IN04	Medicare - Statewide Corp.				3. Date:	11/2/2010

	Insurance P'mnt	Patient Payment		Adjustments	Balance Due
4. P'mnt Type:	PAYINS	7.	10. Adjust:	ADJINS	13. $8.75
5. Reference #:	98222	8.	11. Adj. Amt:	$36.23	
6. Amount Paid:	$35.02	9. $0.00	12. Deductible:	$0.00	
14. Note:					

Post	Cancel	Select/Edit	View Ledger	Close

Source: Delmar/Cengage Learning

FIGURE 29-4

Check your work for Step 2e

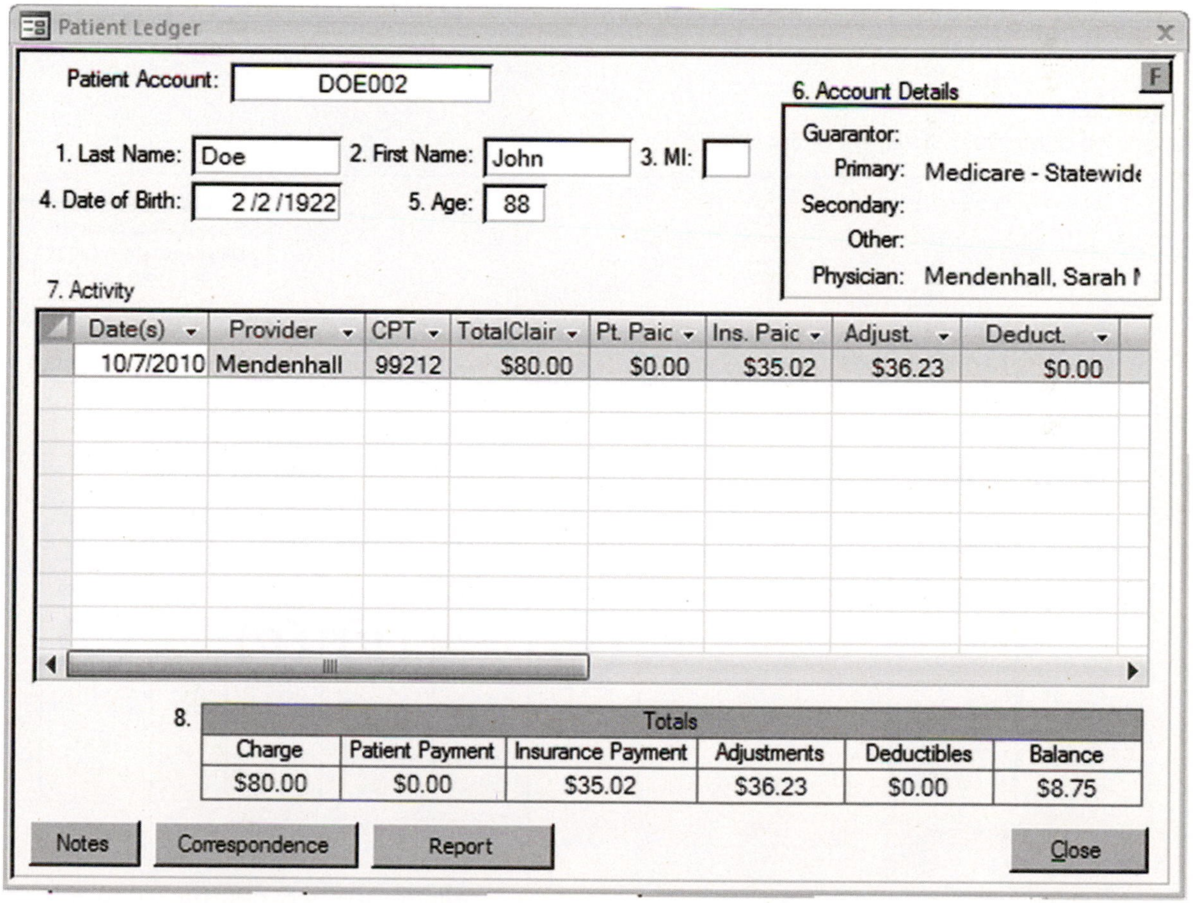

Patient Ledger

Patient Account: DOE002

6. Account Details

1. Last Name: Doe 2. First Name: John 3. MI:

4. Date of Birth: 2/2/1922 5. Age: 88

Guarantor:
Primary: Medicare - Statewide
Secondary:
Other:
Physician: Mendenhall, Sarah

7. Activity

Date(s)	Provider	CPT	TotalClair	Pt. Paic	Ins. Paic	Adjust.	Deduct.
10/7/2010	Mendenhall	99212	$80.00	$0.00	$35.02	$36.23	$0.00

8. Totals

Charge	Patient Payment	Insurance Payment	Adjustments	Deductibles	Balance
$80.00	$0.00	$35.02	$36.23	$0.00	$8.75

Notes	Correspondence	Report		Close

Source: Delmar/Cengage Learning

FIGURE 29-5
Check your work for Step 3b

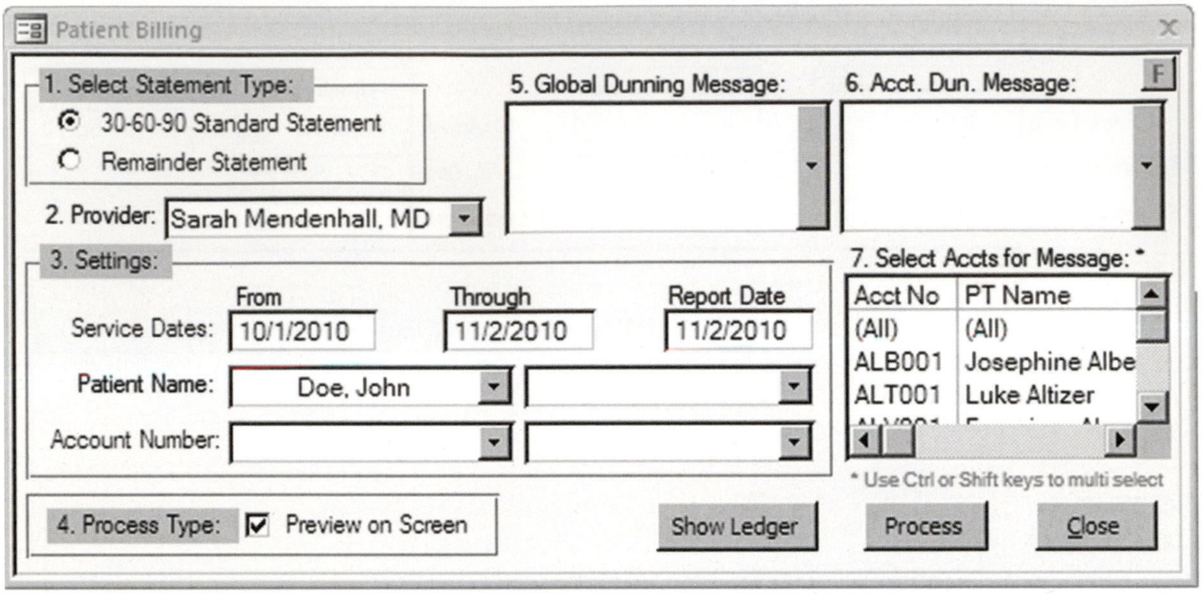

Source: Delmar/Cengage Learning

FIGURE 29-6
Top portion of Mr. Doe's statement of account

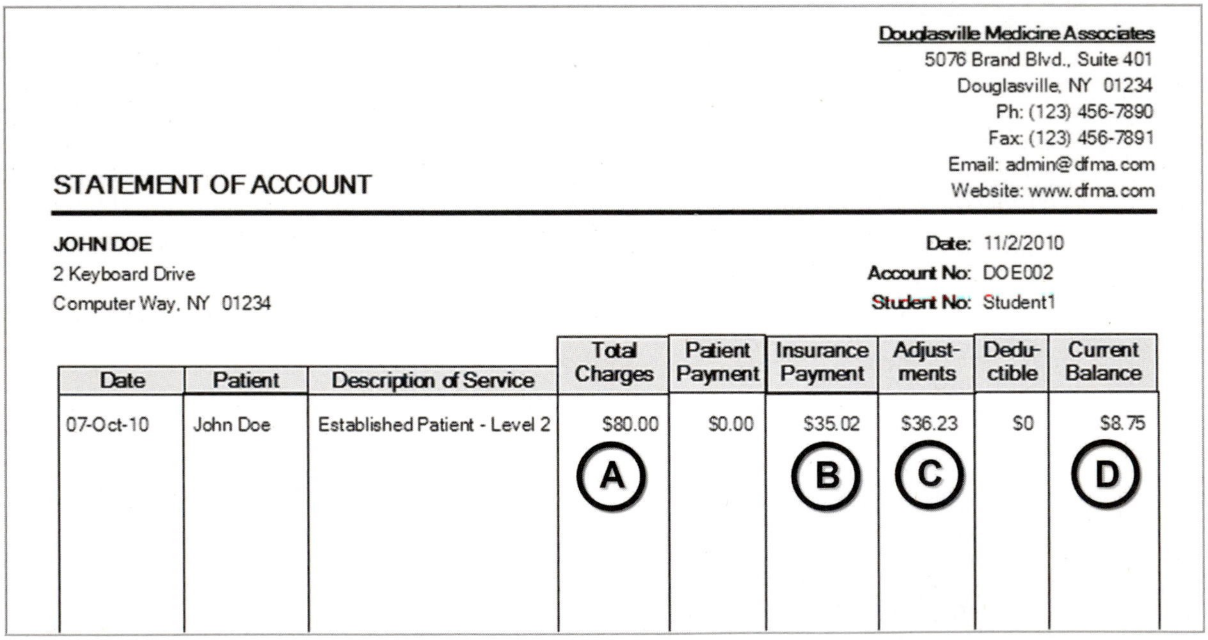

Douglasville Medicine Associates
5076 Brand Blvd., Suite 401
Douglasville, NY 01234
Ph: (123) 456-7890
Fax: (123) 456-7891
Email: admin@dfma.com
Website: www.dfma.com

STATEMENT OF ACCOUNT

JOHN DOE
2 Keyboard Drive
Computer Way, NY 01234

Date: 11/2/2010
Account No: DOE002
Student No: Student1

Date	Patient	Description of Service	Total Charges	Patient Payment	Insurance Payment	Adjust-ments	Dedu-ctible	Current Balance
07-Oct-10	John Doe	Established Patient - Level 2	$80.00 (A)	$0.00	$35.02 (B)	$36.23 (C)	$0	$8.75 (D)

Source: Delmar/Cengage Learning

c. Mr. Doe's Statement of Account will be generated on screen (Figure 29-6). Note the total charge of $80 for his Level 2 office visit (A), the insurance payment of $35.02 (B), the adjustment made for the difference between the allowable amount and the total amount (C), and Mr. Doe's current account balance (what he owes on his account—D).

d. Click the print icon to print out a copy of Mr. Doe's Statement of Account. Set it aside to be handed in to Mrs. Fleet at the end of this tutorial. Click Close until you return to the Main Menu.

SCENARIO #2

Jane Doe was seen by Dr. Heath on October 11, 2010, as a new patient for issues involving her diabetes, hypertension, and depression. On the day of her office visit, Dr. Heath ordered a blood sugar, which she had drawn immediately following her appointment. Ms. Doe was charged for cost of the office visit ($283), blood sugar ($19), and the venipuncture ($18), which totaled $320. She paid $100 in the form of a check that day.

Today you receive an insurance payment of $222 from Aetna, her insurance provider, accompanied by an EOB. Her EOB shows that Aetna paid only $203 of the $283 charged for the office visit. Additionally, Aetna's allowable for the blood sugar was $10, and the venipuncture allowable was $9.

Since there are differences between the billable amounts and the allowable amounts, adjustments will need to be made to the patient's account after procedure and payment posting have been made.

Posting Procedures

1. Start by posting the procedures to Jane Doe's account. From the Main Menu, click Procedure Posting. Find Jane

Doe's name and click Add, since you are adding charges to her account.

2. Complete the following fields to post the *first* charge (office visit); then click Post.
   - Field 1: 11111
   - Field 3: 11
   - Field 5: 10/11/2010
   - Field 8: 99204
   - Field 12a: 250.02
   - Field 12b: 401.9
   - Field 12c: 311

3. Complete the following fields to post the *second* charge (blood sugar); then click Post.
   - Field 1: 11111
   - Field 8: 82947
   - Field 12: 250.02

4. Complete the following fields to post the *third* charge (venipuncture); then click Post.
   - Field 1: 11111
   - Field 8: 36415
   - Field 12a: 250.02

5. Compare your screen with Figure 29-7 before proceeding. Make any necessary changes prior to moving on to Posting Payments.

Posting Payments

1. As you may recall, Ms. Doe made a payment of $100 in the form of a check the day of her office visit. You can post this payment from the

FIGURE 29-7
Posting detail for Jane Doe

Posting Detail							
Date(s) ▾	Bil ▾	Prov ▾	CPT ▾	ICD ▾	Unit ▾	Pt Charge ▾	Ins. Chari ▾
10/11/2010	IN08	D3	99204	250.02 + 401.9 +	1	$0.00	$283.00
10/11/2010	IN08	D3	82947	250.02	1	$0.00	$19.00
10/11/2010	IN08	D3	36415	250.02	1	$0.00	$18.00

Source: Delmar/Cengage Learning

Procedure Posting screen. Click on Post Payment, on the bottom of the screen. (It is unnecessary to return to the Main Menu when immediately posting a payment on a patient account.)

2. Post Ms. Doe's payment:

   a. Highlight the office visit charge (99204) and click Select/Edit. (In this case, procedure 99204 is the most costly; therefore, the $100 payment will go toward this procedure first.)

   b. Enter the following information:

      - Field 3: 10/11/2010
      - Field 7: PATCHECK
      - Field 8: 202
      - Field 9: $100.00

   c. Click Post to record the payment.

   d. Click on View Ledger, and compare your screen to Figure 29-8. Note that the patient's payment is shown in two places—in the Activity area (Field 7) and at the bottom in the Totals (Field 8).

   e. Click Close until you return to the Main Menu.

3. Since Ms. Doe's insurance payment came today (November 2, 2010) through the mail, click on Posting Payments from the Main Menu to access her account since you are posting a check ROA (received on account) rather than at the time of service.

   a. Access Jane Doe's account and click Apply Payment. You will be posting Ms. Doe's insurance payment from Aetna in three steps.

FIGURE 29-8
Patient ledger for Jane Doe

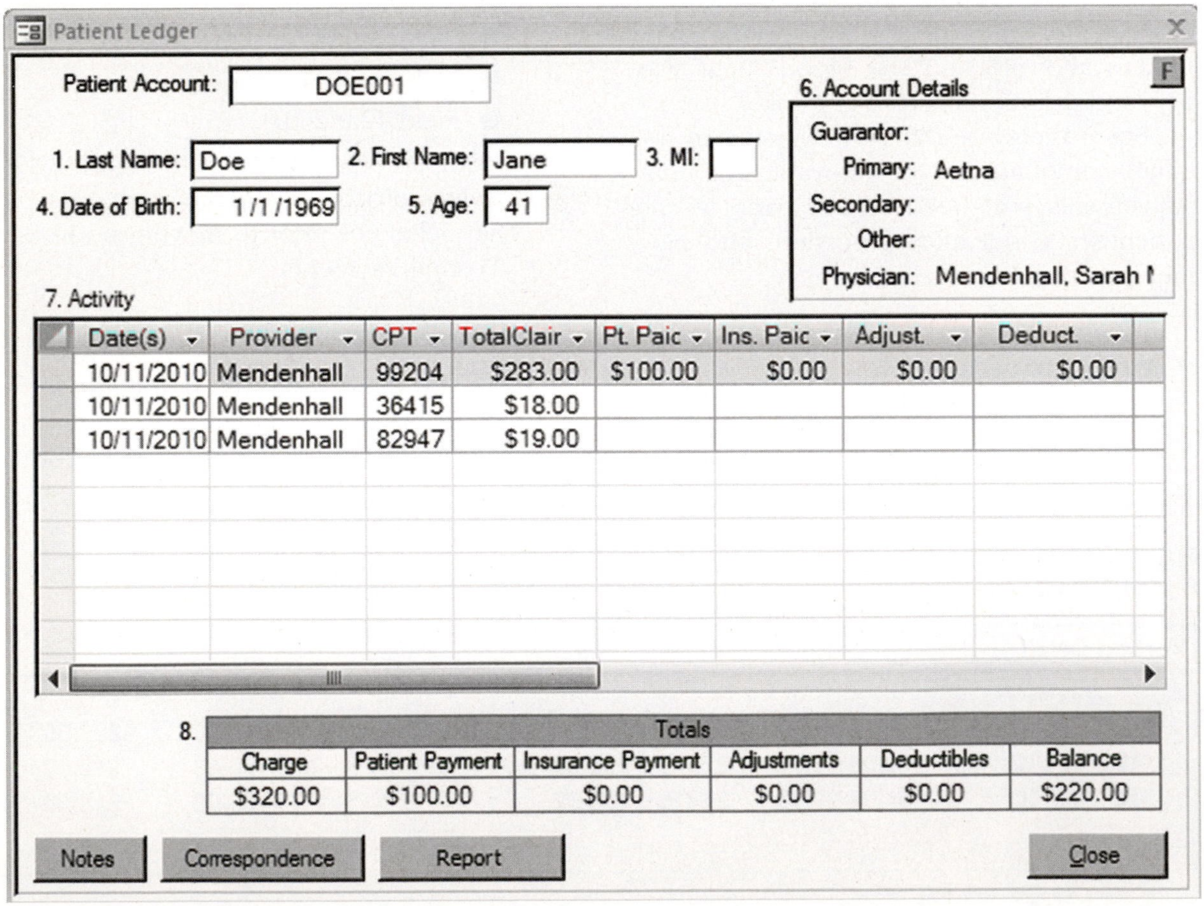

Date(s)	Provider	CPT	TotalClair	Pt. Paic	Ins. Paic	Adjust.	Deduct.
10/11/2010	Mendenhall	99204	$283.00	$100.00	$0.00	$0.00	$0.00
10/11/2010	Mendenhall	36415	$18.00				
10/11/2010	Mendenhall	82947	$19.00				

8. Totals

Charge	Patient Payment	Insurance Payment	Adjustments	Deductibles	Balance
$320.00	$100.00	$0.00	$0.00	$0.00	$220.00

Source: Delmar/Cengage Learning

First, remember that the total amount of the check was $222. However, the EOB outlined the allowable amount of each of the procedures Ms. Doe was charged for; therefore, you will be posting each of the allowable amounts separately.

b. In the Posting Payments screen, highlight the office charge (99204) and click Select/Edit. Enter the following:

- Field 3: 11/02/2010 (you will need to overwrite the previous date)
- Field 4: PAYINS
- Field 5: 22902
- Field 6: $203

c. Click Post. After posting correctly, the Balance field should show a negative $20.00 balance, which is indicated by the amount in parentheses ($20.00).

d. Now post the payment for the blood sugar charge (82947).

Highlight the 82947 row and click Select/Edit.

- Field 3: 11/02/2010
- Field 4: PAYINS
- Field 5: 22902
- Field 6: $10.00

e. Click Post. After posting correctly, the balance shown for procedure 82947 should be $9.00.

f. Now post the payment for the venipuncture charge (36415). Highlight the 36415 row and click Select/Edit.

- Field 3: 11/02/2010
- Field 4: PAYINS
- Field 5: 22902
- Field 6: $9.00

g. Click Post. After posting correctly, the balance shown for procedure 36415 should be $9.00.

h. Click on View Ledger and compare your screen with Figure 29-9.

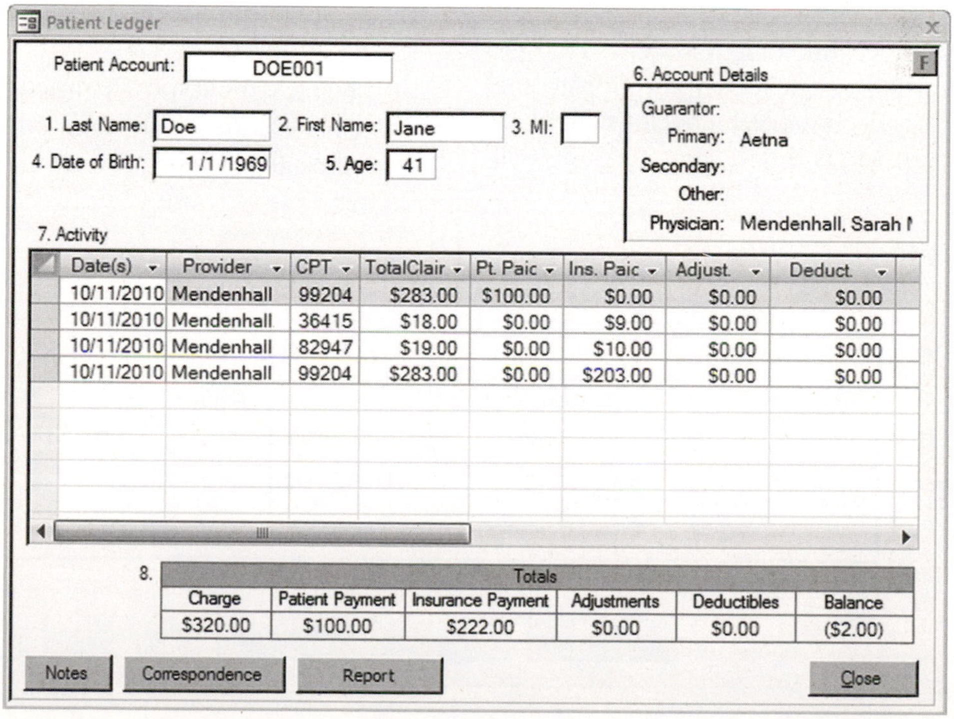

FIGURE 29-9

Patient ledger for Jane Doe, after payments have been posted

Patient Account:	DOE001					6. Account Details			F

Guarantor:
Primary: Aetna
Secondary:
Other:
Physician: Mendenhall, Sarah I

1. Last Name: Doe 2. First Name: Jane 3. MI:
4. Date of Birth: 1/1/1969 5. Age: 41

7. Activity

Date(s)	Provider	CPT	TotalClair	Pt. Paic	Ins. Paic	Adjust.	Deduct.
10/11/2010	Mendenhall	99204	$283.00	$100.00	$0.00	$0.00	$0.00
10/11/2010	Mendenhall	36415	$18.00	$0.00	$9.00	$0.00	$0.00
10/11/2010	Mendenhall	82947	$19.00	$0.00	$10.00	$0.00	$0.00
10/11/2010	Mendenhall	99204	$283.00	$0.00	$203.00	$0.00	$0.00

8. Totals

Charge	Patient Payment	Insurance Payment	Adjustments	Deductibles	Balance
$320.00	$100.00	$222.00	$0.00	$0.00	($2.00)

Notes   Correspondence   Report   Close

Source: Delmar/Cengage Learning

i. As you can see from Ms. Doe's ledger, there is a $2.00 credit on her account. This amount could either be refunded to her in the form of a check, or it could be absorbed by future charges.

j. Click Close until you return to the Main Menu.

> *Make any necessary adjustments before proceeding to the next part of the tutorial. If you determine that you are unable to find your error during this tutorial, you may choose to go into Procedure Posting and delete each procedure separately. This will also delete each charge and payment posted, which will allow you to start over from the beginning.*

SCENARIO #3

Mrs. Fleet informs you that a check received from Jane Doe was returned due to nonsufficient funds (NSF). This happens to be the check she wrote to pay for services rendered on October 11, 2010, at the time of her initial office visit.

Douglasville Medicine Associates charges a $25 returned check fee in addition to the amount of her bounced check, which, in Ms. Doe's case, is $100. Her account will need to be adjusted for both the $100 NSF and the $25 returned check fee.

1. From the Main Menu, click Posting Payments. Select Jane Doe from the patient list and click Apply Payment.

2. Next, click on View Ledger. Note that Ms. Doe's $100 payment was posted to procedure 99204. Therefore, you will make the first adjustment of her NSF check to that procedure line. Click Close to return to the Posting Payment screen.

3. Back on the Posting Payment screen, highlight the 99204 charge in the Procedure Charge History area and click Select/Edit. (When you do this, the Balance Due field should say ($20.00).)

4. Fill in the following fields, to make the adjustment:

- Field 3: (you will overwrite the date to today's date)
- Field 7: OTHER
- Field 8: 202 (this is the check number)
- Field 9: (100.00) (be sure to include the parentheses around the amount; this indicates a negative amount)
- Field 14: Type "Returned check, NSF"

5. Check your screen with Figure 29-10. Click Post.

FIGURE 29-10
Check your work for Step 5

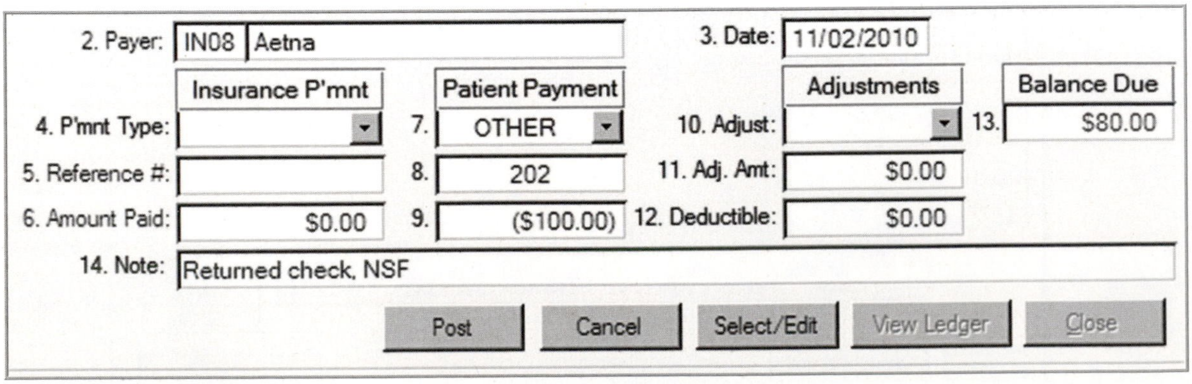

2. Payer: IN08 Aetna			3. Date: 11/02/2010	
	Insurance P'mnt	Patient Payment	Adjustments	Balance Due
4. P'mnt Type:		7. OTHER	10. Adjust:	13. $80.00
5. Reference #:		8. 202	11. Adj. Amt: $0.00	
6. Amount Paid:	$0.00	9. ($100.00)	12. Deductible: $0.00	
14. Note: Returned check, NSF				

Post   Cancel   Select/Edit   View Ledger   Close

Source: Delmar/Cengage Learning

6. We will now record NSF fee of $25. Return to the Procedure Charge History area and highlight 99204 (again—to record the returned check fee). Click Select/Edit.
   - Field 3: 11/02/2010
   - Field 10: ADJDBT
   - Field 11: $25.00
   - Field 14: Type "Returned check fee, NSF"

7. Click Post.

8. Click Close until you return to the Main Menu.

SCENARIO #4

Mrs. Fleet has asked you to print out an Aging Report by Account Number. This will allow you to see which patient accounts are past due, and in what amounts. She explains that there are three patients who need refund checks processed, and she would like you to take care of this today. You will be able to identify these patients on the Aging Report.

1. From the Main Menu, click Report Generation. The Reports Panel allows you to choose and view a specific type of monthly financial report. It is important before proceeding here to type in the Aging Date; that is, the *end* date of the report. Type in 10/31/2010 as the aging date, and click on Aging Report by Patient Account Number (Figure 29-11).

2. Maximize your screen and enlarge your font if necessary. Print out the Aging Report for your reference.

3. You will notice that the patient account numbers are listed alphabetically by last name. Additionally, each patient's balance is listed as either

FIGURE 29-11

The reports panel, showing an aging Date of 10/31/2010

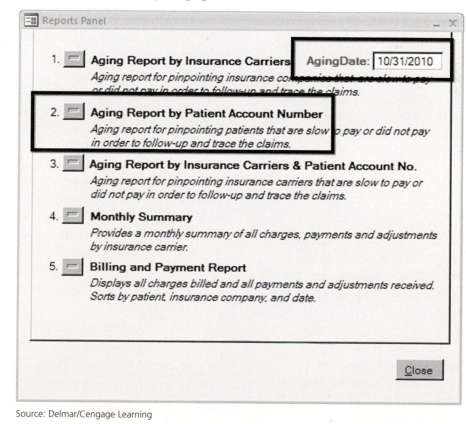

Source: Delmar/Cengage Learning

FIGURE 29-12
Josephine Albertson has a credit balance, as shown on the aging report by patient account number

Account Number	Patient Name	0 to 30 Days Current	31 to 60 Days Past Due	61 to 90 Days Past Due	91+ Days Past Due	Total Due
ALB001	Josephine A. Albertson	$0.00	$0.00	$0.00	($20.00)	($20.00)

Aging Report by Account No. for Student1 — Aging Date: 10/31/2010

Source: Delmar/Cengage Learning

current or past due. If the patient's balance is past due, it is noted by column whether it is 31 to 60 days past due, 61 to 90 days past due, or 91+ days past due. This is known as "aging" a patient's account. Some patient accounts actually have a credit balance, and that is usually indicated in parenthesis in the Total Due column.

4. Josephine Albertson is one of the patients with a credit balance, a $20 credit on her account (see Figure 29-12). Today you will process a refund check for her.

5. From the Main Menu, click Posting Payments. Access Josephine Albertson's account and click Apply Payment.

6. Highlight the row for procedure code 99212 and click Select/Edit.

7. Enter the following:
   - Field 3: 11/02/2010
   - Field 10: REFUND
   - Field 11: $20.00

8. Click Post. In a real office, a refund check would be generated in the amount of $20 and sent to the patient. Click Close and return to the Main Menu.

9. Using the Aging Report and the example from above, process all patient refunds, then close all open screens and return to the Main Menu.

SCENARIO #5

Mrs. Fleet has received a collection agency check (#14587) in the amount of $205 for patient Rusty Potter. She would like you to post this check to his account.

1. From the Main Menu, click Posting Payments. Access Mr. Potter's account and click Apply Payment.

2. Post the collection agency check as an insurance check. Remember to note the check number. Additionally, in the Note field, type "Collection agency check" (see Figure 29-13).

3. Click View Ledger. Mr. Potter's account balance should now be zero. Click Close until you return to the Main Menu.

The final step in this tutorial is to print out a prebilling worksheet for each physician for the month of October 2010. (We will include November 1 and 2 since payments were made to patient accounts today for the purposes of this tutorial.) The prebilling worksheet is an overall picture of what is going to be billed to the insurance company. At this point, changes to the patient's account are still able to be made. It is important to look at the prebilling worksheet prior to transmitting claims to the insurance company.

1. From the Main Menu, click Insurance Billing.

2. On the Claims Preparation window, enter the following:
   - Field 1: Service Dates
   - Field 2, select Bill (not rebill)
   - Field 2, Provider: Heath

FIGURE 29-13
Check your work for Step 2

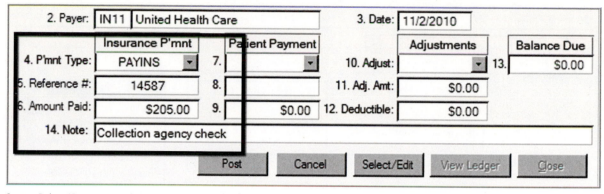

Source: Delmar/Cengage Learning

- ■ Field 2, Services Date: 10/01/2010 through 11/02/2010
- ■ Field 2, Patient Name: (All)
- ■ Field 5: (All)

3. Click Prebilling Worksheet. Print out the Prebilling Worksheet.

4. Repeat this procedure for Dr. Schwartz and Dr. Mendenhall.

You have completed the tutorial! You have done a great job! Submit all printed forms to Mrs. Fleet for examination or file in your Completed Work folder.

JOB 30
Managed Care/ Insurance—Processing Insurance Claims

MATERIALS AND SUPPLIES

- ■ Medical Office Simulation Software CD-ROM

TIME ALLOTMENT

15 minutes

NOVEMBER 3, 2010

At the end of every month, insurance claims are submitted electronically to the various insurance companies for reimbursement. This is easily done, and electronic submission has made reimbursement timelier, provided that information has been submitted *accurately*. Prior to claims submission, a prebilling worksheet is reviewed to look for any errors in patient accounts that can be corrected. Once a claim is submitted, errors cannot be fixed. The claim will likely be denied, and a new claim will have to be submitted. This will delay payment to the physician. Today Mrs. Fleet will guide you through the electronic claims process.

INSTRUCTIONS

1. From the Main Menu of MOSS, click Insurance Billing. The Claims Preparation window will appear.

2. In Field 1, click on the drop-down menu to see the three sort choices: you can prepare a claim to be submitted by patient name, account number, or service date. We are billing for the entire month of October, so choose Service Dates.

3. Field 2 lets you choose various settings for claims billing. The first choice is which provider(s) to bill for. Since Douglasville Medicine Associates has

FIGURE 30-1
Check your work for Step 9

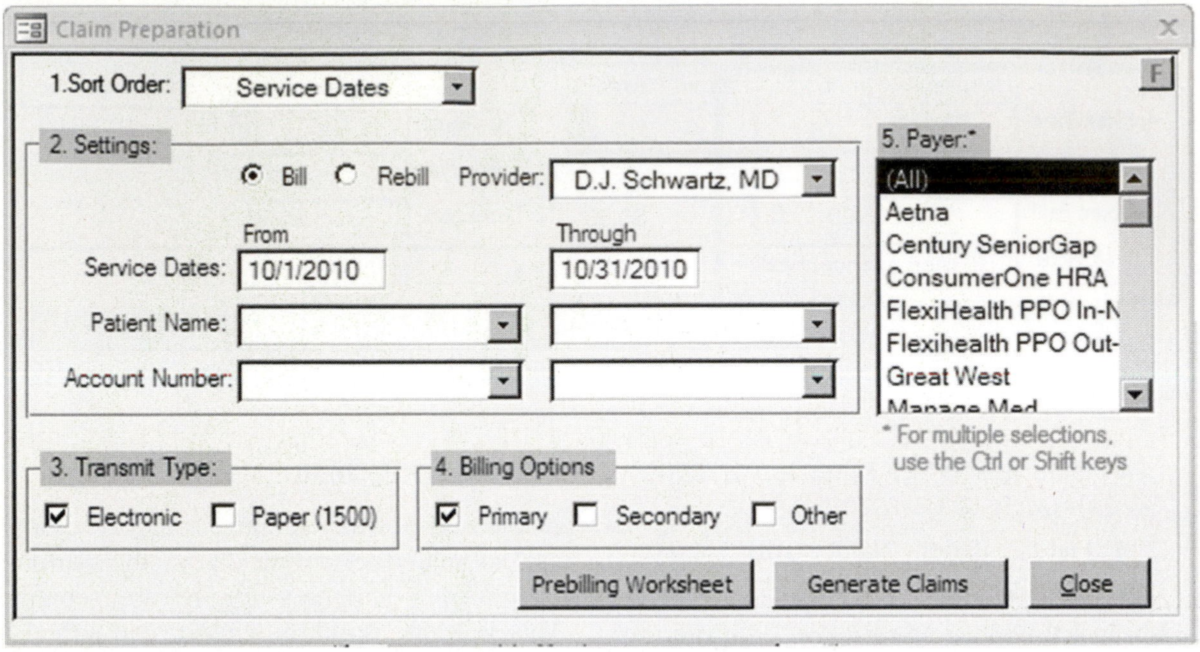

Source: Delmar/Cengage Learning

many providers (not all the physicians listed), we will need to choose one physician at a time. Using the drop-down menu, choose Dr. Schwartz first.

4. Under Service Dates, type 10/01/2010 to 10/31/2010.

5. Tab through Patient Name and Account Number. These fields could be used if you were submitting a claim for only one patient at a time.

6. For Field 3, we will be transmitting claims electronically. This is the default setting, and it is already checked for you.

7. Field 4 lists your billing options. You can choose to bill primary insurances, secondary insurances, or other (tertiary) insurances. We will be billing Dr. Schwartz's primary insurance companies. Primary is already checked as it is also a default.

8. In Field 5, all insurance companies are listed. We want to bill all of Dr. Schwartz's patients' insurance companies for the month of October so that we can secure reimbursement. Click (All).

9. Check your work with Figure 30-1.

10. At the bottom, you have a choice to view a Prebilling Worksheet or Generate Claims. Remember that it is important to view the Prebilling Worksheet to check for errors. Click on Prebilling Worksheet and click once using the magnifying lens to increase the size of the document (Figure 30-2). The Prebilling Worksheet reveals that one insurance company will be billed this month for services rendered by Dr. Schwartz (FlexiHealth). (In a real office setting, there would be many patients and insurance companies.)

11. Print out Dr. Schwartz's Prebilling Worksheet. Your instructor may wish to review this with you prior to claims submission.

12. If your Prebilling Worksheet is correct, click on the X in the upper right-hand corner to return to the Claim Preparation screen.

13. Click Generate Claims at the bottom of the screen. You will see that an insurance claim appears for Denise Guest.

If there were multiple claims, you could use the Record bar at the bottom left side of the screen to scroll through to review prior to transmitting.

14. The final step in electronic claims submission is to transmit the claim. Click Transmit EMC (Electronic Medical Claim), located on the bottom right of your screen. You should see evidence of claims transmission occurring on your screen, followed by a transmission status report (Figure 30-3). Print out your transmission report as evidence of successful completion.

FIGURE 30-2

Dr. Schwartz's prebilling worksheet for the month of October

INSURANCE PREBILLING WORKSHEET
Student1

Dates of Service	Diag Code	Proc Code	POS	Units	Dr	As	Bill Amt	Receipts	Net
FlexiHealth PPO In-Network									
Guest, Denise									
10/29/2010	780.79	87086	11	1.00	D2	Y	$24.00	$0.00	$24.00
10/29/2010	780.79	36415	11	1.00	D2	Y	$18.00	$0.00	$18.00
10/29/2010	780.79	80053	11	1.00	D2	Y	$47.00	$0.00	$47.00
10/29/2010	780.79	85031	11	1.00	D2	Y	$11.00	$0.00	$11.00
10/29/2010	780.79	99204	11	1.00	D2	Y	$283.00	$20.00	$263.00
					Totals		$383.00	$20.00	$363.00
		TOTAL TO BE BILLED FOR FlexiHealth PPO In-Network							$363.00
Grand Total		Grand Total							$363.00

Source: Delmar/Cengage Learning

FIGURE 30-3

Claims transmission report for Dr. Schwartz

Claims Submission Report
Student1

FlexiHealth PPO In-Network

Patient Name
Denise Guest

Account No GUE001	*DOS*	*Procedure*	*Charges*	*Result*
	10/29/2010	99204	$283.00	A
	10/29/2010	85031	$11.00	A
	10/29/2010	80053	$47.00	A
	10/29/2010	36415	$18.00	A
	10/29/2010	87086	$24.00	A
Patient Totals			$383.00	

Source: Delmar/Cengage Learning

15. Repeat the process for Drs. Heath and Mendenhall for the month of October. Print out Prebilling Worksheets for both physicians, as well as evidence of claims transmission.

16. When you have completed your assignment, submit all printouts to your instructor or file in your Completed Work folder.

JOB 31
Procedural and Diagnostic Coding

MATERIAL AND SUPPLIES

- Form: Job 31—Worksheet: Procedural and Diagnostic Coding Practice
- Current CPT (Current Procedural Terminology) book (if available)
- ICD-9 (International Classification of Disease) book (if available)
- The Internet

TIME ALLOTMENT

45 minutes

NOVEMBER 4, 2010

Throughout your experience at Douglasville Medicine Associates, you have had some exposure to both procedure and diagnostic codes, specifically during procedure posting. You have learned the difference between a CPT code and an ICD-9 code, as well as the relationship between the two, and you are well aware of the importance of ensuring that the diagnostic codes support and match the procedure code in order to receive proper reimbursement by the insurance company.

Mrs. Fleet approaches you today with an exercise she gives all new employees as a method of helping them become more comfortable with the process of procedural and diagnostic coding. She informs you that procedure codes change each year in the fall and that the new codes are implemented at the beginning of the following year. Therefore, it is important to keep abreast of the changes and to update all forms and all codes in the computer system as quickly as possible in order to avoid denied claims.

Furthermore, claims can be denied, or payment to the provider can be delayed, due to incorrect procedure codes, absence of modifiers, overuse of modifiers, or any number of issues. It is important to know as much as possible about this ever-changing subject and how and where to find updated information.

INSTRUCTIONS

1. Gather all materials. If you have access to a CPT manual and ICD-9 book, you may choose to complete this worksheet without the Internet. If you do not have access to these books, you *can* complete this assignment without the manuals; however, it is important to know how to code properly, and finding codes in both manuals can be overwhelming without some practice. If this is the case, go ahead and complete this assignment using the Internet, but try to gain access to both the CPT manual and the ICD-9 book so that you can learn how to use them properly.

2. Complete the Procedural and Diagnostic Coding Practice Worksheet to the best of your ability. When you have finished, file the worksheet in your Completed Work folder.

JOB 32
Protective Practices— Identifying Community Resources

MATERIALS AND SUPPLIES

- Computer with Internet access or use of a telephone book—or both

TIME ALLOTMENT

60 minutes

NOVEMBER 4, 2010

Mrs. Fleet has asked you to update the Emergency Preparedness Manual. All physicians and staff of Douglasville Medicine Associates must be familiar with the contents of this manual in the event of an emergency, such as a natural disaster, fire, or patient emergency beyond our capacity.

Your assignment today is to utilize all available references to locate the following information:

A. Specific names and telephone numbers of the following local emergency facilities (aside from 911):

- Fire company
- Ambulance
- Police
- County Emergency Management Agency
- Crisis Intervention
- Poison Control Center
- Area hospitals
- Children and youth
- ChildLine

B. Additionally, Mrs. Fleet would like you to take this opportunity to familiarize yourself with other *nonemergency* agencies that are available to our patients, as a patient may ask you for assistance in locating a specific service that he or she may otherwise be unaware. Your second assignment is to find the name and telephone number of a specific local agency or service who provides, or who supplies, the following:

- Colostomy care items
- Bras for women who are postmastectomy
- Meals delivered to the homes of the elderly
- Wigs for cancer patients
- Depression support group
- Transportation to the physician
- Narcotics/alcoholic anonymous
- Free or reduced medication

INSTRUCTIONS

1. When you have located all of the information, type your information in alphabetic order in two sections (Emergency Numbers and Nonemergency Numbers). Be sure to include the name of the agency or organization, the telephone number, and—in the case of nonemergency numbers—the service they provide.

2. File this in your Completed Work folder.

JOB 33
Concepts of Effective Communication—Scheduling Admission to a Hospital; Preparing Patient for Procedure

MATERIALS AND SUPPLIES

- Medical Office Simulation Software
- Form: Job 33—Preadmission Questionnaire
- Form: Job 33—Progress Note

TIME ALLOTMENT

20 minutes

NOVEMBER 4, 2010

This morning, Ernesto Santana called in for an appointment with Dr. Mendenhall. It seems that he has a history of inflamed tonsils and adenoids, and today he is miserable, missing yet another day of work. As this has been going on for some time now and appears to be worsening, Dr. Mendenhall has advised Mr. Santana to have a tonsillectomy and adenoidectomy as soon as possible.

You have been asked to schedule Mr. Santana's outpatient surgery at Community General Hospital.

INSTRUCTIONS

1. Open MOSS and pull up Ernesto Santana's demographic information via the Patient Registration screen. (You will need to reference this information when scheduling his surgery.)

   As this is a simulation, you will not have an opportunity to actually schedule Mr. Santana's admission. *Therefore, you will role-play the process by pairing up with a classmate. Using the Preadmission Questionnaire, role-play the part of the medical office assistant and the hospital admissions representative. Be sure to have the answers to the questions readily available before "calling."*

   If you are playing the part of the admissions representative, schedule Mr. Santana for his surgery ten days from today. It will be your responsibility also to research his pre-op instructions for a tonsillectomy and adenoidectomy so that you may inform the medical office assistant of this important information to then be given to the patient.

2. When you have completed the role-play simulation, reflect on your conversation. What went well? What seemed awkward? If you were Mr. Santana receiving instructions from the medical office assistant, would you feel informed about your surgery?

3. Write down your thoughts about the above as a pair and submit to your instructor or place in your Completed Work folder.

JOB 34
Administrative Functions—Proofreading and Preparing Final Copies from Draft Copies

MATERIALS AND SUPPLIES

- Flash Drive
- Form *on flash drive*: Job 34— Discharge summary (Gormann)

■ Form *on flash drive*: Job 34—History and physical examination record (Delgado)

TIME ALLOTMENT

1 hour

NOVEMBER 5, 2010

From time to time, Mrs. Fleet supervises a trainee who is completing an externship as a medical assistant in our office. One of the trainees has keyed two medical reports in draft form, a discharge summary for Edward Gormann and a history and physical examination for Manuel Delgado. As part of your training, Mrs. Fleet has asked you to proofread, revise, and produce final copies in proper format.

She asks that you read each one carefully for accuracy of content and mechanics (spelling, punctuation, capitalization, terminology, spacing, presentation, etc.). Make corrections as needed, using all available references, including patient files, and Appendix A: Reference Materials.

INSTRUCTIONS

1. Open your flash drive and find the forms for this job (Job 34—Discharge Summary: Gormann) and (Job 34—History and Physical Examination Record: Delgado).

2. Edit each rough draft carefully.

3. Prepare the final copies in the style preferred at Douglasville Medicine Associates. Save your finished work on your flash drive.

4. Print copies of the finished documents and place them in your Completed Work folder.

JOB 35
Legal Implications—Creating or Updating Resume and Preparing for Job Interview

MATERIALS AND SUPPLIES

■ Flash drive
■ Word processing software
■ Resume (if already created)

TIME ALLOTMENT

Variable

NOVEMBER 5, 2010

Today is the last day of your paid internship at Douglasville Medicine Associates! Mrs. Fleet and the staff at Douglasville are very proud of your accomplishments, and now it is time for you to update your resume accordingly. You have learned some valuable skills and knowledge here, and it is important to market yourself on paper (i.e., resume) fittingly in order to secure your first job as a Medical Office Assistant.

Mrs. Fleet has given you time this morning to complete this task. Additionally, for completing your "internship" successfully, you will be given a Certificate of Completion to add to your portfolio.

INSTRUCTIONS

1. With your instructor's assistance, create or update your resume to include the skills you have successfully mastered during this *Medical Office Practice* experience.

2. When you have finished, print out your resume for your instructor's review, or file in your Completed Work folder.

CONGRATULATIONS!!!

Reference Materials

Important Information

DOUGLASVILLE MEDICINE ASSOCIATES

5076 Brand Boulevard, Suite 401
Douglasville, NY 01234
Phone (123) 456-7890
Fax (123) 456-7800
Website: www.dfma.com

PHYSICIANS

L.D. Heath, MD
SS#: 999-00-1111
UPIN: B81111
NPI: 9995010111
Medicare No: 999501

Sarah O. Mendenhall, MD
SS#: 999-00-2222
UPIN: B81113
NPI: 9995030313
Medicare No: 999503

D.J. Schwartz, MD
SS#: 999-00-1235
UPIN: B81112
NPI: 9995020212
Medicare No: 999502

OFFICE STAFF

Flora Mae Fleet, RN
Office Manager

Wanda N. Balash, RN

Joseph T. Hasara, CMA

Mei Ling Chun, RMA

Emily Parker, Medical Assistant

Student, Medical Office Assistant

OUTSIDE FACILITIES

NEW YORK COUNTY HOSPITAL

1402 Northern Drive
King Park, NY 01238
Phone (123) 555-8745

COMMUNITY GENERAL HOSPITAL

4000 Brand Boulevard
Douglasville, NY 01234
Phone (123) 555-2587

RETIREMENT INN NURSING HOME

890 Millennium Way
Douglasville, NY 01234
Phone (123) 555-2345

BIOPACE LABORATORY

1600 Midway Avenue, Suite 100
Douglasville, NY 01234
Phone (123) 555-3334

QUALI-CARE CLINIC

5076 Brand Boulevard, Suite 300
Douglasville, NY 01234
Phone (123) 456-1019

REFERRING PHYSICIANS

MIDWAY SPECIALTY ASSOCIATES
Cynthia Brennen, MD (Obstetrics/ Gynecology)
1600 Midway Boulevard, Suite 102
Douglasville, NY 01234
Phone (123) 555-1302
Fax (123) 555-1322

Samantha Green, MD (Neurology)
1600 Midway Avenue, Suite 102
Douglasville, NY 01234
Phone (123) 555-1302
Fax (123) 555-1322

Joseph Reed, MD (Cardiology)
1600 Midway Avenue, Suite 102
Douglasville, NY 01234
Phone (123) 555-1302
Fax (123) 555-1322

QUALI-CARE CLINIC

5076 Brand Boulevard, Suite 300
Douglasville, NY 01234
Phone (123) 456-1019
Fax (123) 456-1020

Lee Westfail, MD (Orthopedics)

David Childs, MD (Gastroenterology)

Jack Zullig, MD (Orthopedics)

Eric Lopez, MD (Oncology)

INSURANCE INFORMATION

Century SeniorGap
4500 Old Town Way
Lowville, NY 01453
Phone (800) 555-6699

ConsumerOne HRA
1230 Main Street
Missoula, MT 08896
Phone (800) 555-8887

FlexiHealth PPO
30 West Fifth Avenue, Suite 100
New York, NY 10002
Phone (800) 555-1256

Medicaid
POB 345
Albany, NY 12201

Medicare – Statewide Corp.
200 Tech Center
Queens City, NY 01135
Phone (800) 555-2447

Signal HMO
4500 Old Town Way
Lowville, NY 01453
Phone (800) 555-2121

Partial Patient List

Francisco B. Alvarez
410 Hyde Park
Douglasville, NY 01234
(123) 457-6610

Francois Blanc
890 Millennium Way
Retirement INN
Douglasville, NY 01234
(123) 528-0012

Maria L. Carvajal
845 Fifth Street
Douglasville, NY 01234
(123) 457-2325

Xao Chang
890 Millennium Way
Retirement INN
Douglasville, NY 01234
(123) 528-0012

Jordan S. Connell
803 Slate Drive, Apt. 103
Douglasville, NY 01234
(123) 457-8123

Edward Gormann
485 Slate Drive
Douglasville, NY 01234
(123) 457-1122

Carla Jacobi
50 Logan Street
Douglasville, NY 01234
(123) 457-2160

David F. James
11690 Marble Way
Douglasville, NY 01234
(123) 457-1188

Stanley R. Kramer
58682 Pebble Trail, Apt. 20
Douglasville, NY 01234
(123) 456-1118

Theresa F. Lingard
2455 Valencia Drive
Douglasville, NY 01234
(123) 457-7123

Richard L. Manaly
116 Granite Street
Douglasville, NY 01234
(123) 457-8724

Vito A. Mangano
8123 Slate Court, Apt. 31
Douglasville, NY 01234
(123) 457-3108

Raymond A. Nolte
4720 Linwood Lane
Douglasville, NY 01234
(123) 457-8000

Daniel M. Oliver
10075 Princess Circle
Douglasville, NY 01234
(123) 457-6600

Diane R. Parker
1424 Candlelight Drive
Douglasville, NY 01234
(123) 457-2414

Miriam Pinnerwell
690 Park Rose Avenue
Douglasville, NY 01234
(123) 528-0121

Caroline A. Pratt
1268 Gravel Way
Douglasville, NY 01234
(123) 457-2166

Harold M. Prosser
1433 Forest Run Drive
Douglasville, NY 01234
(123) 457-8100

Manuel S. Ramirez
211 Gravel Way
Douglasville, NY 01234
(123) 457-1113

Julia T. Richard
1922 Webber Street
Douglasville, NY 01234
(123) 457-7701

Ernesto F. Santana
1950 Sunset Drive
Douglasville, NY 01234
(123) 457-7124

Paula M. Shektar
58682 Pebble Trail, Apt. 20
Douglasville, NY 01234
(123) 456-1118

Robert B. Shinn
5821 Pebble Trail
Douglasville, NY 01234
(123) 457-2100

Christopher A. Snider
1853 Felker Road
Douglasville, NY 01234
(123) 456-6281

Wilma A. Stearn
2116 Slate Drive, Apt. 202
Douglasville, NY 01234
(123) 457-6215

Eugene M. Sykes
5201 Marble Way
Douglasville, NY 01234
(123) 457-2252

John J. Wittmer
5070 Prospect Road
Douglasville, NY 01234
(123) 457-6216

Cynthia Worthington
5857 Granite Street
Douglasville, NY 01234
(123) 457-1123

Elaine A. Ybarra
1156 Pebble Trail
Douglasville, NY 01234
(123) 457-2133

SOAP Notes Format

Patient Name: **PCP:**

Date of Birth: **Age:**   **Sex:**

Date of Evaluation:

SUBJECTIVE:

OBJECTIVE:

ASSESSMENT:

PLAN:

_____

Physician's name
Specialty

(XX:xx) **Physician's initials in caps; your initials in lower case

D: (date dictated)
T: (date transcribed)

C:

Transcription Terms

ablation

adenopathy

affect

angina

anorexia

antalgic

arthralgia

atraumatic

Avonex

axillary

barium

bolus

Bright disease

carcinoma

carotid

cholesterol

cholestyramine

conjunctiva(e)

cyanosis

dyspepsia

dysphagia

dyspnea

Effexor

empyema

endoscopy

epistaxis

esophageal

funduscopic

gait

gallop

Gemzar

hematochezia

hematologic

hematuria

hemoccult

hemoptysis

hemorrhoids

hernia(e)

heterogeneity

homogeneous

leucovorin

Lipitor

Lomotil

melena

metastasis

metastatic

multiple sclerosis

nares

neoplasm

neurologic

normocephalic

Novantrone

orophayrnx

orthopnea

palpitations

penicillin

peptic

peptide

picograms/mL

polydipsia

polyuria

psoriasis

psychiatric

pubic ramus

reflux

regurgitate

rigors

stricture

substernal

symptomatology

Tegretol

tinnitus

trigeminal

neuralgia

triglyceride

vasoactive

vertigo

vipoma

wellbutrin

Whipple procedure

Abbreviations

5-FU	5 fluorouracil (chemotherapy drug)	mg/m2	milligrams per square meter
A&P	auscultation and percussion	MRI	magnetic resonance imaging
AP	anteroposterior	MS	multiple sclerosis
CBC	complete blood count	MVA	motor vehicle accident
CPT-11	Irinotecan (chemotherapy drug)	NKDA	no known drug allergies
CT	computed tomography	PCP	primary care provider
CV	cardiovascular	PE	physical exam
CVA	cerebrovascular accident	plts	platelets
DTRs	deep tendon reflexes	PMI	point of maximal impulse
GI	gastrointestinal	PND	paroxysmal nocturnal dyspnea
GU	genitourinary	q3	every 3
GYN	gynecologist	q4	every 4
HEENT	head, eyes, ears, nose, and throat	ROM	range of motion
HPI	history of present illness	ROS	review of systems
L&W	living and well	TMs	tympanic membranes
IV	intravenous	S/P	status post
mcg	micrograms	x4	times four
mg	milligrams		

Oncology Consult Format (1)

Patient Name: **PCP:**

Date of Birth: **Age:**   **Sex:**

Date of Exam:

PAST HISTORY:

MEDICATIONS: *(All allergies must be typed in all caps and bold)*

SOCIAL HISTORY:

FAMILY HISTORY:

ROS: *(Type in single-space. Capitalize all subheadings, followed by a colon and one space.) Example: NECK: No pain or adenopathy.*

PE: *(Use the same format as above.)*

IMPRESSION
   1.
   2.

PLAN
   1.
   2.
   3.

Eric J. Lopez, MD
Oncology

EJL:xxx

D: 10/15/XX
T: date transcribed

C:

Oncology Consult Format (2)

Patient Name: PCP:

Date of Birth: Age: Sex:

Date of Exam:

HISTORY:

PAST HISTORY:

ALLERGIES:

SOCIAL HISTORY:

FAMILY HISTORY:

REVIEW OF SYSTEMS
CONSTITUTIONAL:
EYES:
EARS, NOSE, MOUTH, THROAT:
RESPIRATORY:
GI:
GU:
MS:
SKIN:
BREASTS:
NEUROLOGICAL:
PSYCHIATRIC:
ENDOCRINE:
HEMATOLOGIC AND LYMPHATIC:
EXTREMITIES:

PHYSICAL EXAM
VITAL SIGNS:
GENERAL APPEARANCE:
HENT AND NECK:
EYES:
CHEST:
CV:
BREASTS:
ABDOMEN:
GU AND RECTAL:

(continued)

Oncology Consult Format (2) (continued)

Patient Name:
PCP:
Date of Exam:
page 2

LYMPHATIC:
EXTREMITIES:
SKIN:
NEUROLOGIC:
PSYCHIATRIC:

IMPRESSION

1.

2.

3.

PLAN

1.

2.

COMMENT:

_____

Jesse E. McCracken, MD
Oncology

JEM:xx
D:
T:

C: Jean W. Mooney, MD

Charting Guidelines

Documentation should always be done:

- After performing a procedure (such as a lab test or EKG) on a patient;
- After giving patient education per physician protocol;
- If the patient fails to show for an appointment;
- When calling in a medication refill;
- After administration of medication;
- When a risk management issue occurs (such as when the patient fails to follow medical advice).

Some things to remember when charting:

1. Progress notes should always be brief, accurate, and legible.
2. Ensure that the patient's name is always on the top of the progress note sheet.
3. Use phrases and approved abbreviations, and use third person. (Example: Pt c/o migraine headache on the left side x 6 hours.)
4. Use only black or blue ink—never pencil or erasable pen.
5. Use proper punctuation to avoid confusion.
6. Pay careful attention to spelling—when in doubt, look it up.
7. Always include both date and time in the progress note.
8. Chart immediately after patient contact (to avoid forgetting essential information).
9. Correct errors properly (a single line through the wrong word, initial it, write "error," and date it). Never erase, white out, or scribble through the error.
10. Chart notes directly below one another. Never skip lines or leave large, blank spaces within a note. Draw a line through blank space.
11. Always authenticate your progress note with your name or initials, as well as your credentials.

Web Sites for Drug Information

Some helpful web sites for obtaining information on medications:

- Drug information on the FDA web site: www.fda.gov/Drugs/
- Drugs@FDA: www.accessdata.fda.gov/Scripts/cder/DrugsatFDA/
- RxList: www.rxlist.com
- Drugs.com: www.drugs.com
- SafeMedication.com: www.safemedication.com/
- DrugDigest: www.drugdigest.com/
- MedicineNet: http://www.medicinenet.com/medications/article.htm
- mediLexicon: http://www.medilexicon.com/drugsearch.php
- PDRHealth: http://www.pdrhealth.com/drugs/altmed/altmed-a-z.aspx

Creating a Travel Itinerary

The purpose of a travel itinerary is to have quick access to information on dates, times, and places for lodging, flights, and other forms of transportation (such as car rental or train). A travel itinerary makes it easy for physicians to ensure that their trips go smoothly by creating a synopsis of important travel information.

When creating a travel itinerary for physicians, it is important to acknowledge the interests of the physician. Some of the considerations include: Do they prefer flying? Will they fly first class or coach? Will they be renting a car? If so, what kind of car do they prefer—compact, mid-size, luxury? How many miles will they be travelling? Do they prefer a nonsmoking hotel room? Would they prefer a suite? What size bed?

Dr. Schwartz prefers to fly coach class and does not mind having a layover flight. However, he would prefer getting into San Antonio the night before the convention begins so that he can be well rested for the first morning session. He would like to rent a car at the airport terminal in San Antonio, if possible. He is looking specifically to rent a mid-size car with unlimited mileage. As Dr. Schwartz does not smoke, he would prefer a nonsmoking room at the Hyatt with a queen or king size bed.

Dr. Schwartz would also like to sightsee during his free time in the evenings. His interests include the symphony and cultural events, as well as historical sites. He enjoys dining at Italian restaurants and sushi bars, but likes all kinds of food.

Some of the web sites you will find to be most helpful in the creation of his travel itinerary are listed below:

- www.kayak.com
- www.igougo.com
- www.aaa.com
- www.mapquest.com

You can also use one of the major search engines (such as Google, Bing, or Yahoo) to locate the Hyatt Regency San Antonio. Just type in www.google.com (for example) and then type in the keywords (such as Hyatt Regency San Antonio). From there, you will be able to find information on hotel policies (such as cancellation policy, check in/out times, and whether or not there is a restaurant on the premises). You can print this information out, highlight it, and attach it to your typed itinerary. You also have the option of rekeying the important points onto a separate, attached sheet. (However, be sure to reference any attachment directly within the itinerary, such as "See Attachment A.")

In a real office setting, you may also be responsible for making the actual reservations for lodging, flight, and car rental. It is important to include all confirmation numbers obtained during the reservation on the travel itinerary. Many hotels send out confirmation letters or emails prior to a trip. In this case, you would also attach the letter or email to the itinerary.

In addition, a copy of the itinerary would be kept at the physician's office, and the original would be given to the physician.

Checking and Proofreading Your Work

1. Proofread your transcripts for content and understanding.

2. Consult other documents in this Appendix for the correct spelling of names and medical terms.

3. Refer to an office style manual, such as *The Book of Style for Medical Transcription* from the Association for Healthcare Documentation Integrity (AHDI), for rules of number usage, punctuation, capitalization, and so forth.

4. Use standard proofreaders' marks (see figure below) to indicate changes to be made.

5. Revise your work. Eliminate mechanical errors (e.g., spelling, typographical errors, or punctuation).

SYMBOL	EXAMPLE	CORRECTION
‖	Align this line with the next line.	Align this line with the next line.
cap or ≡	capitalize	Capitalize
⌒	clo se up	close up
✗	delete this	delete
∧	ins e rt	insert
⌃	insert comma	insert comma,
⊙	insert period	insert period.
lc	Lowercase	lowercase
⊏	move left	move left
⊐	move right	move right
¶	¶Paragraph	Paragraph
#	add space	add space
O sp	spell out & sp	spell out and
tr or ∩	transpose	transpose

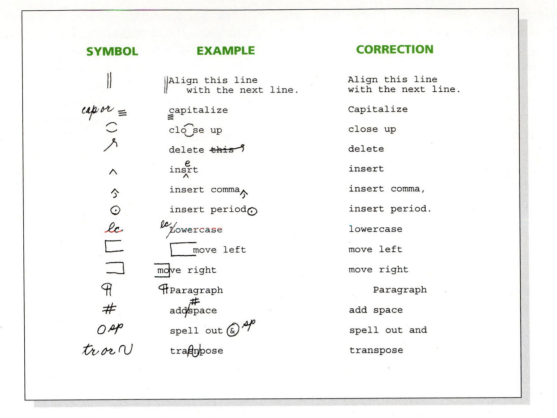

Wage Bracket Table for Income Tax Withholding (Circular E)

SINGLE Persons—MONTHLY Payroll Period
(For Wages Paid Through December 2009)

| Wages | | Number of Withholding Allowances | | | | | | | | | | |
At least	But less than	0	1	2	3	4	5	6	7	8	9	10
		The amount of income tax withheld shall be:										
$0	$220	0	0	0	0	0	0	0	0	0	0	0
220	230	0	0	0	0	0	0	0	0	0	0	0
230	240	0	0	0	0	0	0	0	0	0	0	0
240	250	0	0	0	0	0	0	0	0	0	0	0
250	260	0	0	0	0	0	0	0	0	0	0	0
260	270	0	0	0	0	0	0	0	0	0	0	0
270	280	0	0	0	0	0	0	0	0	0	0	0
280	290	0	0	0	0	0	0	0	0	0	0	0
290	300	0	0	0	0	0	0	0	0	0	0	0
300	320	0	0	0	0	0	0	0	0	0	0	0
320	340	0	0	0	0	0	0	0	0	0	0	0
340	360	0	0	0	0	0	0	0	0	0	0	0
360	380	0	0	0	0	0	0	0	0	0	0	0
380	400	0	0	0	0	0	0	0	0	0	0	0
400	420	0	0	0	0	0	0	0	0	0	0	0
420	440	0	0	0	0	0	0	0	0	0	0	0
440	460	0	0	0	0	0	0	0	0	0	0	0
460	480	0	0	0	0	0	0	0	0	0	0	0
480	500	0	0	0	0	0	0	0	0	0	0	0
500	520	0	0	0	0	0	0	0	0	0	0	0
520	540	0	0	0	0	0	0	0	0	0	0	0
540	560	0	0	0	0	0	0	0	0	0	0	0
560	580	0	0	0	0	0	0	0	0	0	0	0
580	600	0	0	0	0	0	0	0	0	0	0	0
600	640	2	0	0	0	0	0	0	0	0	0	0
640	680	6	0	0	0	0	0	0	0	0	0	0
680	720	10	0	0	0	0	0	0	0	0	0	0
720	760	14	0	0	0	0	0	0	0	0	0	0
760	800	18	0	0	0	0	0	0	0	0	0	0
800	840	22	0	0	0	0	0	0	0	0	0	0
840	880	26	0	0	0	0	0	0	0	0	0	0
880	920	32	0	0	0	0	0	0	0	0	0	0
920	960	38	4	0	0	0	0	0	0	0	0	0
960	1000	44	8	0	0	0	0	0	0	0	0	0
1000	1040	50	12	0	0	0	0	0	0	0	0	0
1040	1080	56	16	0	0	0	0	0	0	0	0	0
1080	1120	62	20	0	0	0	0	0	0	0	0	0
1120	1160	68	24	0	0	0	0	0	0	0	0	0
1160	1200	74	28	0	0	0	0	0	0	0	0	0
1200	1240	80	34	1	0	0	0	0	0	0	0	0
1240	1280	86	40	5	0	0	0	0	0	0	0	0
1280	1320	92	46	9	0	0	0	0	0	0	0	0
1320	1360	98	52	13	0	0	0	0	0	0	0	0
1360	1400	104	58	17	0	0	0	0	0	0	0	0
1400	1440	110	64	21	0	0	0	0	0	0	0	0
1440	1480	116	70	25	0	0	0	0	0	0	0	0
1480	1520	122	76	31	0	0	0	0	0	0	0	0
1520	1560	128	82	37	3	0	0	0	0	0	0	0
1560	1600	134	88	43	7	0	0	0	0	0	0	0
1600	1640	140	94	49	11	0	0	0	0	0	0	0

(continued)

Wage Bracket Table for Income Tax Withholding (Circular E)

SINGLE Persons-MONTHLY Payroll Period
(For Wages Paid Through December 2009)

Wages		Number of Withholding Allowances										
At least	But less than	0	1	2	3	4	5	6	7	8	9	10
		The amount of income tax withheld shall be:										
1640	1680	146	100	55	15	0	0	0	0	0	0	0
1680	1720	152	106	61	19	0	0	0	0	0	0	0
1720	1760	158	112	67	23	0	0	0	0	0	0	0
1760	1800	164	118	73	27	0	0	0	0	0	0	0
1800	1840	170	124	79	33	1	0	0	0	0	0	0
1840	1880	176	130	85	39	5	0	0	0	0	0	0
1880	1920	182	136	91	45	9	0	0	0	0	0	0
1920	1960	188	142	97	51	13	0	0	0	0	0	0
1960	2000	194	148	103	57	17	0	0	0	0	0	0
2000	2040	200	154	109	63	21	0	0	0	0	0	0
2040	2080	206	160	115	69	25	0	0	0	0	0	0
2080	2120	212	166	121	75	29	0	0	0	0	0	0
2120	2160	218	172	127	81	35	2	0	0	0	0	0
2160	2200	224	178	133	87	41	6	0	0	0	0	0
2200	2240	230	184	139	93	47	10	0	0	0	0	0
2240	2280	236	190	145	99	53	14	0	0	0	0	0
2280	2320	242	196	151	105	59	18	0	0	0	0	0
2320	2360	248	202	157	111	65	22	0	0	0	0	0
2360	2400	254	208	163	117	71	26	0	0	0	0	0
2400	2440	260	214	169	123	77	32	0	0	0	0	0
2440	2480	266	220	175	129	83	38	4	0	0	0	0
2480	2520	272	226	181	135	89	44	8	0	0	0	0
2520	2560	278	232	187	141	95	50	12	0	0	0	0
2560	2600	284	238	193	147	101	56	16	0	0	0	0
2600	2640	290	244	199	153	107	62	20	0	0	0	0
2640	2680	296	250	205	159	113	68	24	0	0	0	0
2680	2720	302	256	211	165	119	74	28	0	0	0	0
2720	2760	308	262	217	171	125	80	34	1	0	0	0
2760	2800	314	268	223	177	131	86	40	5	0	0	0
2800	2840	320	274	229	183	137	92	46	9	0	0	0
2840	2880	326	280	235	189	143	98	52	13	0	0	0
2880	2920	332	286	241	195	149	104	58	17	0	0	0
2920	2960	338	292	247	201	155	110	64	21	0	0	0
2960	3000	344	298	253	207	161	116	70	25	0	0	0
3000	3040	350	304	259	213	167	122	76	30	0	0	0
3040	3080	360	310	265	219	173	128	82	36	3	0	0
3080	3120	370	316	271	225	179	134	88	42	7	0	0
3120	3160	380	322	277	231	185	140	94	48	11	0	0
3160	3200	390	328	283	237	191	146	100	54	15	0	0
3200	3240	400	334	289	243	197	152	106	60	19	0	0
3240	3280	410	340	295	249	203	158	112	66	23	0	0
3280	3320	420	346	301	255	209	164	118	72	27	0	0
3320	3360	430	354	307	261	215	170	124	78	33	0	0
3360	3400	440	364	313	267	221	176	130	84	39	4	0
3400	3440	450	374	319	273	227	182	136	90	45	8	0
3440	3480	460	384	325	279	233	188	142	96	51	12	0
3480	3520	470	394	331	285	239	194	148	102	57	16	0
3520	3560	480	404	337	291	245	200	154	108	63	20	0
3560	3600	490	414	343	297	251	206	160	114	69	24	0
3600	3640	500	424	349	303	257	212	166	120	75	29	0

(continued)

Wage Bracket Table (Single Persons) (continued)

Wage Bracket Table for Income Tax Withholding (Circular E)

SINGLE Persons-MONTHLY Payroll Period
(For Wages Paid Through December 2009)

Wages At least	But less than	0	1	2	3	4	5	6	7	8	9	10
		The amount of income tax withheld shall be:										
3640	3680	510	434	358	309	263	218	172	126	81	35	2
3680	3720	520	444	368	315	269	224	178	132	87	41	6
3720	3760	530	454	378	321	275	230	184	138	93	47	10
3760	3800	540	464	388	327	281	236	190	144	99	53	14
3800	3840	550	474	398	333	287	242	196	150	105	59	18
3840	3880	560	484	408	339	293	248	202	156	111	65	22
3880	3920	570	494	418	345	299	254	208	162	117	71	26
3920	3960	580	504	428	352	305	260	214	168	123	77	32
3960	4000	590	514	438	362	311	266	220	174	129	83	38
4000	4040	600	524	448	372	317	272	226	180	135	89	44
4040	4080	610	534	458	382	323	278	232	186	141	95	50
4080	4120	620	544	468	392	329	284	238	192	147	101	56
4120	4160	630	554	478	402	335	290	244	198	153	107	62
4160	4200	640	564	488	412	341	296	250	204	159	113	68
4200	4240	650	574	498	422	347	302	256	210	165	119	74
4240	4280	660	584	508	432	356	308	262	216	171	125	80
4280	4320	670	594	518	442	366	314	268	222	177	131	86
4320	4360	680	604	528	452	376	320	274	228	183	137	92
4360	4400	690	614	538	462	386	326	280	234	189	143	98
4400	4440	700	624	548	472	396	332	286	240	195	149	104
4440	4480	710	634	558	482	406	338	292	246	201	155	110
4480	4520	720	644	568	492	416	344	298	252	207	161	116
4520	4560	730	654	578	502	426	350	304	258	213	167	122
4560	4600	740	664	588	512	436	360	310	264	219	173	128
4600	4640	750	674	598	522	446	370	316	270	225	179	134
4640	4680	760	684	608	532	456	380	322	276	231	185	140
4680	4720	770	694	618	542	466	390	328	282	237	191	146
4720	4760	780	704	628	552	476	400	334	288	243	197	152
4760	4800	790	714	638	562	486	410	340	294	249	203	158
4800	4840	800	724	648	572	496	420	346	300	255	209	164
4840	4880	810	734	658	582	506	430	354	306	261	215	170
4880	4920	820	744	668	592	516	440	364	312	267	221	176
4920	4960	830	754	678	602	526	450	374	318	273	227	182
4960	5000	840	764	688	612	536	460	384	324	279	233	188
5000	5040	850	774	698	622	546	470	394	330	285	239	194
5040	5080	860	784	708	632	556	480	404	336	291	245	200

Wage Bracket Table for Income Tax Withholding (Married Persons)

Wage Bracket Table for Income Tax Withholding (Circular E)

MARRIED Persons -- MONTHLY Payroll Period

(For Wages Paid Through December 2009)

Wages		Number of Withholding Allowances										
At least	But less than	0	1	2	3	4	5	6	7	8	9	10
		The amount of income tax withheld shall be:										
$0	$540	0	0	0	0	0	0	0	0	0	0	0
540	560	0	0	0	0	0	0	0	0	0	0	0
560	580	0	0	0	0	0	0	0	0	0	0	0
580	600	0	0	0	0	0	0	0	0	0	0	0
600	640	0	0	0	0	0	0	0	0	0	0	0
640	680	0	0	0	0	0	0	0	0	0	0	0
680	720	0	0	0	0	0	0	0	0	0	0	0
720	760	0	0	0	0	0	0	0	0	0	0	0
760	800	0	0	0	0	0	0	0	0	0	0	0
800	840	0	0	0	0	0	0	0	0	0	0	0
840	880	0	0	0	0	0	0	0	0	0	0	0
880	920	0	0	0	0	0	0	0	0	0	0	0
920	960	0	0	0	0	0	0	0	0	0	0	0
960	1000	0	0	0	0	0	0	0	0	0	0	0
1000	1040	0	0	0	0	0	0	0	0	0	0	0
1040	1080	0	0	0	0	0	0	0	0	0	0	0
1080	1120	0	0	0	0	0	0	0	0	0	0	0
1120	1160	0	0	0	0	0	0	0	0	0	0	0
1160	1200	0	0	0	0	0	0	0	0	0	0	0
1200	1240	0	0	0	0	0	0	0	0	0	0	0
1240	1280	0	0	0	0	0	0	0	0	0	0	0
1280	1320	0	0	0	0	0	0	0	0	0	0	0
1320	1360	3	0	0	0	0	0	0	0	0	0	0
1360	1400	7	0	0	0	0	0	0	0	0	0	0
1400	1440	11	0	0	0	0	0	0	0	0	0	0
1440	1480	15	0	0	0	0	0	0	0	0	0	0
1480	1520	19	0	0	0	0	0	0	0	0	0	0
1520	1560	23	0	0	0	0	0	0	0	0	0	0
1560	1600	27	0	0	0	0	0	0	0	0	0	0
1600	1640	31	0	0	0	0	0	0	0	0	0	0
1640	1680	35	4	0	0	0	0	0	0	0	0	0
1680	1720	39	8	0	0	0	0	0	0	0	0	0
1720	1760	43	12	0	0	0	0	0	0	0	0	0
1760	1800	47	16	0	0	0	0	0	0	0	0	0
1800	1840	51	20	0	0	0	0	0	0	0	0	0
1840	1880	55	24	0	0	0	0	0	0	0	0	0
1880	1920	59	28	0	0	0	0	0	0	0	0	0
1920	1960	63	32	2	0	0	0	0	0	0	0	0
1960	2000	67	36	6	0	0	0	0	0	0	0	0
2000	2040	71	40	10	0	0	0	0	0	0	0	0
2040	2080	76	44	14	0	0	0	0	0	0	0	0
2080	2120	82	48	18	0	0	0	0	0	0	0	0
2120	2160	88	52	22	0	0	0	0	0	0	0	0
2160	2200	94	56	26	0	0	0	0	0	0	0	0
2200	2240	100	60	30	0	0	0	0	0	0	0	0
2240	2280	106	64	34	4	0	0	0	0	0	0	0
2280	2320	112	68	38	8	0	0	0	0	0	0	0
2320	2360	118	72	42	12	0	0	0	0	0	0	0
2360	2400	124	78	46	16	0	0	0	0	0	0	0
2400	2440	130	84	50	20	0	0	0	0	0	0	0

Source: ©2009 IRS.gov, Internal Revenue Service, Department of the U.S. Treasury

(continued)

Wage Bracket Table (Married Persons) (continued)

Wage Bracket Table for Income Tax Withholding (Circular E)

MARRIED Persons -- MONTHLY Payroll Period

(For Wages Paid Through December 2009)

Wages		Number of Withholding Allowances										
At least	But less than	0	1	2	3	4	5	6	7	8	9	10
		The amount of income tax withheld shall be:										
2440	2480	136	90	54	24	0	0	0	0	0	0	0
2480	2520	142	96	58	28	0	0	0	0	0	0	0
2520	2560	148	102	62	32	1	0	0	0	0	0	0
2560	2600	154	108	66	36	5	0	0	0	0	0	0
2600	2640	160	114	70	40	9	0	0	0	0	0	0
2640	2680	166	120	75	44	13	0	0	0	0	0	0
2680	2720	172	126	81	48	17	0	0	0	0	0	0
2720	2760	178	132	87	52	21	0	0	0	0	0	0
2760	2800	184	138	93	56	25	0	0	0	0	0	0
2800	2840	190	144	99	60	29	0	0	0	0	0	0
2840	2880	196	150	105	64	33	3	0	0	0	0	0
2880	2920	202	156	111	68	37	7	0	0	0	0	0
2920	2960	208	162	117	72	41	11	0	0	0	0	0
2960	3000	214	168	123	77	45	15	0	0	0	0	0
3000	3040	220	174	129	83	49	19	0	0	0	0	0
3040	3080	226	180	135	89	53	23	0	0	0	0	0
3080	3120	232	186	141	95	57	27	0	0	0	0	0
3120	3160	238	192	147	101	61	31	0	0	0	0	0
3160	3200	244	198	153	107	65	35	4	0	0	0	0
3200	3240	250	204	159	113	69	39	8	0	0	0	0
3240	3280	256	210	165	119	73	43	12	0	0	0	0
3280	3320	262	216	171	125	79	47	16	0	0	0	0
3320	3360	268	222	177	131	85	51	20	0	0	0	0
3360	3400	274	228	183	137	91	55	24	0	0	0	0
3400	3440	280	234	189	143	97	59	28	0	0	0	0
3440	3480	286	240	195	149	103	63	32	2	0	0	0
3480	3520	292	246	201	155	109	67	36	6	0	0	0
3520	3560	298	252	207	161	115	71	40	10	0	0	0
3560	3600	304	258	213	167	121	76	44	14	0	0	0
3600	3640	310	264	219	173	127	82	48	18	0	0	0
3640	3680	316	270	225	179	133	88	52	22	0	0	0
3680	3720	322	276	231	185	139	94	56	26	0	0	0
3720	3760	328	282	237	191	145	100	60	30	0	0	0
3760	3800	334	288	243	197	151	106	64	34	3	0	0
3800	3840	340	294	249	203	157	112	68	38	7	0	0
3840	3880	346	300	255	209	163	118	72	42	11	0	0
3880	3920	352	306	261	215	169	124	78	46	15	0	0
3920	3960	358	312	267	221	175	130	84	50	19	0	0
3960	4000	364	318	273	227	181	136	90	54	23	0	0
4000	4040	370	324	279	233	187	142	96	58	27	0	0
4040	4080	376	330	285	239	193	148	102	62	31	1	0
4080	4120	382	336	291	245	199	154	108	66	35	5	0
4120	4160	388	342	297	251	205	160	114	70	39	9	0
4160	4200	394	348	303	257	211	166	120	75	43	13	0
4200	4240	400	354	309	263	217	172	126	81	47	17	0
4240	4280	406	360	315	269	223	178	132	87	51	21	0
4280	4320	412	366	321	275	229	184	138	93	55	25	0
4320	4360	418	372	327	281	235	190	144	99	59	29	0
4360	4400	424	378	333	287	241	196	150	105	63	33	3
4400	4440	430	384	339	293	247	202	156	111	67	37	7

(continued)

Wage Bracket Table (Married Persons) (continued)

Wage Bracket Table for Income Tax Withholding (Circular E)

MARRIED Persons -- MONTHLY Payroll Period

(For Wages Paid Through December 2009)

Wages		Number of Withholding Allowances										
At least	But less than	0	1	2	3	4	5	6	7	8	9	10
		The amount of income tax withheld shall be:										
4440	4480	436	390	345	299	253	208	162	117	71	41	11
4480	4520	442	396	351	305	259	214	168	123	77	45	15
4520	4560	448	402	357	311	265	220	174	129	83	49	19
4560	4600	454	408	363	317	271	226	180	135	89	53	23
4600	4640	460	414	369	323	277	232	186	141	95	57	27
4640	4680	466	420	375	329	283	238	192	147	101	61	31
4680	4720	472	426	381	335	289	244	198	153	107	65	35
4720	4760	478	432	387	341	295	250	204	159	113	69	39
4760	4800	484	438	393	347	301	256	210	165	119	73	43
4800	4840	490	444	399	353	307	262	216	171	125	79	47
4840	4880	496	450	405	359	313	268	222	177	131	85	51
4880	4920	502	456	411	365	319	274	228	183	137	91	55
4920	4960	508	462	417	371	325	280	234	189	143	97	59
4960	5000	514	468	423	377	331	286	240	195	149	103	63
5000	5040	520	474	429	383	337	292	246	201	155	109	67
5040	5080	526	480	435	389	343	298	252	207	161	115	71
5080	5120	532	486	441	395	349	304	258	213	167	121	76
5120	5160	538	492	447	401	355	310	264	219	173	127	82
5160	5200	544	498	453	407	361	316	270	225	179	133	88
5200	5240	550	504	459	413	367	322	276	231	185	139	94
5240	5280	556	510	465	419	373	328	282	237	191	145	100
5280	5320	562	516	471	425	379	334	288	243	197	151	106
5320	5360	568	522	477	431	385	340	294	249	203	157	112
5360	5400	574	528	483	437	391	346	300	255	209	163	118
5400	5440	580	534	489	443	397	352	306	261	215	169	124
5440	5480	586	540	495	449	403	358	312	267	221	175	130
5480	5520	592	546	501	455	409	364	318	273	227	181	136
5520	5560	598	552	507	461	415	370	324	279	233	187	142
5560	5600	604	558	513	467	421	376	330	285	239	193	148
5600	5640	610	564	519	473	427	382	336	291	245	199	154
5640	5680	616	570	525	479	433	388	342	297	251	205	160
5680	5720	622	576	531	485	439	394	348	303	257	211	166
5720	5760	628	582	537	491	445	400	354	309	263	217	172
5760	5800	634	588	543	497	451	406	360	315	269	223	178
5800	5840	640	594	549	503	457	412	366	321	275	229	184
5840	5880	646	600	555	509	463	418	372	327	281	235	190

New York State Special Tables for Deduction and Exemption Allowances (T-12, T-13, T-14)

T-12 (1/06)

New York State
Special Tables for Deduction and Exemption Allowances

Applicable to Method II, Exact Calculation Method
for New York State; see pages T-13 and T-14

Applicable to Dollar to Dollar Withholding Tables
for New York State; see pages T-15 and T-16

Using the tables below, compute the total deduction and exemption allowance to subtract from wages.

Table A
Combined Deduction and Exemption Allowance (full year)

Using Payroll Type, Marital Status, and the Number of Exemptions, locate the combined deduction and exemption allowance amount in the chart below and subtract that amount from wages, before using the exact calculation method (or dollar to dollar withholding tables) to determine the amount to be withheld.

(Use Tables B and C below if more than 10 exemptions are claimed.)

Payroll Type	Marital Status	Number of Exemptions										
		0	1	2	3	4	5	6	7	8	9	10
Daily or	Single	$26.85	$30.70	$34.55	$38.40	$42.25	$46.10	$49.95	$53.80	$57.65	$61.50	$65.35
Miscellaneous	Married	28.75	32.60	36.45	40.30	44.15	48.00	51.85	55.70	59.55	63.40	67.25
Weekly	Single	134.15	153.40	172.65	191.90	211.15	230.40	249.65	268.90	288.15	307.40	326.65
	Married	143.75	163.00	182.25	201.50	220.75	240.00	259.25	278.50	297.75	317.00	336.25
Biweekly	Single	268.30	306.80	345.30	383.80	422.30	460.80	499.30	537.80	576.30	614.80	653.30
	Married	287.50	326.00	364.50	403.00	441.50	480.00	518.50	557.00	595.50	634.00	672.50
Semimonthly	Single	290.60	332.25	373.90	415.55	457.20	498.85	540.50	582.15	623.80	665.45	707.10
	Married	311.45	353.10	394.75	436.40	478.05	519.70	561.35	603.00	644.65	686.30	727.95
Monthly	Single	581.25	664.55	747.85	831.15	914.45	997.75	1,081.05	1,164.35	1,247.65	1,330.95	1,414.25
	Married	622.90	706.20	789.50	872.80	956.10	1,039.40	1,122.70	1,206.00	1,289.30	1,372.60	1,455.90
Annual	Single	6,975	7,975	8,975	9,975	10,975	11,975	12,975	13,975	14,975	15,975	16,975
	Married	7,475	8,475	9,475	10,475	11,475	12,475	13,475	14,475	15,475	16,475	17,475

Table B
Deduction Allowance

Use payroll period and marital status of employee to find the deduction allowance. Then see Table C.

Payroll Period	Marital Status	Deduction Amount
Daily or	Single	$26.85
Miscellaneous	Married	28.75
Weekly	Single	134.15
	Married	143.75
Biweekly	Single	268.30
	Married	287.50
Semimonthly	Single	290.60
	Married	311.45
Monthly	Single	581.25
	Married	622.90
Annual	Single	6,975
	Married	7,475

Table C
Exemption Allowance

Based on a full year exemption of $1,000.

Multiply the number of exemptions claimed by the applicable amount from the table below and add the result to the deduction amount from Table B.

Payroll Period	Value of one exemption
Daily/miscellaneous	$3.85
Weekly	19.25
Biweekly	38.50
Semimonthly	41.65
Monthly	83.30
Annual	1,000

Table D
Adjustment for Difference Between Federal* and New York State Exemption Allowances

For employers who elect to use the federal exemption amounts* in computing wages after exemptions, the following adjustments correct for the difference between the federal exemption of $3,200* and the New York State exemption of $1,000 according to the particular payroll period.

To correct for the lower New York State exemption allowances:
Multiply the amount below for one exemption by the number of exemptions claimed. Add the product to the federally computed wages after exemptions.

Payroll Period	Adjustment for each federal exemption
Daily/miscellaneous	$8.45
Weekly	42.25
Biweekly	84.50
Semimonthly	91.75
Monthly	183.50
Quarterly	550.00
Semiannual	1,100.00
Annual	2,200.00

* The adjustments in Table D are based on the 2005 federal exemption amount of $3,200. The federal exemption amount may be adjusted for inflation as prescribed by the Internal Revenue Code. For an annual payroll period, the adjustment for each federal exemption should be changed by subtracting $1,000 from the current federal exemption amount. Other payroll periods should be recalculated accordingly.

(continued)

New York State Special Tables for Deduction and Exemption Allowances (T-12, T-13, T-14) (continued)

Method II Exact Calculation Method **New York State Single** T-13 (1/06)

Table II - A Weekly Payroll

If the amount of net wages (after subtracting deductions and exemptions) is:

Line	At Least (Column 1)	But less than (Column 2)	Subtract Column 3 amount from net wages (Column 3)	Multiply the result by Column 4 amount (Column 4)	Add the result to Column 5 amount. Withhold the resulting sum. (Column 5)
1	$0	$154	$0	0.0400	$0
2	154	212	154	0.0450	6.15
3	212	250	212	0.0525	8.75
4	250	385	250	0.0590	10.77
5	385	1,731	385	0.0685	18.71
6	1,731	1,923	1,731	0.0764	110.92
7	1,923	2,885	1,923	0.0814	125.62
8	2,885	....	2,885	0.0735	203.92

Table II - B Biweekly Payroll

If the amount of net wages (after subtracting deductions and exemptions) is:

Line	At Least (Column 1)	But less than (Column 2)	Subtract Column 3 amount from net wages (Column 3)	Multiply the result by Column 4 amount (Column 4)	Add the result to Column 5 amount. Withhold the resulting sum. (Column 5)
1	$0	$308	$0	0.0400	$0
2	308	423	308	0.0450	12.31
3	423	500	423	0.0525	17.50
4	500	769	500	0.0590	21.54
5	769	3,462	769	0.0685	37.42
6	3,462	3,846	3,462	0.0764	221.85
7	3,846	5,769	3,846	0.0814	251.23
8	5,769	....	5,769	0.0735	407.85

Table II - C Semimonthly Payroll

If the amount of net wages (after subtracting deductions and exemptions) is:

Line	At Least (Column 1)	But less than (Column 2)	Subtract Column 3 amount from net wages (Column 3)	Multiply the result by Column 4 amount (Column 4)	Add the result to Column 5 amount. Withhold the resulting sum. (Column 5)
1	$0	$333	$0	0.0400	$0
2	333	458	333	0.0450	13.33
3	458	542	458	0.0525	18.96
4	542	833	542	0.0590	23.33
5	833	3,750	833	0.0685	40.54
6	3,750	4,167	3,750	0.0764	240.33
7	4,167	6,250	4,167	0.0814	272.17
8	6,250	....	6,250	0.0735	441.83

Table II - D Monthly Payroll

If the amount of net wages (after subtracting deductions and exemptions) is:

Line	At Least (Column 1)	But less than (Column 2)	Subtract Column 3 amount from net wages (Column 3)	Multiply the result by Column 4 amount (Column 4)	Add the result to Column 5 amount. Withhold the resulting sum. (Column 5)
1	$0	$667	$0	0.0400	$0
2	667	917	667	0.0450	26.67
3	917	1,083	917	0.0525	37.92
4	1,083	1,667	1,083	0.0590	46.67
5	1,667	7,500	1,667	0.0685	81.08
6	7,500	8,333	7,500	0.0764	480.67
7	8,333	12,500	8,333	0.0814	544.33
8	12,500	....	12,500	0.0735	883.67

Table II - E Daily Payroll

If the amount of net wages (after subtracting deductions and exemptions) is:

Line	At Least (Column 1)	But less than (Column 2)	Subtract Column 3 amount from net wages (Column 3)	Multiply the result by Column 4 amount (Column 4)	Add the result to Column 5 amount. Withhold the resulting sum. (Column 5)
1	$0	$31	$0	0.0400	$0
2	31	42	31	0.0450	1.23
3	42	50	42	0.0525	1.75
4	50	77	50	0.0590	2.15
5	77	346	77	0.0685	3.74
6	346	385	346	0.0764	22.18
7	385	577	385	0.0814	25.12
8	577	....	577	0.0735	40.78

Annual Tax Rate Schedule

If annual wages (after subtracting deductions and exemptions) are:

Line	At Least (Column 1)	But less than (Column 2)	Subtract Column 3 amount from taxable portion of annualized pay (Column 3)	Multiply the result by Column 4 amount (Column 4)	Add the result to Column 5 amount. The resulting sum is the annualized tax. (Column 5)
1	$0	$8,000	$0	0.0400	$0
2	8,000	11,000	8,000	0.0450	320.00
3	11,000	13,000	11,000	0.0525	455.00
4	13,000	20,000	13,000	0.0590	560.00
5	20,000	90,000	20,000	0.0685	973.00
6	90,000	100,000	90,000	0.0764	5,768.00
7	100,000	150,000	100,000	0.0814	6,532.00
8	150,000	....	150,000	0.0735	10,604.00

Steps for computing the amount of tax to be withheld:

Step 1 If the number of exemptions claimed is ten or fewer, look up the total exemption and deduction amount in Table A on page T-12, according to the payroll period and marital status claimed. (If there are more than 10 exemptions, multiply the number by the exemption amount in Table C on page T-12 and add it to the deduction amount from Table B.) Subtract the total exemption and deduction amount from the wages to get net wages.

For weekly payroll periods, if the amount of net wages is $600 or less, you may use the simplified Dollar to Dollar Withholding Table beginning on page T-15 to find the amount to withhold. Otherwise, continue with Step 2.

Step 2 Locate the table on this page for the appropriate payroll period. Find the line on which the net wages fall between the amounts in Columns 1 and 2.

Step 3 Following across on the line you found in Step 2, subtract the amount in Column 3 from the net wages.

Step 4 Following across the same line, multiply the result from Step 3 by the amount in Column 4.

Step 5 Following across on the same line, add the result from Step 4 to the amount in Column 5. The resulting sum is the amount to withhold from wages.

See page T-14-A for withholding calculation examples using Method II.

(continued)

New York State Special Tables for Deduction and Exemption Allowances (T-12, T-13, T-14) (continued)

T-14 (1/06) New York State **Married** **Method II Exact Calculation Method**

Table II - A Weekly Payroll

Line	At Least (Column 1)	But less than (Column 2)	Subtract Column 3 amount from net wages (Column 3)	Multiply the result by Column 4 amount (Column 4)	Add the result to Column 5 amount. Withhold the resulting sum. (Column 5)
1	$0	$154	$0	0.0400	$0
2	154	212	154	0.0450	6.15
3	212	250	212	0.0525	8.75
4	250	385	250	0.0590	10.77
5	385	1,731	385	0.0685	18.71
6	1,731	1,923	1,731	0.0764	110.92
7	1,923	2,885	1,923	0.0814	125.62
8	2,885	....	2,885	0.0735	203.92

Table II - D Monthly Payroll

Line	At Least (Column 1)	But less than (Column 2)	Subtract Column 3 amount from net wages (Column 3)	Multiply the result by Column 4 amount (Column 4)	Add the result to Column 5 amount. Withhold the resulting sum. (Column 5)
1	$0	$667	$0	0.0400	$0
2	667	917	667	0.0450	26.67
3	917	1,083	917	0.0525	37.92
4	1,083	1,667	1,083	0.0590	46.67
5	1,667	7,500	1,667	0.0685	81.08
6	7,500	8,333	7,500	0.0764	480.67
7	8,333	12,500	8,333	0.0814	544.33
8	12,500	....	12,500	0.0735	883.67

Table II - B Biweekly Payroll

Line	At Least (Column 1)	But less than (Column 2)	Subtract Column 3 amount from net wages (Column 3)	Multiply the result by Column 4 amount (Column 4)	Add the result to Column 5 amount. Withhold the resulting sum. (Column 5)
1	$0	$308	$0	0.0400	$0
2	308	423	308	0.0450	12.31
3	423	500	423	0.0525	17.50
4	500	769	500	0.0590	21.54
5	769	3,462	769	0.0685	37.42
6	3,462	3,846	3,462	0.0764	221.85
7	3,846	5,769	3,846	0.0814	251.23
8	5,769	....	5,769	0.0735	407.85

Table II - E Daily Payroll

Line	At Least (Column 1)	But less than (Column 2)	Subtract Column 3 amount from net wages (Column 3)	Multiply the result by Column 4 amount (Column 4)	Add the result to Column 5 amount. Withhold the resulting sum. (Column 5)
1	$0	$31	$0	0.0400	$0
2	31	42	31	0.0450	1.23
3	42	50	42	0.0525	1.75
4	50	77	50	0.0590	2.15
5	77	346	77	0.0685	3.74
6	346	385	346	0.0764	22.18
7	385	577	385	0.0814	25.12
8	577	....	577	0.0735	40.78

Table II - C Semimonthly Payroll

Line	At Least (Column 1)	But less than (Column 2)	Subtract Column 3 amount from net wages (Column 3)	Multiply the result by Column 4 amount (Column 4)	Add the result to Column 5 amount. Withhold the resulting sum. (Column 5)
1	$0	$333	$0	0.0400	$0
2	333	458	333	0.0450	13.33
3	458	542	458	0.0525	18.96
4	542	833	542	0.0590	23.33
5	833	3,750	833	0.0685	40.54
6	3,750	4,167	3,750	0.0764	240.33
7	4,167	6,250	4,167	0.0814	272.17
8	6,250	....	6,250	0.0735	441.83

Annual Tax Rate Schedule

Line	At Least (Column 1)	But less than (Column 2)	Subtract Column 3 amount from taxable portion of annualized pay (Column 3)	Multiply the result by Column 4 amount (Column 4)	Add the result to Column 5 amount. The resulting sum is the annualized tax. (Column 5)
1	$0	$8,000	$0	0.0400	$0
2	8,000	11,000	8,000	0.0450	320.00
3	11,000	13,000	11,000	0.0525	455.00
4	13,000	20,000	13,000	0.0590	560.00
5	20,000	90,000	20,000	0.0685	973.00
6	90,000	100,000	90,000	0.0764	5,768.00
7	100,000	150,000	100,000	0.0814	6,532.00
8	150,000	....	150,000	0.0735	10,604.00

Steps for computing the amount of tax to be withheld:

Step 1 If the number of exemptions claimed is ten or fewer, look up the total exemption and deduction amount in Table A on page T-12, according to the payroll period and marital status claimed. (If there are more than 10 exemptions, multiply the number by the exemption amount in Table C on page T-12 and add it to the deduction amount from Table B.) Subtract the total exemption and deduction amount from the wages to get net wages.

For weekly payroll periods, if the amount of net wages is $600 or less, you may use the simplified Dollar to Dollar Withholding Table beginning on page T-15 to find the amount to withhold. Otherwise, continue with Step 2.

Step 2 Locate the table on this page for the appropriate payroll period. Find the line on which the net wages fall between the amounts in Columns 1 and 2.

Step 3 Following across on the line you found in Step 2, subtract the amount in Column 3 from the net wages.

Step 4 Following across the same line, multiply the result from Step 3 by the amount in Column 4.

Step 5 Following across on the same line, add the result from Step 4 to the amount in Column 5. The resulting sum is the amount to withhold from wages.

See page T-14-A for withholding calculation examples using Method II.

Source: ©2006 www.tax.state.ny.us, New York State Department of Taxation and Finance

New York State Income Tax Method I, Single (T-2)

T-2 (1/06)

Method I

Table I

NY STATE

Income Tax

SINGLE

WEEKLY

Payroll Period

WAGES		EXEMPTIONS CLAIMED										10
At Least	But Less Than	0	1	2	3	4	5	6	7	8	9	or more
		TAX TO BE WITHHELD										
$0	$100	$0.00										
100	105	0.00										
105	110	0.00										
110	115	0.00	$0.00									
115	120	0.00	0.00									
120	125	0.00	0.00									
125	130	0.00	0.00									
130	135	0.00	0.00	$0.00								
135	140	0.10	0.00	0.00								
140	145	0.30	0.00	0.00								
145	150	0.50	0.00	0.00								
150	160	0.80	0.10	0.00	$0.00							
160	170	1.20	0.50	0.00	0.00							
170	180	1.60	0.90	0.10	0.00	$0.00						
180	190	2.00	1.30	0.50	0.00	0.00						
190	200	2.40	1.70	0.90	0.10	0.00	$0.00					
200	210	2.80	2.10	1.30	0.50	0.00	0.00					
210	220	3.20	2.50	1.70	0.90	0.20	0.00	$0.00				
220	230	3.60	2.90	2.10	1.30	0.60	0.00	0.00				
230	240	4.00	3.30	2.50	1.70	1.00	0.20	0.00	$0.00			
240	250	4.40	3.70	2.90	2.10	1.40	0.60	0.00	0.00	$0.00		
250	260	4.80	4.10	3.30	2.50	1.80	1.00	0.20	0.00	0.00		
260	270	5.20	4.50	3.70	2.90	2.20	1.40	0.60	0.00	0.00	$0.00	
270	280	5.60	4.90	4.10	3.30	2.60	1.80	1.00	0.30	0.00	0.00	
280	290	6.00	5.30	4.50	3.70	3.00	2.20	1.40	0.70	0.00	0.00	$0.00
290	300	6.50	5.70	4.90	4.10	3.40	2.60	1.80	1.10	0.30	0.00	0.00
300	310	6.90	6.10	5.30	4.50	3.80	3.00	2.20	1.50	0.70	0.00	0.00
310	320	7.40	6.50	5.70	4.90	4.20	3.40	2.60	1.90	1.10	0.30	0.00
320	330	7.80	7.00	6.10	5.30	4.60	3.80	3.00	2.30	1.50	0.70	0.00
330	340	8.30	7.40	6.50	5.70	5.00	4.20	3.40	2.70	1.90	1.10	0.30
340	350	8.70	7.90	7.00	6.10	5.40	4.60	3.80	3.10	2.30	1.50	0.70
350	360	9.20	8.30	7.40	6.60	5.80	5.00	4.20	3.50	2.70	1.90	1.10
360	370	9.80	8.80	7.90	7.00	6.20	5.40	4.60	3.90	3.10	2.30	1.50
370	380	10.30	9.30	8.30	7.50	6.60	5.80	5.00	4.30	3.50	2.70	1.90
380	390	10.80	9.80	8.80	7.90	7.10	6.20	5.40	4.70	3.90	3.10	2.30
390	400	11.40	10.30	9.30	8.40	7.50	6.60	5.80	5.10	4.30	3.50	2.70
400	410	12.00	10.90	9.80	8.80	8.00	7.10	6.20	5.50	4.70	3.90	3.10
410	420	12.60	11.50	10.40	9.40	8.40	7.50	6.70	5.90	5.10	4.30	3.50
420	430	13.20	12.00	10.90	9.90	8.90	8.00	7.10	6.30	5.50	4.70	3.90
430	440	13.80	12.60	11.50	10.40	9.40	8.40	7.60	6.70	5.90	5.10	4.30
440	450	14.40	13.20	12.10	11.00	9.90	8.90	8.00	7.20	6.30	5.50	4.70
450	460	15.00	13.80	12.70	11.50	10.50	9.40	8.50	7.60	6.70	5.90	5.10
460	470	15.50	14.40	13.30	12.10	11.00	10.00	9.00	8.10	7.20	6.30	5.50
470	480	16.10	15.00	13.90	12.70	11.60	10.50	9.50	8.50	7.60	6.80	5.90
480	490	16.70	15.60	14.50	13.30	12.20	11.00	10.00	9.00	8.10	7.20	6.40
490	500	17.30	16.20	15.00	13.90	12.80	11.60	10.50	9.50	8.50	7.70	6.80
500	510	17.90	16.80	15.60	14.50	13.40	12.20	11.10	10.00	9.00	8.10	7.30
510	520	18.50	17.40	16.20	15.10	14.00	12.80	11.70	10.60	9.60	8.60	7.70
520	530	19.10	17.90	16.80	15.70	14.50	13.40	12.30	11.10	10.10	9.10	8.20
530	540	19.80	18.50	17.40	16.30	15.10	14.00	12.90	11.70	10.60	9.60	8.60
540	550	20.50	19.20	18.00	16.90	15.70	14.60	13.50	12.30	11.20	10.10	9.10
550	560	21.20	19.90	18.60	17.40	16.30	15.20	14.00	12.90	11.80	10.70	9.60
560	570	21.90	20.60	19.20	18.00	16.90	15.80	14.60	13.50	12.40	11.20	10.20
570	580	22.60	21.20	19.90	18.60	17.50	16.40	15.20	14.10	13.00	11.80	10.70
580	590	23.20	21.90	20.60	19.30	18.10	16.90	15.80	14.70	13.50	12.40	11.30
590	600	23.90	22.60	21.30	20.00	18.70	17.50	16.40	15.30	14.10	13.00	11.90
600	610	24.60	23.30	22.00	20.70	19.40	18.10	17.00	15.90	14.70	13.60	12.50
610	620	25.30	24.00	22.70	21.40	20.00	18.70	17.60	16.40	15.30	14.20	13.00
620	630	26.00	24.70	23.40	22.00	20.70	19.40	18.20	17.00	15.90	14.80	13.60
630	640	26.70	25.40	24.00	22.70	21.40	20.10	18.80	17.60	16.50	15.40	14.20
640	650	27.40	26.00	24.70	23.40	22.10	20.80	19.50	18.20	17.10	15.90	14.80

$650 & over	Use Method II, "Exact Calculation Method," on page T-13 of this booklet

Source: ©2006 www.tax.state.ny.us, New York State Department of Taxation and Finance

New York State Income Tax Method I, Married (T-2)

T-3 (1/06)

WAGES		EXEMPTIONS CLAIMED										10
At	But	0	1	2	3	4	5	6	7	8	9	or more
Least	Less Than	TAX TO BE WITHHELD										
$0	$100	$0.00										
100	105	0.00										
105	110	0.00										
110	115	0.00	$0.00									
115	120	0.00	0.00									
120	125	0.00	0.00									
125	130	0.00	0.00									
130	135	0.00	0.00	$0.00								
135	140	0.00	0.00	0.00								
140	145	0.00	0.00	0.00								
145	150	0.20	0.00	0.00								
150	160	0.50	0.00	0.00	$0.00							
160	170	0.90	0.10	0.00	0.00							
170	180	1.30	0.50	0.00	0.00	$0.00						
180	190	1.70	0.90	0.10	0.00	0.00						
190	200	2.10	1.30	0.50	0.00	0.00	$0.00					
200	210	2.50	1.70	0.90	0.10	0.00	0.00					
210	220	2.90	2.10	1.30	0.50	0.00	0.00	$0.00				
220	230	3.30	2.50	1.70	0.90	0.20	0.00	0.00				
230	240	3.70	2.90	2.10	1.30	0.60	0.00	0.00	$0.00			
240	250	4.10	3.30	2.50	1.70	1.00	0.20	0.00	0.00	$0.00		
250	260	4.50	3.70	2.90	2.10	1.40	0.60	0.00	0.00	0.00		
260	270	4.90	4.10	3.30	2.50	1.80	1.00	0.20	0.00	0.00	$0.00	
270	280	5.30	4.50	3.70	2.90	2.20	1.40	0.60	0.00	0.00	0.00	
280	290	5.70	4.90	4.10	3.30	2.60	1.80	1.00	0.30	0.00	0.00	$0.00
290	300	6.10	5.30	4.50	3.70	3.00	2.20	1.40	0.70	0.00	0.00	0.00
300	310	6.50	5.70	4.90	4.10	3.40	2.60	1.80	1.10	0.30	0.00	0.00
310	320	6.90	6.10	5.30	4.50	3.80	3.00	2.20	1.50	0.70	0.00	0.00
320	330	7.40	6.50	5.70	4.90	4.20	3.40	2.60	1.90	1.10	0.30	0.00
330	340	7.80	7.00	6.10	5.30	4.60	3.80	3.00	2.30	1.50	0.70	0.00
340	350	8.30	7.40	6.60	5.70	5.00	4.20	3.40	2.70	1.90	1.10	0.40
350	360	8.70	7.90	7.00	6.10	5.40	4.60	3.80	3.10	2.30	1.50	0.80
360	370	9.30	8.30	7.50	6.60	5.80	5.00	4.20	3.50	2.70	1.90	1.20
370	380	9.80	8.80	7.90	7.00	6.20	5.40	4.60	3.90	3.10	2.30	1.60
380	390	10.30	9.30	8.40	7.50	6.60	5.80	5.00	4.30	3.50	2.70	2.00
390	400	10.80	9.80	8.80	7.90	7.10	6.20	5.40	4.70	3.90	3.10	2.40
400	410	11.40	10.40	9.30	8.40	7.50	6.70	5.80	5.10	4.30	3.50	2.80
410	420	12.00	10.90	9.90	8.90	8.00	7.10	6.20	5.50	4.70	3.90	3.20
420	430	12.60	11.50	10.40	9.40	8.40	7.60	6.70	5.90	5.10	4.30	3.60
430	440	13.20	12.10	10.90	9.90	8.90	8.00	7.10	6.30	5.50	4.70	4.00
440	450	13.80	12.70	11.50	10.40	9.40	8.50	7.60	6.70	5.90	5.10	4.40
450	460	14.40	13.20	12.10	11.00	9.90	8.90	8.00	7.20	6.30	5.50	4.80
460	470	15.00	13.80	12.70	11.60	10.50	9.50	8.50	7.60	6.80	5.90	5.20
470	480	15.60	14.40	13.30	12.20	11.00	10.00	9.00	8.10	7.20	6.30	5.60
480	490	16.20	15.00	13.90	12.70	11.60	10.50	9.50	8.50	7.70	6.80	6.00
490	500	16.70	15.60	14.50	13.30	12.20	11.10	10.00	9.00	8.10	7.20	6.40
500	510	17.30	16.20	15.10	13.90	12.80	11.70	10.60	9.50	8.60	7.70	6.80
510	520	17.90	16.80	15.70	14.50	13.40	12.20	11.10	10.10	9.10	8.10	7.30
520	530	18.50	17.40	16.20	15.10	14.00	12.80	11.70	10.60	9.60	8.60	7.70
530	540	19.20	18.00	16.80	15.70	14.60	13.40	12.30	11.20	10.10	9.10	8.20
540	550	19.90	18.60	17.40	16.30	15.20	14.00	12.90	11.80	10.60	9.60	8.60
550	560	20.50	19.20	18.00	16.90	15.70	14.60	13.50	12.30	11.20	10.10	9.10
560	570	21.20	19.90	18.60	17.50	16.30	15.20	14.10	12.90	11.80	10.70	9.70
570	580	21.90	20.60	19.30	18.10	16.90	15.80	14.70	13.50	12.40	11.30	10.20
580	590	22.60	21.30	20.00	18.60	17.50	16.40	15.20	14.10	13.00	11.80	10.70
590	600	23.30	22.00	20.60	19.30	18.10	17.00	15.80	14.70	13.60	12.40	11.30
600	610	24.00	22.60	21.30	20.00	18.70	17.60	16.40	15.30	14.20	13.00	11.90
610	620	24.60	23.30	22.00	20.70	19.40	18.10	17.00	15.90	14.70	13.60	12.50
620	630	25.30	24.00	22.70	21.40	20.10	18.70	17.60	16.50	15.30	14.20	13.10
630	640	26.00	24.70	23.40	22.10	20.70	19.40	18.20	17.10	15.90	14.80	13.70
640	650	26.70	25.40	24.10	22.70	21.40	20.10	18.80	17.70	16.50	15.40	14.20

$650 & over	Use Method II, "Exact Calculation Method," on page T-14 of this booklet

Method I

Table I

NY STATE

Income Tax

MARRIED

WEEKLY

Payroll Period

Source: ©2006 www.tax.state.ny.us, New York State Department of Taxation and Finance

Partial List of CPT Code List and Fee Schedule

CPT Code	Description	Charge	Medicare Allowable
20600	Arthrocentesis Small Joint	$61.00	$47.00
36415	Routine Venipuncture	$3.00	$0.00
45378	Colonoscopy	$315.00	$237.00
71020	X-ray, Chest PA/LAT	$54.00	$42.00
80053	Metabolic Panel, Comprehensive	$20.00	$0.00
81000	UA, Routine with Microscopy	$6.00	$0.00
81002	UA, Routine w/out Microscopy	$5.00	$0.00
82465	Cholesterol	$8.00	$0.00
82710	Wet Prep	$32.00	$0.00
82947	Blood Sugar	$7.00	$0.00
84132	Potassium	$8.00	$0.00
84550	Uric Acid	$9.00	$0.00
84702	Pregnancy Test, Quantitative	$28.00	$0.00
85014	Hematocrit	$10.00	$0.00
85031	CBC w/differential	$11.00	$0.00
85651	ESR (erythrocyte sedimentation rate)	$7.00	$0.00
86308	Mono Screen	$9.00	$0.00
87081	VDRL (Venereal Disease Research Laboratory)—test for syphilis	$8.00	$0.00
87081	Strep Screen	$12.00	$0.00
88150	PAP Smear	$14.00	$0.00
90050	Pelvic Exam—Routine	$75.99	$50.99
90659	Influenza Virus Vaccine	$8.00	$7.00
90703	Tetanus Toxoid	$9.00	$8.00
90732	Pneumococcal Vaccine	$14.00	$13.00
93000	EKG w/interpretation	$50.00	$90.99
99058	First Aid Care	$10.99	$5.99
99070	Dressing of Wound	$10.99	$5.99
99201	New Patient—Level 2—Problem focused; problem focused; straight forward	$53.00	$40.00
99202	New Patient—Level 2—Expanded problem focused; expanded problem focused	$95.00	$72.00

(continued)

Partial List of CPT Code List and Fee Schedule (continued)

CPT Code	Description	Charge	Medicare Allowable
99203	New Patient—Level 3—Detailed; detailed; low complexity	$142.00	$108.00
99204	New Patient—Level 4—Comprehensive; comprehensive; moderate complexity	$200.00	$153.00
99205	New Patient—Level 5—Comprehensive; comprehensive; high complexity	$253.00	$193.00
99211	Established Patient—Level 1—Minimal; minimal; minimal (nurse or lab visit)	$32.00	$24.00
99212	Established Patient—Level 2—Problem focused; problem focused; straight forward	$56.00	$43.00
99213	Established Patient—Level 3—Expanded problem focused; expanded problem focused; low	$78.00	$59.00
99214	Established Patient—Level 4—Detailed; detailed; moderate complexity	$121.00	$92.00
99215	Established Patient—Level 5—Comprehensive; comprehensive; high complexity	$176.00	$135.00
99221	Hospital Care, Detailed, 30 minutes	$97.00	$74.00
99231	Hospital, Subsequent Care	$48.00	$37.00
99238	Hospital, Discharge Services	$98.00	$75.00
99282	Emergency Room	$35.00	$30.00
99291	Critical Care 30–74 minutes	$312.00	$238.00
99292	Critical Care, each subsequent 30 minutes	$162.0	$124.00
99311	Est. Pt., subsequent care, problem focused	$60.00	$60.00
99312	Est. Pt., subsequent care, Expanded, nursing	$78.00	$74.00
99313	Est. Pt., subsequent care, Detailed, nursing	$97.00	$47.00
99322	New Pt., Expanded, nursing home	$96.00	$73.00
99323	New Pt., Detailed, nursing home	$124.00	$94.00

Note: This list of Current Procedural Terminology (CPT) codes represents the codes used in Medical Office Simulation Software (MOSS) 2.0 and should be used for this simulation only; the American Medical Association updates codes annually. The Charge and Medicare Allowable columns represent the fee schedule of Douglasville Medicine Associates.

Partial List of ICD-9-CM Code List

034.0	Pharyngitis, Strep
070.1	Hepatitis A, Infectious
075	Mononucleosis
079.99	Viral Syndrome
250.00	Diabetes Mellitus, Non-Insulin Dependent
250.02	Diabetes Mellitus, Insulin Dependent
251.2	Hypoglycemia, Nondiabetic, Unspecified
272.0	Hypercholesterolemia, Pure
276.5	Dehydration
276.8	Hypokalemia
280.9	Anemia, Iron Deficiency, Unspecified
281.0	Anemia, Pernicious
285.9	Anemia, NOS (not otherwise specified)
289.3	Lymphadenitis, Unspecified
310.9	Organic Brain Syndrome
311	Depression, NOS
380.10	Otitis Externa, Acute
381.10	Serous Otitis Media, Chronic
381.4	Otitis Media
401.9	Hypertension, Unspecified
410.9	Myocardial Infarction, Acute, NOS
413.9	Angina Pectoris, Unspecified
416.9	Cardiopulmonary Disease
427.31	Atrial Fibrillation
427.5	Cardiac Arrest
427.69	PVC (premature ventricular contractions)
428.0	Congestive Heart Failure
429.2	ASCVD (arteriosclerotic cardiovascular disease)
436	CVA, Acute, NOS
438	CVA, Old or Healed
443.9	Peripheral Vascular Insufficiency
461.9	Sinusitis, Unspecified
462	Pharyngitis, Acute
463	Tonsillitis, Purulent

(continued)

Partial List of ICD-9-CM Code List (continued)

465.9	Upper Respiratory Infection, Acute
466.0	Bronchitis, Acute
466.1	Bronchiolitis
477.9	Allergic Rhinitis, Unspecified
486	Pneumonia
490	Bronchitis, NOS
493.90	Asthmatic Bronchitis
493.92	Asthma w/exacerbation
496	COPD (chronic obstructive pulmonary disease)
530.81	Gastroesophageal Reflux
535.0	Gastritis
536.9	Peptic Ulcer Disease
558.9	Gastroenteritis, NOS
599.0	Urinary Tract Infection
601.9	Prostatitis, NOS
682.9	Cellulitis, NOS
684	Impetigo
691.0	Diaper Rash
692	Contact Dermatitis
692.2	Eczema
708.9	Urticaria
715.9	Degenerative Arthritis (specify site)
780.0	Abdominal Pain
780.3	Seizure Disorder
780.4	Vertigo, Acute
780.6	Fever, Unknown Origin
780.79	Weakness, Generalized
782.1	Rash, Nonspecific
782.3	Peripheral Edema
783.21	Weight Loss
786.50	Atypical Chest Pain, Unspecified
788.1	Dysuria
995.2	Drug Reaction

Note: This list of International Classification of Diseases, 9th Revision (ICD-9) codes represents the codes used in Medical Office Simulation Software (MOSS) 2.0 and should be used for this simulation only; ICD-9 codes are updated annually by the National Center for Health Statistics (NCHS), a part of the Centers for Disease Control and Prevention (CDC).

Job Reference Table

Job #	Date of Job	Job Name	Time Allotment	File Placement	MOSS	Internet	Flash Drive
Getting Started	10/5	**Administrative Functions—** Organizing Work Files	30 min	*Medical Office Practice* package			
1	10/5	**Legal Implications—** Introduction to HIPAA and Signing a Confidentiality Statement	30 min	Completed Work Folder Supplies			
2	10/6	**Concepts of Effective Communication—** Revising a Patient Information Brochure	45 min	Completed Work Folder			X
3	10/7	**Administrative Functions—**Blocking the Schedule Using MOSS	75 min	Completed Work Folder	X		
4	10/8	**Administrative Functions—**Filing Procedures	45 min	Completed Work Folder			
5	10/8	**Administrative Functions and Managed Care/ Insurance—** Preparing Patient Files	60 min	*Medical Office Practice* package			
6	10/11	**Administrative Functions—** Scheduling Patient Appointments	1.5 hours	Completed Work Folder	X		
7	10/12	**Administrative Functions—**Patient Registration	45 min	Completed Work Folder Supplies Folder	X		
8	10/13	**Legal Implications—** Request for Release of Medical Information	20 min	Completed Work Folder			

Job #	Date of Job	Job Name	Time Allotment	File Placement	MOSS	Internet	Flash Drive
9	10/14	**Concepts of Effective Communication—** Transcription: SOAP Notes	60 min	Completed Work Folder			X
10	10/15	**Concepts of Effective Communication—** Telephone Messages	30 min	Completed Work Folder			
11	10/18	**Concepts of Effective Communication—** Looking up a Patient Appointment, Scheduling Patient Appointments; Creating Daily Appointment Patient List, and Making New Patient Reminder Calls	60 min	Completed Work Folder	X		
12	10/19	**Concepts of Effective Communication and Ethical Considerations—** Patient Scenarios	30 min	Completed Work Folder			
13	10/19	**Administrative Functions—** Scheduling Special Procedures (Mammogram)	15–30 min		X		
14	10/20	**Concepts of Effective Communication—** Transcription: Oncology Consult	60 min	Completed Work Folder			X
15	10/21	**Concepts of Effective Communication—** Making a Referral to a Specialist	30 min	Richard medical record Completed Work Folder			
16	10/22	**Administrative Functions—** Researching Drug Information	60 min	Completed Work Folder		X	
17	10/25	**Administrative Functions—**Creating a Travel Itinerary	1.5 hours	Completed Work Folder		X	X
18	10/25	**Administrative Functions—**Blocking the Physicians Schedule	30 min		X		

Job #	Date of Job	Job Name	Time Allotment	File Placement	MOSS	Internet	Flash Drive
19	10/26	**Concepts of Effective Communication—** Transcription: Oncology Consult	1 hour	Completed Work Folder			X
20	10/27	**Concepts of Effective Communication—** Completing Finished Copy from Rough Draft	30 min	Completed Work Folder			X
21	10/28	**Safety and Emergency Practices/Legal Implications—** Preparing Occupational Exposure Incident Report	15 min	Completed Work Folder			
22	10/28	**Administrative Functions—**Ordering Office Supplies and Preparing a Purchase Order	1 hour	Completed Work Folder		X	X
23	10/29	**Administrative Functions—**Manual Appointment Scheduling	45 min	Completed Work Folder			
24	10/29	**Basic Practice Finances—**Posting Entries on a Day Sheet	60 min	Supplies Folder Encounter Forms Folder Completed Work Folder			
25	11/1	**Basic Practice Finances—** Computerized Procedure Posting	60 min	Encounter Forms Folder Completed Work Folder Supplies Folder	X		
26	11/1	**Basic Practice Finances—** Computerized Payment Posting	30 min	Encounter Forms Folder	X		
27	11/2	**Employee Payroll—** Completing Work Record and Preparing and Proving Totals on Payroll Register	60 min	Completed Work Folder			
28	11/2	**Protective Practices—**Material Safety Data Sheet (MSDS)	30 min	Completed Work Folder			

Job #	Date of Job	Job Name	Time Allotment	File Placement	MOSS	Internet	Flash Drive
29	11/3	**Basic Practice Finances**—Posting Adjustments and Collection Agency Payments and Processing Refunds	1.5 hours	Completed Work Folder	X		
30	11/3	**Managed Care/ Insurance**— Processing Insurance Claims	15 min	Completed Work Folder	X		
31	11/4	**Procedural and Diagnostic Coding**	45 min	Completed Work Folder	X	X	
32	11/4	**Protective Practices**— Identifying Community Resources	60 min	Completed Work Folder		X	
33	11/4	**Concepts of Effective Communication**— Scheduling Admission to a Hospital; Preparing Patient for Procedure	20 min	Completed Work Folder	X		
34	11/5	**Administrative Functions**— Proofreading and Preparing Final Copies from Draft Copies	1 hour	Completed Work Folder			X
35	11/5	**Legal Implications**— Creating or Updating Resume and Preparing for Job Interview	Varies	Completed Work Folder			X

Medical Office Simulation Software (MOSS) 2.0

About Medical Office Simulation Software (MOSS) 2.0

Medical Office Simulation Software (MOSS) 2.0 is generic practice management software, realistic in its look and functionality, which helps users prepare to work with any commercial software used in medical offices today. With a friendly, highly graphical interface, MOSS allows users to learn the fundamentals of medical office software packages in an educational environment. It is designed to be used with many of the jobs in this Job Training Manual.

MOSS Support and Companion Site

For technical support related to MOSS 2.0, please contact Delmar Technical Support, Monday to Friday, from 8:30 a.m. to 6:30 p.m., Eastern Standard Time:

- Phone: 1-800-648-7450
- E-mail: Delmar.help@cengage.com

Software support and additional resources and tutorials can be found on our Student Companion Site. To access, go to www.cengagebrain.com, enter "Timme" in the search bar and click Find. Click on this book's title to bring up the Product page, then click the Access Now button.

Installation and Setup Instructions

These are the installation instructions to install the MOSS 2.0 program from the CD in your *Medical Office Practice* package:

1. Close all open programs and documents.
2. Place the MOSS 2.0 CD into your CD-ROM drive.
3. MOSS 2.0 should begin setup automatically. Follow the on-screen prompts to install MOSS and Microsoft Access Runtime:
   - Click "Next"
   - Click "I Accept" the terms of the license agreement
   - Click "Next"
   - Click the button next to "TYPICAL" as the setup type
   - Click "Install"
4. If MOSS does not begin setup automatically, follow these instructions:
   - Double click on My Computer.
   - Double click the Control Panel icon.
   - Utilize the Add/Remove Programs feature (for specific instructions on how to use, please reference the User Manual for your Operating System).
   - Click the Install button, and follow the prompts as indicated in Step 3.
5. When you finish installing MOSS, it will be accessible through the Start menu:

   Start > Programs > MOSS 2.0

Using MOSS in Multiple Locations: User Scenarios

Scenario #1: MOSS is used on a home computer only

Follow the installation instructions to install MOSS 2.0 single-user version onto the home computer. Once MOSS is installed, the user logs in with the username "Student1" and default password "Student1." Changing the password is not necessary. All work is saved on the home computer.

Scenario #2: MOSS is used in a school computer lab only

If MOSS will be used exclusively in a school computer lab, the best option is to use MOSS 2.0 Network Version. As part of the Network Version, a classroom management Instructor's Console is available to provide comprehensive monitoring of individual students or entire classes. Some of the additional features included in the Network Version are the following:

- Security levels for students, instructors, administrators, and superadministrator.

- Reporting for student data, to immediately show incorrect entries.

- Reporting for time spent in the program by student and by class.

Scenario #3: MOSS is used in a school computer lab (the Network Version is not used)

In a school computer lab, the best option is to use MOSS 2.0 Network Version; however, if it cannot be used, it is possible to use the single-user version. The following routine will need to be performed each time MOSS is used:

- MOSS single-user version needs to be installed on each computer in the lab.

- The first time a user works in the program: At the end of the session, the user needs to create a Backup File when he or she leaves that computer. The Backup utility is found in the File Maintenance section of the program (the next section, Getting Started with MOSS, contains step-by-step instructions).

- That Backup File should be saved onto a flash drive.

- The next time the user works on MOSS, insert the flash drive to restore the Backup File that was created at the previous session. The Restore utility is also found in the File Maintenance section of the program (step-by-step instructions are provided in the next section).

- Each user will need to follow this same routine when working in a classroom lab, if the Network Version is not used.

- To summarize: At the end of each session, the user will create a Backup File saving all work accomplished, and at the beginning of each session, the user will restore the most recent Backup File to continue at the spot where he or she left off.

Scenario #4: MOSS is used in both a home computer and a school computer lab

Users can work at home and at school using the single-user version, provided that MOSS is installed on every computer on which the user will work. The routine is similar to using MOSS in a school computer lab:

- MOSS single-user version needs to be installed on the user's home computer and on each computer in the lab.

- The first time a user works in the program: At the end of the session, the user needs to create a Backup File when he or she leaves that computer. The Backup utility is found in the File Maintenance section of the program (the next section, Getting Started with MOSS, contains step-by-step instructions).

- That Backup File should be saved onto a flash drive.

- The next time the user works on MOSS, insert the flash drive and restore the Backup File that was created at the previous session. The Restore utility is also found in the File Maintenance section of the program (step-by-step instructions are provided in the next section).

- Each user will need to follow this same routine when working in a classroom lab.

- To summarize: At the end of each session, the user will create a Backup File saving all work accomplished, and at the beginning of each session, the user will restore the most recent Backup File to continue at the spot where he or she left off.

Getting Started with MOSS 2.0

Log on Instructions (Single-User Version)

1. When MOSS is launched, it brings up a logon window. See Figure C-1.

FIGURE C-1
Logging in to MOSS

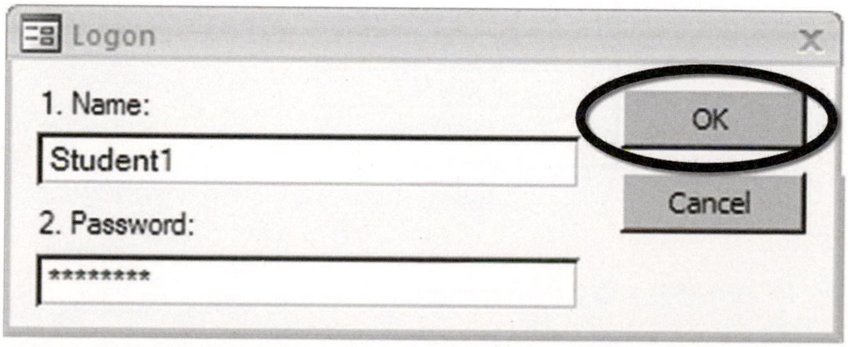

Source: Delmar/Cengage Learning

2. The default user name and password are already loaded for you. (The default user name and password is "Student1.")

3. Click **OK**.

4. You are now at the Main Menu screen of MOSS.

Log on Instructions (Network Version)

If you are using the Network Version of MOSS, you will have a username and initial password assigned to you by your instructor *(it will not be "Student1" as in the single-user version)*.

1. When MOSS Network Version is launched, it brings up a logon window.

2. If not already selected, set the login level to Student by using the drop-down menu.

3. Enter the logon name and password given to you by your instructor in Fields 1 and 2. (Directions to change your initial password are given in a later section.)

4. Click **OK**.

5. You are now at the Main Menu screen of MOSS.

Navigating within the Program

The Main Menu screen orients you to the general functions of most practice management software programs and includes buttons that provide access to specific areas (see Figure C-2). Clicking on a specific button will allow you to work in that area of the program. Alternatively, there is an icon bar along the top left to quickly access the areas of the software, or the user may choose to navigate the software by using the pull-down menus below the software title bar.

■ **Patient Registration:** This feature allows you to input information about each patient in the practice, including demographic, HIPAA, and medical insurance information. From the Main Menu screen, click on the Patient Registration button to search for a patient, or to add a new patient, using the command buttons along the bottom of the patient selection dialog box.

■ **Appointment Scheduling:** This feature allows you to make appointments and also cancel, reschedule, and search for appointments. MOSS allows for block

scheduling, as well as several print features including appointment cards and daily schedules.

■ **Procedure Posting:** This feature allows you to apply patient fees for services. When procedures are input into the procedure posting system, the software assigns the fee to be charged according to the fee schedule for the patient's insurance.

■ **Insurance Billing:** This feature allows you to prepare claims to be sent to insurance companies for the medical office to receive payment for services provided. You can generate and print a paper claim or simulate sending the claim electronically.

■ **Claims Tracking:** This simulates receiving an electronic explanation of benefits or remittance advice from an insurance carrier.

■ **Posting Payments:** This feature allows you to input payments received by the practice from

FIGURE C-2
The main menu screen

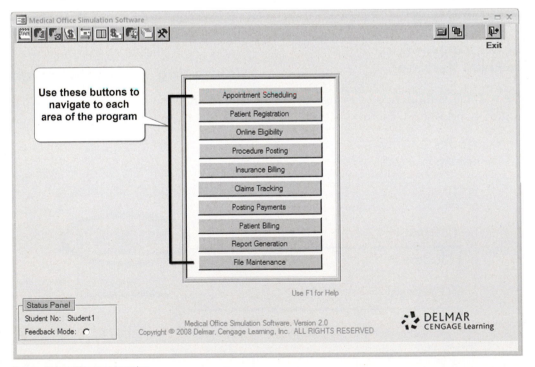

Source: Delmar/Cengage Learning

patients or insurance companies, as well as enter adjustments to the account.

- **Patient Billing:** This feature allows you to generate a bill to be sent directly to the patient to collect any outstanding balances.

- **File Maintenance:** This is a utility area of the program that contains common information used by various systems within the software. In this area, you can create and restore Backup Files, change your password, turn Feedback Mode and Balloon Help on and off, and more. *In the Network Version, please note you will not have these options, as they are controlled by the Instructor's Console.*

Creating Backup Files (Single-User Version)

Backing up your MOSS database is just like saving a document or other file on your computer. Creating a backup file allows you to save all of the work you have completed up until that point. You may create a backup

file of the work you have completed in the program at any time.

Backup files are very useful; for example, if you realize you have made a mistake and cannot correct it, you could restore a previous backup file and start the exercise over again. (Directions for restoring backup files are in the next section.)

We recommend creating a backup file after each Job requiring MOSS.

Follow these steps to create a backup file:

1. Click on File Maintenance, and then click the button next to **2. Backup Database.**

2. Click Yes at the prompt.

3. Now, select a location to save your backup file. We recommend that you save the file on a flash drive (in most computers, this is your E:/ or F:/ computer drive). When saving your file, you may also choose to rename the file. You may rename the file to anything you choose; **however, you must keep the file extension (.mde) in the file name. See Figure C-3.**

FIGURE C-3

Naming your backup file—keep the file extension (.mde) in the file name

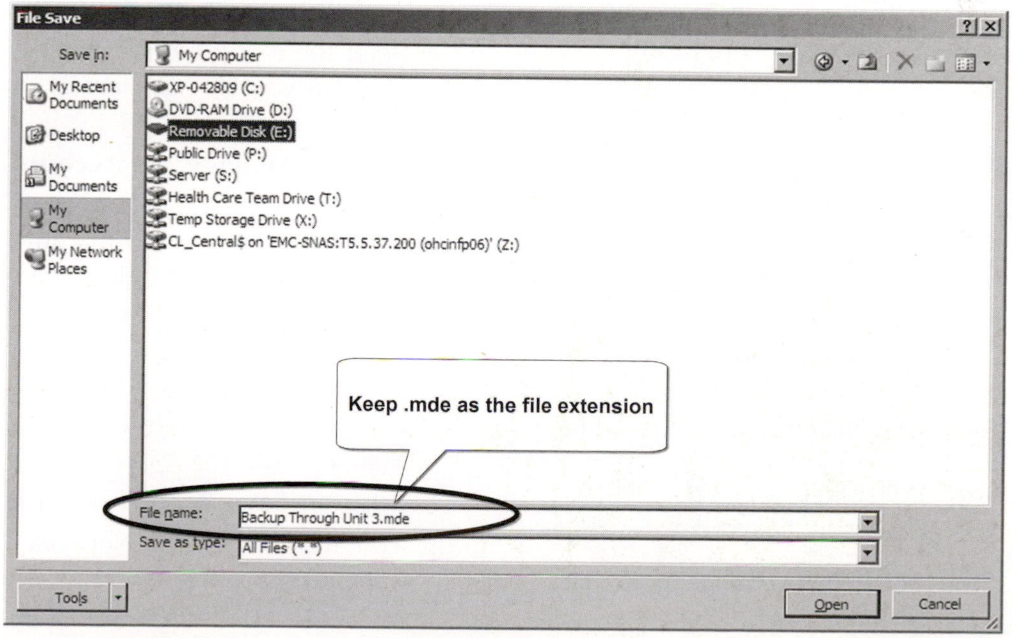

Source: Delmar/Cengage Learning

4. Click **Save** when you are finished. You will receive a prompt telling you that your file was completed successfully. Click **OK**.

Please note: if you are using the Network Version, the network administrator or instructor follows a different routine to back up your database.

Restoring Backup Files (Single-User Version)

The restore function allows you to return to a previous point in the program. For instance, if you realize you have made a mistake and cannot correct it, you could restore a previous backup file and start the exercise over again. You may restore a backup file of previous work you have saved in the program at any time. Please note that restoring a backup file is permanent; all entries you have entered after creating that backup file will no longer appear in the program.

Follow these steps to restore a backup file:

1. Click on File Maintenance, and then click the button next to **3. Restore Database**. Note that restoring a back up file is an irreversible process.

2. Click **Yes** at the prompt.

3. Click **Restore MOSS from Database** at the next prompt.

4. Click **Yes** at the following prompt. (Remember that restoring a backup file is an irreversible process.)

5. Find the backup file that you have created, click once to highlight it, and then click **OK**.

6. Click **Yes** at the following prompt.

7. Click the button **Return to MOSS**.

8. You have successfully restored your back up database. You will need to log in to the new database to start working.

Changing Your Password in the Single-User Version

You are not required to change your password; it is advisable to always use the default password. If you choose to change your password, it can be done in the File Maintenance area of the program.

1. Click File Maintenance from the Main Menu screen.

2. Click on the button next to **1. Change Password**.

3. Enter the current password ("Student1") and then your new password.

4. Click **Change Password** when you are finished.

If you change your password, write your new password down and keep it in a secure place. If lost, the new password cannot be retrieved. Thus, it is recommended that the default password is always used.

Changing Your Password in the Network Version

If you are using the Network Version, you will follow a slightly different routine. You will have a username and initial password assigned to you by your instructor (it will not be "Student1" as in the single-user version). Follow these instructions:

5. Open MOSS Network Version.

6. A logon dialog box will open. If not already selected, set the login level to Student by using the drop-down menu.

7. Enter the logon name and password given to you by your instructor in Fields 1 and 2.

8. Click on **Manage My Account**. See Figure C-4.

9. Move your cursor into the Student Password field and delete the existing password. Enter a new password of your choice.

10. Retype the new password in the Re-Enter Password field. See Figure C-5.

11. Click on **Save Record** when finished.

12. You are back on the Network Version logon screen. Type your new password and click **OK** to enter the program.

FIGURE C-4

The network version logon screen

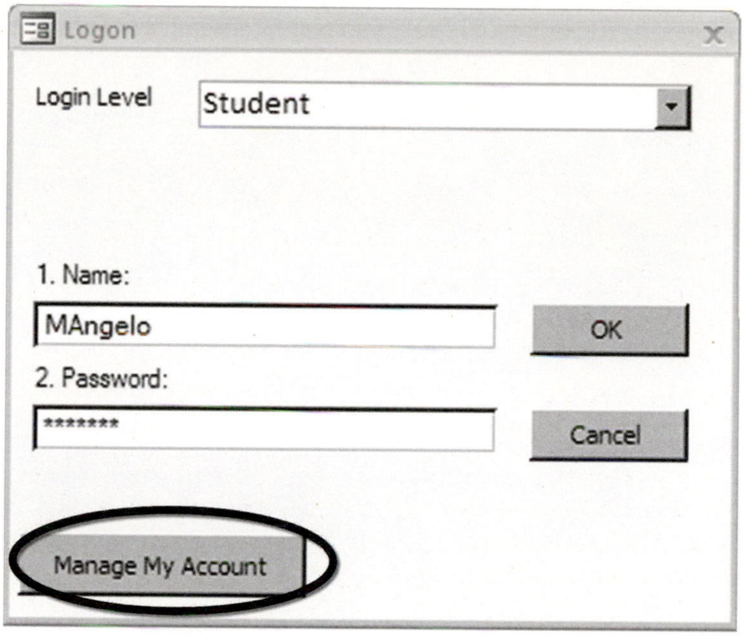

Source: Delmar/Cengage Learning

FIGURE C-5

Click save record to change your password

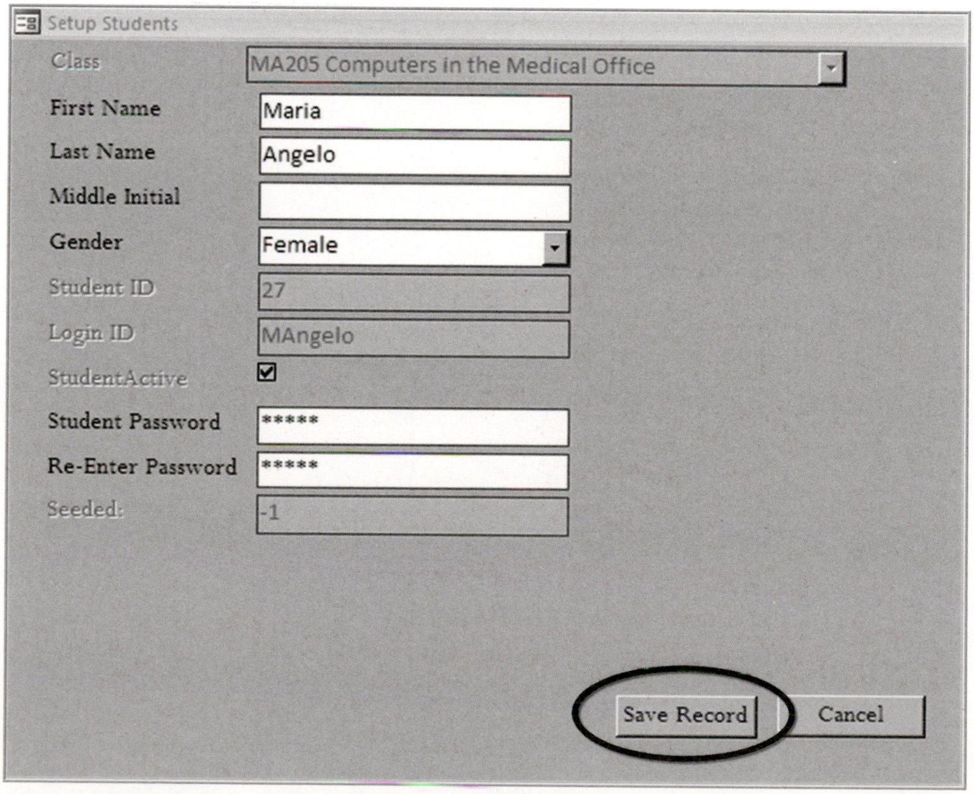

Source: Delmar/Cengage Learning

Forms

Getting Started—Welcome Letter

Job 1—HIPAA Privacy Module

Job 1—Confidentiality Statement

Job 2—Patient Information Sheet

Job 4—Alphabetic Filing Guidelines

Job 4—Filing Order Worksheet

Job 5—Patient Information Form (Harold Prosser)

Job 5—Patient Information Form (Raymond Nolte)

Job 5—Patient Information Form (Theresa Lingard)

Job 5—Patient Information Form (Julia Richard)

Job 5—Patient Information Form (Francisco Alvarez)

Job 5—Patient Information Form (John Wittmer)

Job 5—Progress Note (Harold Prosser)

Job 5—History & Physical Examination Record (Harold Prosser)

Job 5—History & Physical Examination Record (Francisco Alvarez)

Job 5—History & Physical Examination Record (John Wittmer)

Job 7—Patient Information Form (Thomas Furtaw)

Job 7—Patient Information Form (Raul Perez)

Job 7—Patient Information Form (Elmer Freno)

Job 7—Patient Information Form (Karen Boyd)

Job 7—Patient Information Form (Edward Brewer)

Job 8—Authorization to Release Medical Information

Job 9—Quali-Care Clinic Letterhead

Job 10—Message Forms (Patients Coleman, Richard, Santana, Shektar)

Job 12—Patient Scenario Sheet

Job 14—Quali-Care Clinic Letterhead

Job 15—Telephone Referral Information Form

Job 15—Fax Cover Sheet

Job 15—Progress Note

Job 15—History & Physical Examination Record (Julia Richard)

Job 15—Appointment Card

Job 19—Quali-Care Clinic Letterhead

Job 20—Draft: Procedure-Vasectomy

Job 21—Occupational Exposure Incident Report

Job 22—Purchase Order

Job 23—Appointment Cards

Job 24—Encounter Form (John Wittmer)

Job 24—Encounter Form (Thomas Furtaw)

Job 24—Encounter Form (Raul Perez)

Job 24—Encounter Form (Denise Guest)

Douglasville Medicine Associates

5076 Brand Boulevard, Suite 401 • Douglasville, NY 01234 • (123) 456-7890

Sarah O. Mendenhall, MD—Family Practice

L.D. Heath, MD—Family Practice

D.J. Schwartz, MD—Family Practice

October 5, 2010

WELCOME TO DOUGLASVILLE MEDICINE ASSOCIATES

You have been hired as a student medical office assistant for Douglasville Medicine Associates. A medical office assistant assists physicians in many ways, both in the front and back offices. Your function here at Douglasville Medicine Associates is to assist in the front office. As you gain experience in transcribing dictation, you will function more as a medical secretary. Although a medical secretary has advanced transcription skills, it is important for you, the medical office assistant, to be able to perform this vital front office duty.

You have joined a closely-knit group of people who work together to provide quality health care for our patients. All three of us see private, managed health care, and on-site nursing home patients. Private patients are able to make appointments with a doctor of their choice. Managed health care patients who participate in the Signal HMO network may select any one of our three doctors as their Primary Care Physician. Residents of the nearby Retirement Inn Nursing Home are seen by our doctors on a rotation basis.

Your first responsibility will be to us, Doctors Mendenhall, Heath, and Schwartz, through supervision by Flora Mae Fleet, RN, who is our office manger. As a medical office assistant, you will be assigned responsibilities and tasks by the office manager, but you are also expected to use initiative in meeting the daily tasks that evolve in our very active medical office.

You will quickly develop an understanding of our medical office procedures, such as preparing patient files, making appointments, billing patients, handling telephone messages, and completing other business activities. You will complete insurance forms for our patients. You will also transcribe dictations for our affiliate, Quali-Care Clinic.

We look forward to a rewarding working relationship, and we hope that your employment as a medical office assistant at Douglasville Medicine Associates will be a valuable experience.

Sincerely,

Sarah O. Mendenhall

Sarah O. Mendenhall, MD

L.D. Heath

L.D. Heath, MD

D.J. Schwartz

D.J. Schwartz, MD

Douglasville Medicine Associates
HIPAA Privacy Module

General Guidelines

As an employee of Douglasville Medicine Associates, you are responsible to keep patients' health information confidential. Patients have a right to the protection of their confidential information in their files, whether that information be hard copy (the actual physical medical record), electronic media (electronic medical records or online medical records), or even verbal communication that takes place throughout the course of the day between providers concerning them. According to HIPAA guidelines, if you have access or availability to information regarding a patient, you may use and/or disclose only the minimum information that is needed to perform your job duties.

HIPAA Background

HIPAA stands for the Health Information Portability and Accountability Act, which was created by Congress as a means to provide more uniformity to the security and privacy of healthcare rules and regulations throughout the country. Prior to HIPAA being passed on August 21, 1996, each state had differing rules and regulations. Rules and regulations varied even between healthcare organizations, making things very confusing for healthcare providers and even more difficult for patients in understanding the system.

What this meant for healthcare providers was that administrative tasks would now become much simpler with the advent of standardized forms and electronic billing and claims submission. Of course, with the electronic submission came increased security concerns as to the safety of the patient data being transferred. Therefore, HIPAA guidelines require that only those employees who have a "need to know" be given access to a patient's protected health information (PHI) and that access is further restricted to the minimum necessary to do their job.

Covered Entities & Business Associates

According to the Health Insurance Portability and Accountability Act of 1996, certain categories are considered "covered entities" and must abide by HIPAA rules and regulations. They include the following:

- A health plan
- A health care clearinghouse
- A health care provider who transmits any health information in electronic form (electronic form includes internet transmission, phone transmission, and fax)

Dr. Sarah Mendenhall of Douglasville Medicine Associates participates with Medicare and transmits all claims electronically. Therefore, Douglasville Medicine Associates is considered a covered entity and must abide by all HIPAA rules and regulations.

Additionally, Douglasville Medicine Associates shares protected health information with business associates, such as accountants, collection firms, and occasionally a medical transcription company. Under HIPAA, these people must sign a confidentiality agreement.

Notice of Privacy Practices

When a new patient comes to Douglasville Medicine Associates, a Notice of Privacy Practices is given, and their signature is obtained and recorded. The Notice of Privacy Practices details what our practices and procedures are regarding the use and disclosure of their protected health information. This is also done when an established patient comes to the office who has not yet received a Notice of Privacy Practices (check the chart for verification).

Requests for Information

Douglasville Medicine Associates requires that signed authorization forms be received for all requests for information except for those involving treatment, payment, or healthcare operations in accordance with HIPAA guidelines.

Incidental Use and Disclosure

Under the HIPAA Privacy Rule, it is recognized that incidental use and disclosure of protected health information may occur as a result of normal day-to-day operations within a healthcare facility. However, Douglasville Medicine Associates has put in place reasonable safeguards and necessary policies to ensure the privacy of our patients. It is our expectation that all employees of Douglasville Medicine Associates speak quietly while in public patient areas so as to maintain confidentiality. Additionally, the patient sign-in sheet will only contain patient names, not the reason for the visit. Furthermore, once the patient is signed in and recognized by the staff, the patient's name will be blacked out with a permanent marker. Front desk staff members will be careful to close the glass while talking on the phone to patients in the reception area.

Douglasville Medicine Associates recognizes that disclosure of some protected health information is unavoidable (such as using a patient's name when calling them back to the exam room). However, it is your responsibility to be cognizant of the fact that others are listening to your conversations and to limit them to "hello" and "goodbye" while in the presence of other patients.

According to HIPAA, protected health information (PHI) includes such things as:

- Name
- Address
- Phone/fax
- Dates (birth/death/admission/discharge)
- Important numbers (i.e., social security number, medical record number, account numbers)
- E-mail address
- Biometrics
- Full facial images
- Patient's medical history

PHI is not only limited to the patient but also the patient's relatives, employees, or household members.

When in doubt, don't give information out!

One Last Thing . . .

While HIPAA was passed by Congress on August 21,1996, it took some time to finalize all the rules and regulations. The final version actually went into effect on April 14, 2001, but there was a two-year "grace period" during which employers had an opportunity to train their employees and become HIPAA compliant. The HIPAA Privacy Act went into effect as law on April 14, 2003, and is now enforced by the Department of Health and Human Services.

Douglasville Medicine Associates
Confidentiality Statement

      I, _____, an employee of Douglasville Medicine Associates, have completed and reviewed the Health Insurance Portability and Accountability Act (HIPAA) privacy module. I understand that I may encounter protected health information (PHI) as defined by HIPAA during my employment with Douglasville Medicine Associates through access and/or availability and that it is my responsibility to maintain confidentiality of this information to the highest standards in accordance with HIPAA regulations and Douglasville Medicine Associates' policy. I further understand that any breach of confidentiality could result in legal action against Douglasville Medicine Associates, disciplinary action against me, or possible termination of employment.

_____   _____

Signature   Date

_____

Printed Name

_____   _____

Witness   Date

WELCOME TO OUR OFFICE

Douglasville Medicine Associates
5076 Brand Boulevard, Suite 401
Douglasville, NY 01234
Phone: (123) 456-7890
Fax: (123) 456-7800

Sarah O. Mendenhall, MD
Family Practice

L.D. Health, MD
Family Practice

Flora Mae Fleet, RN
Office Manager

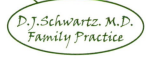

D.J.Schwartz. M.D. Family Practice

Wanda N. Balash, RN
Joseph T. Hasara, CMA (AAMA)
Mei Ling Chun, RMA
Emily Parker, Medical Assistant
~~Lidia S. Valdez,~~ Medical Office Assistant

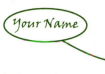

Your Name

Appointments

Please call for an appointment before coming to the office. Briefly describe your problem so that the proper time may be set aside for your visit. This will shorten your waiting time.

We will try to keep your waiting time to a minimum. However, emergencies do arise and your appointment may be delayed. If you are unable to wait, arrangements can be made for another appointment at your convenience.

If you are unable to keep your appointment, we ask that you kindly give us 24 hours notice so that we may accommodate another patient.

Office Hours

Call (123) 456-7890

*Student: Dr. Mendenhall's column should appear after Dr. Schwartz's *see office Hours notes (on second page) ***

Day	Dr. Mendenhall	Dr. Heath	Dr. Schwartz
Monday	9:00 – 12:00 ~~10:00 – 5:00~~ 1:00 – 5:00	9:00 – 12:00 ~~10:00 – 5:00~~ 1:00 – 6:00	12:00 10:00 – ~~4:00~~ 1:00 – 5:00
Tuesday	9:00 – 12:00 ~~10:00 – 2:30~~ 1:00 – 5:00	9:00 – 12:00 ~~9:00 – 5:00~~ 1:00 – 6:00	1:00 – 5:00* ~~10:00 – 3:00~~
Wednesday	9:00 – 12:00 ~~OFF~~ 1:00 – 5:00	12:00 * 9:00 – ~~5:00~~	10:00 – 12:00 ~~12:00 – 5:00~~ 1:00 – 5:00
Thursday	9:00 – 12:00 ~~10:00 – 12:00~~ 1:00 – 5:00	12:00 9:00 – ~~6:00~~ 1:00 – 6:00	10:00 – 12:00 ~~9:00 – 5:00~~ 1:00 – 5:00
Friday	OFF * ~~10:00 – 5:00~~	12:00 9:00 – ~~6:00~~ 1:00 – 6:00	10:00 – 12:00 ~~OFF~~ 1:00 – 5:00

Insurance

As a courtesy to you, we will submit insurance claims to your insurance company. However, you will be responsible for prompt payment of any unpaid balances by your insurance company. **Douglasville Medical Associates will charge $25.00 for all returned checks.** Questions or problems with your insurance should be directed to the office manager. Financial benefits from insurance or government agencies are a matter of settlement solely between you and your insurance carrier or governmental agency involved.

Hospitalization

If hospitalization is necessary, you will be admitted to:

New York County Hospital
1042 Northern Drive
King Park, NY 01238
(123) 555-8745

Community General Hospital
4000 Brand Boulevard
Douglasville, NY 01234
(123) 555-2587

Referrals

If you need to see a specialist, we will be happy to refer you. After the specialist examines you, he/she will be discuss findings with us so that we may share in your health care.

After Hours Problems   *non-life-threatening*

In the event of an emergency, our answering service will contact us (or the physician who may be covering for us) to respond to your call.

In all instances of life-threatening emergencies. please dial 911. For all other medical concernrs after normal business hours, please dial (123) 456-7890.

Billing and Collecting

Payment for medical services is expected at the time of your visit. This includes payment for co-payments, co-insurances, and payment for services rendered if you do not have medical insurance. If you are unable to pay at the time of your visit, a payment plan may be arranged with the office staff. Additionally, we accept cash payments, MasterCard and VISA, and personal checks. In the event of nonsufficient funds (NSF), a $25.00 fee will be added to your account balance.

* *Office Hours Notes*

   Dr. Mendenhall-morning rounds at New York country Hospital from 9:00 a.m.-12:00 p.m., then off in afternoon.
   Dr. Heath-afternoon rounds at Retirement Inn Nursing Home from 1:00 p.m.-6:00 p.m
   Dr. Schwartz-morning rounds at Community General Hospital from 10:00 a.m.-12:00 p.m.

Alphabetic Filing Guidelines

The following guidelines are used with permission from ARMA International. *Establishing Alphabetic, Numeric and Subject Filing System.* Lenexa, KS: ARMA International, 2005.

1. Patient names are *indexed as units.* With regard to medical records, indexing means separating a patient's full name into its parts or **units** (i.e., last name, first name, middle name or initial) and, when properly performed, allows for consistency throughout the system.

    Example: Victoria G. Appleby would be indexed as

Unit 1	Unit 2	Unit 3
Appleby	Victoria	G

2. Nothing always comes before something.

    Examples: Nicholas T. Karn

    Nicholas T. Karns

Unit 1	Unit 2	Unit 3
Karn	Nicholas	T
Karns	Nicholas	T
Vondersahl	Charles	M

3. Ignore all punctuation when indexing (hyphens, periods, apostrophes, etc). Additionally, when a last name includes a prefix with a space, the space is ignored, and the entire last name filed as one unit.

    Examples: O'Keefe, Gina M.

    Olinger-Brown, Kelly A

    Von der Sahl, Charles M

Unit 1	Unit 2	Unit 3
OKeefe	Gina	M
OlingerBrown	Kelly	A

4. Use the patient's preferred name, such as a nickname, or the name by which they wish to be addressed when indexing.

    Example: Long, Maggie A.

    **In this case, the patient prefers to be called "Maggie," but her first name is actually Margaret. Her chart is actually filed using the name "Maggie Long";

however, if there were another Maggie Long (first name actually Maggie), it may then be necessary to use cross-referencing to avoid confusion.

Example: Long, Maggie C.

Unit 1	Unit 2	Unit 3
Long	Maggie	A
Long	Maggie	C
Long (see Long, Maggie A)	Margaret	A

5.   Index abbreviated names as written.

Examples: Peters, Wm.

Thompson, Pat

**In this example, one cannot correctly identify whether "Pat" is short for Patricia or Patrick. Since Pat is the preferred name, once again, it must be indexed as written.*

6.   Numbers are indexed before letters. This includes both Arabic and Roman numerals, which can be used as the fourth or final indexing unit if needed to determine correct filing order. If both Arabic and Roman numerals are present, Arabic numbers are indexed first.

Examples: Wagner, Zachariah A I

Wagner, Zachariah A II

Wagner, Zachariah A Jr.

Unit 1	Unit 2	Unit 3	Unit 4
Wagner	Zachariah	A	I
Wagner	Zachariah	A	II
Wagner	Zachariah	A	Jr.

7.   Foreign names are indexed using the same rules as above (last name, first name, middle name).

Example: Laio, Jun

Religious titles are indexed as written.

Example: Sister Mary Theresa

Unit 1	Unit 2	Unit 3
Laio	Jun	Theresa
Sister	Mary	

Indexing Order

Patient Name	Unit 1	Unit 2	Unit 3	Unit 4
D'Angelo, Marcus				
Scheaffer, M				
Hartman, S				
Cox, K D				
Koval, Patricia				
Bender, Anita				
O'Shea, Peter				
Kloepfer, Gregory				
O'Dell, Larry				
Hafer, Ed				
Ross, Michael J Sr				
Cox, Krista				
Scheaffer, Melinda				
Bender, A K				
Koval, P				
Cox, K				
O'Dell-Martin, Linda				
Ross, Michael J (II)				
Harman, S R				
Ross, Michael J Jr				
Klohr, Maryanne				
Cox, L				
Bender, Anita V				
Daniels, Chester				
Ross, Michael J (I)				
Scheaffer, Melinda				
O'Dell, Lloyd				

Filing Order

Pt #	Patient Name
1	
2	
3	
4	
5	
6	
7	
8	
9	
10	
11	
12	
13	
14	
15	
16	
17	
18	
19	
20	
21	
22	
23	
24	
25	
26	
27	

Douglasville Medicine Associates

5076 Brand Boulevard, Suite 401 • Douglasville, NY 01234 • (123) 456-7890

PATIENT INFORMATION FORM

DATE 10/8/2010

Section A

LAST NAME .... Prosser   FIRST NAME .... Harold   MI .. M

SS# .. 999-16-8119   GENDER ☑ MALE ☐ FEMALE   DATE OF BIRTH 6/23/1937

MARITAL STATUS

☐ Single   ☐ Divorced   ☑ Married   ☐ Other (separated, widowed)

HOME ADDRESS .... 1433 Forest Run Drive
                          Street   Apt./Unit

CITY .... Douglasville   STATE .. NY   ZIP CODE .. 01234

HOME PHONE .... (123) 457-8100   WORK PHONE .... EXT ....

EMPLOYMENT STATUS   EMPLOYER/SCHOOL ....

☐ Employed   ☐ Full-time student   ☐ Unemployed   ☑ Retired   ☐ Part-time student

EMPLOYER ADDRESS ....
                   Street   City   State   Zip Code

REFERRAL SOURCE ....   RESPONSIBLE PARTY ☐ SELF ☐ GUARANTOR

Section B – Spouse Information

LAST NAME .... Prosser   FIRST NAME .... Verna   MI .. E

GENDER ☐ MALE ☑ FEMALE   DATE OF BIRTH 6/6/1937

SS# 999-07-7849   Is your spouse the guarantor of the account? ☐ Y ☑ N

Section C – Health Insurance Information

NAME OF INSURANCE PLAN .... Century SeniorGap

PATIENT RELATIONSHIP TO THE POLICYHOLDER ☑ Self ☐ Spouse ☐ Child ☐ Other

POLICYHOLDER INFORMATION: (If same as patient, check box and skip to ID#, If not, complete all information beginning with Last Name.)

☑ Same as patient

LAST NAME ....   FIRST NAME ....   MI ....

GENDER ☐ MALE ☐ FEMALE   DATE OF BIRTH ....

ID# 999248698   POLICY# (If different from ID#) ....

GROUP # ....   EMPLOYER NAME ....

Do you have a secondary insurance plan? If yes, complete information below. ☐ Y ☑ N

NAME OF INSURANCE PLAN ....   ID # ....

POLICY # ....   GROUP # ....

PATIENT RELATIONSHIP TO THE POLICYHOLDER ☐ Self ☐ Spouse ☐ Child ☐ Other

Are you seeing a doctor due to a work-related injury? ☐ Y ☑ N   If yes, date of injury ....

Are you seeing a doctor due to the result of an auto accident? ☐ Y ☑ N   If yes, date of accident ....

Section D – Assignment of Benefits

I hereby authorize the physicians at Douglasville Medicine Associates to release all information necessary concerning my medical condition to secure proper payment, and I hereby assign the physicians payment for services rendered. I understand that I am responsible for all charges whether or not paid by my insurance. This assignment will remain in effect until revoked by me in writing.

SIGNATURE .. Harold M. Prosser   DATE 10/8/2010

Douglasville Medicine Associates

5076 Brand Boulevard, Suite 401 • Douglasville, NY 01234 • (123) 456-7890

PATIENT INFORMATION FORM

DATE 10/8/2010

Section A

LAST NAME .... Nolte   FIRST NAME .... Raymond   MI ...A...

SS# ...999-64-5153... GENDER ☑MALE ☐ FEMALE DATE OF BIRTH ...6/10/1971...

MARITAL STATUS

☐ Single   ☐ Divorced   ☑ Married   ☐ Other (separated, widowed)

HOME ADDRESS .... 4720 Linwood Lane
Street   Apt./Unit

CITY .... Douglasville   STATE ...NY...   ZIP CODE ...01234...

HOME PHONE .... (123) 457-8000   WORK PHONE ...(123) 457-2733... EXT ....

EMPLOYMENT STATUS   EMPLOYER/SCHOOL .... State Bank of NY

☑ Employed   ☐ Full-time student   ☐ Unemployed   ☐ Retired   ☐ Part-time student

EMPLOYER ADDRESS ...9933 Business Way... Douglasville   NY   01234
                              Street   City   State   Zip Code

REFERRAL SOURCE ....   RESPONSIBLE PARTY ☑SELF ☐ GUARANTOR

Section B – Spouse Information

LAST NAME .... Nolte   FIRST NAME .... Amy   MI ....

GENDER ☐ MALE ☑ FEMALE   DATE OF BIRTH 9/5/1970

SS# 488-16-4387   Is your spouse the guarantor of the account? ☐ Y ☑ N

Section C – Health Insurance Information

NAME OF INSURANCE PLAN .... Signal HMO

PATIENT RELATIONSHIP TO THE POLICYHOLDER ☑ Self   ☐ Spouse   ☐ Child   ☐ Other

POLICYHOLDER INFORMATION: (If same as patient, check box and skip to ID#, If not, complete all information beginning with Last Name.)
☑ Same as patient

LAST NAME ....   FIRST NAME .... MI ....

GENDER ☐ MALE ☐ FEMALE   DATE OF BIRTH ....

ID# 99962110302   POLICY# (If different from ID#) ....

GROUP # .... SBNY37   EMPLOYER NAME .... State Bank of NY

Do you have a secondary insurance plan? If yes, complete information below. ☐ Y ☑ N

NAME OF INSURANCE PLAN ....   ID # ....

POLICY # ....   GROUP # ....

PATIENT RELATIONSHIP TO THE POLICYHOLDER ☐ Self   ☐ Spouse   ☐ Child   ☐ Other

Are you seeing a doctor due to a work-related injury? ☐ Y ☑ N   If yes, date of injury ....

Are you seeing a doctor due to the result of an auto accident? ☐ Y ☑ N   If yes, date of accident ....

Section D – Assignment of Benefits

I hereby authorize the physicians at Douglasville Medicine Associates to release all information necessary concerning my medical condition to secure proper payment, and I hereby assign the physicians payment for services rendered. I understand that I am responsible for all charges whether or not paid by my insurance. This assignment will remain in effect until revoked by me in writing.

SIGNATURE ...Raymond A. Nolte...   DATE ...10/8/2010...

Douglasville Medicine Associates

5076 Brand Boulevard, Suite 401 • Douglasville, NY 01234 • (123) 456-7890

PATIENT INFORMATION FORM

DATE 10/8/2010

Section A

LAST NAME .... Lingard   FIRST NAME .... Theresa   MI .... F

SS# 999-36-8766   GENDER ☐ MALE ☑ FEMALE   DATE OF BIRTH 12/3/1966

MARITAL STATUS

☐ Single   ☐ Divorced   ☑ Married   ☐ Other (separated, widowed)

HOME ADDRESS .... 2455 Valencia Drive
                                          Street   Apt./Unit

CITY .... Douglasville   STATE .... NY   ZIP CODE 01234

HOME PHONE .... (123) 457-7123   WORK PHONE .... (123) 457-0005   EXT ....

EMPLOYMENT STATUS   EMPLOYER/SCHOOL .... Douglasville Elementary

☑ Employed   ☐ Full-time student   ☐ Unemployed   ☐ Retired   ☐ Part-time student

EMPLOYER ADDRESS .... 1000 Schoolhouse Lane   Douglasville   NY   01234
                                                    Street   City   State   Zip Code

REFERRAL SOURCE ....   RESPONSIBLE PARTY ☑ SELF   ☐ GUARANTOR

Section B – Spouse Information

LAST NAME .... Lingard   FIRST NAME .... Robin   MI .... A

GENDER ☑ MALE ☐ FEMALE   DATE OF BIRTH 3/12/1964

SS# 999-75-8262   Is your spouse the guarantor of the account? ☑ Y ☐ N

Section C – Health Insurance Information

NAME OF INSURANCE PLAN .... FlexiHealth PPO In-Network

PATIENT RELATIONSHIP TO THE POLICYHOLDER ☐ Self ☑ Spouse ☐ Child ☐ Other

POLICYHOLDER INFORMATION: (If same as patient, check box and skip to ID#, If not, complete all
information beginning with Last Name.)

☐ Same as patient

LAST NAME .... Lingard   FIRST NAME .... Robin   MI .... A

GENDER ☑ MALE ☐ FEMALE   DATE OF BIRTH 3/12/1964

ID# 99975826275   POLICY# (If different from ID#) ....

GROUP # .... DVL43   EMPLOYER NAME .... Rob's Rattan, Inc

Do you have a secondary insurance plan? If yes, complete information below. ☐ Y ☑ N

NAME OF INSURANCE PLAN ....   ID # ....

POLICY # ....   GROUP # ....

PATIENT RELATIONSHIP TO THE POLICYHOLDER ☐ Self ☐ Spouse ☐ Child ☐ Other

Are you seeing a doctor due to a work-related injury? ☐ Y ☑ N   If yes, date of injury ....

Are you seeing a doctor due to the result of an auto accident? ☐ Y ☑ N   If yes, date of accident ....

Section D – Assignment of Benefits

I hereby authorize the physicians at Douglasville Medicine Associates to release all information necessary concerning my medical
condition to secure proper payment, and I hereby assign the physicians payment for services rendered. I understand that I am
responsible for all charges whether or not paid by my insurance. This assignment will remain in effect until revoked by me in writing.

SIGNATURE .... *Theresa Lingard*   DATE 10/8/2010

Douglasville Medicine Associates

5076 Brand Boulevard, Suite 401 • Douglasville, NY 01234 • (123) 456-7890

PATIENT INFORMATION FORM

DATE 01/20/2005

Section A

LAST NAME .... Richard   FIRST NAME............ Julia   MI .... T

SS# .. 999-34-9220   GENDER ☐ MALE ☑ FEMALE   DATE OF BIRTH............ Nov 11, 1944

MARITAL STATUS

☑ Single   ☐ Divorced   ☐ Married   ☐ Other (separated, widowed)

HOME ADDRESS .... 1922 Webber Street
                           Street   Apt./Unit

CITY .... Douglasville   STATE .... NY   ZIP CODE 01234

HOME PHONE .... (123) 457-7701   WORK PHONE .... EXT ....

EMPLOYMENT STATUS   **EMPLOYER/SCHOOL** ....

☐ Employed   ☐ Full-time student   ☐ Unemployed   ☑ Retired   ☐ Part-time student

EMPLOYER ADDRESS ....
                           Street   City   State   Zip Code

REFERRAL SOURCE ....   **RESPONSIBLE PARTY** ☑ SELF ☐ GUARANTOR

Section B – Spouse Information

LAST NAME ....   FIRST NAME............ MI ....

GENDER ☐ MALE ☐ FEMALE   DATE OF BIRTH............

SS# ....   Is your spouse the guarantor of the account? ☐ Y ☐ N

Section C – Health Insurance Information

NAME OF INSURANCE PLAN .... Century SeniorGap

PATIENT RELATIONSHIP TO THE POLICYHOLDER ☑ Self ☐ Spouse ☐ Child ☐ Other

POLICYHOLDER INFORMATION: (If same as patient, check box and skip to ID#, If not, complete all information beginning with Last Name.)

☑ Same as patient

LAST NAME ....   FIRST NAME .... MI ....

GENDER ☐ MALE ☐ FEMALE   DATE OF BIRTH ....

ID# .... 921349220B   POLICY# (If different from ID#) ....

GROUP # ....   EMPLOYER NAME ....

Do you have a secondary insurance plan? If yes, complete information below. ☐ Y ☑ N

NAME OF INSURANCE PLAN ....   ID # ....

POLICY # ....   GROUP # ....

PATIENT RELATIONSHIP TO THE POLICYHOLDER ☐ Self ☐ Spouse ☐ Child ☐ Other

Are you seeing a doctor due to a work-related injury? ☐ Y ☑ N   If yes, date of injury ....

Are you seeing a doctor due to the result of an auto accident? ☐ Y ☑ N   If yes, date of accident ....

Section D – Assignment of Benefits

I hereby authorize the physicians at Douglasville Medicine Associates to release all information necessary concerning my medical condition to secure proper payment, and I hereby assign the physicians payment for services rendered. I understand that I am responsible for all charges whether or not paid by my insurance. This assignment will remain in effect until revoked by me in writing.

SIGNATURE .... Julia T. Richard   DATE 01/20/2005

Douglasville Medicine Associates

5076 Brand Boulevard, Suite 401 • Douglasville, NY 01234 • (123) 456-7890

PATIENT INFORMATION FORM

DATE .... April 17, 2004

Section A

LAST NAME .... Alvarez   FIRST NAME .... Francisco   MI   B

SS# ... 999-26-1748   GENDER ☑ MALE ☐ FEMALE   DATE OF BIRTH .... March 1, 1949

MARITAL STATUS

☑ Single   ☐ Divorced   ☐ Married   ☐ Other (separated, widowed)

HOME ADDRESS .... 410 Hyde Park
                          Street   Apt./Unit

CITY .... Douglasville   STATE ... NY   ZIP CODE ... 01234

HOME PHONE .... (123) 457-6610   WORK PHONE ... (123) 457-4286   EXT ...

EMPLOYMENT STATUS   EMPLOYER/SCHOOL .... Marble and Tile, Inc.

☑ Employed   ☐ Full-time student   ☐ Unemployed   ☐ Retired   ☐ Part-time student

EMPLOYER ADDRESS .... 4070 Sawyer Court   Douglasville   NY   01234
                              Street   City   State   Zip Code

REFERRAL SOURCE ....   RESPONSIBLE PARTY   ☑ SELF ☐ GUARANTOR

Section B – Spouse Information

LAST NAME ....   FIRST NAME ....   MI ....

GENDER ☐ MALE ☐ FEMALE   DATE OF BIRTH ....

SS# ....   Is your spouse the guarantor of the account? ☐ Y ☐ N

Section C – Health Insurance Information

NAME OF INSURANCE PLAN ....   FlexiHealth PPO In-Network

PATIENT RELATIONSHIP TO THE POLICYHOLDER ☑ Self ☐ Spouse ☐ Child ☐ Other

POLICYHOLDER INFORMATION: (If same as patient, check box and skip to ID#, If not, complete all
                                        information beginning with Last Name.)
☑ Same as patient

LAST NAME ....   FIRST NAME ....   MI ....

GENDER ☐ MALE ☐ FEMALE   DATE OF BIRTH ....

ID# ... A791261748   POLICY# (If different from ID#) ....

GROUP # ... 4002200   EMPLOYER NAME ...

Do you have a secondary insurance plan? If yes, complete information below. ☐ Y ☑ N

NAME OF INSURANCE PLAN ....   ID # ....

POLICY # ....   GROUP # ....

PATIENT RELATIONSHIP TO THE POLICYHOLDER ☐ Self ☐ Spouse ☐ Child ☐ Other

Are you seeing a doctor due to a work-related injury? ☐ Y ☑ N If yes, date of injury ....

Are you seeing a doctor due to the result of an auto accident? ☐ Y ☑ N If yes, date of accident ....

Section D – Assignment of Benefits

I hereby authorize the physicians at Douglasville Medicine Associates to release all information necessary concerning my medical condition to secure proper payment, and I hereby assign the physicians payment for services rendered. I understand that I am responsible for all charges whether or not paid by my insurance. This assignment will remain in effect until revoked by me in writing.

SIGNATURE ... Francisco Alvarez   DATE ... April 17, 2004

Douglasville Medicine Associates

5076 Brand Boulevard, Suite 401 • Douglasville, NY 01234 • (123) 456-7890

PATIENT INFORMATION FORM

DATE .... *Sept. 6, 2010*

Section A

LAST NAME .... *Wittmer* FIRST NAME .... *John* MI .... *J.*

SS# .. *999-54-3833* GENDER ☑ MALE ☐ FEMALE DATE OF BIRTH .... *Jan 11, 1957*

MARITAL STATUS

☐ Single ☐ Divorced ☑ Married ☐ Other (separated, widowed)

HOME ADDRESS .... *5070 Prospect Road*
Street Apt./Unit

CITY .... *Douglasville* STATE .... *NY* ZIP CODE *01234*

HOME PHONE .... *(123) 457-6216* WORK PHONE .. *(123) 457-0720* EXT ....

EMPLOYMENT STATUS EMPLOYER/SCHOOL .... *Webber Nursing Home*

☑ Employed ☐ Full-time student ☐ Unemployed ☐ Retired ☐ Part-time student

EMPLOYER ADDRESS .... *1900 Mayes Street* *Douglasville* *NY* *01234*
Street City State Zip Code

REFERRAL SOURCE .... RESPONSIBLE PARTY ☑ SELF ☐ GUARANTOR

Section B – Spouse Information

LAST NAME .... *Wittmer* FIRST NAME .... *Vera* MI ....

GENDER ☐ MALE ☑ FEMALE DATE OF BIRTH .... *May 22, 1957*

SS# .... Is your spouse the guarantor of the account? ☐ Y ☐ N

Section C – Health Insurance Information

NAME OF INSURANCE PLAN .... *Medicaid*

PATIENT RELATIONSHIP TO THE POLICYHOLDER ☑ Self ☐ Spouse ☐ Child ☐ Other

POLICYHOLDER INFORMATION: (If same as patient, check box and skip to ID#, If not, complete all information beginning with Last Name.)

☑ Same as patient

LAST NAME .... FIRST NAME .... MI ....

GENDER ☐ MALE ☐ FEMALE DATE OF BIRTH ....

ID# .... *546465107* POLICY# (If different from ID#) ....

GROUP # .... EMPLOYER NAME ....

Do you have a secondary insurance plan? If yes, complete information below. ☐ Y ☑ N

NAME OF INSURANCE PLAN .... ID # ....

POLICY # .... GROUP # ....

PATIENT RELATIONSHIP TO THE POLICYHOLDER ☐ Self ☐ Spouse ☐ Child ☐ Other

Are you seeing a doctor due to a work-related injury? ☐ Y ☑ N If yes, date of injury ....

Are you seeing a doctor due to the result of an auto accident? ☐ Y ☑ N If yes, date of accident ....

Section D – Assignment of Benefits

I hereby authorize the physicians at Douglasville Medicine Associates to release all information necessary concerning my medical condition to secure proper payment, and I hereby assign the physicians payment for services rendered. I understand that I am responsible for all charges whether or not paid by my insurance. This assignment will remain in effect until revoked by me in writing.

SIGNATURE *John J. Wittmer* DATE .... *Sept. 6, 2010*

Douglasville Medicine Associates

5076 Brand Boulevard, Suite 401 • Douglasville, NY 01234 • (123) 456-7890

Sarah O. Mendenhall, MD—Family Practice

L.D. Heath, MD—Family Practice

D.J. Schwartz, MD—Family Practice

PROGRESS NOTE

9/5/10   Harold Prosser

Patient presented for follow-up gastroenterology care since recommending long-term Tagamet 400 mg q.d. in June of this year. In the last month, patient has felt generally well with only one brief flare-up of abdominal discomfort that lasted several days and was promptly relieved with Maalox. He is tolerating the Tagamet without difficulty. His physical examination was unchanged from that performed six months ago. As he seems to be reasonably comfortable on this regimen, I have asked him to continue taking the Tagamet at bedtime and Maalox as needed. He is to return in one month.

Sarah O. Mendenhall, MD

SOM:pa

Douglasville Medicine Associates

5076 Brand Boulevard, Suite 401 • Douglasville, NY 01234 • (123) 456-7890

Sarah O. Mendenhall, MD—Internal Practice

L.D.Heath, MD—Family Practice

D.J. Schwartz, MD—Family Practice

PATIENT: Prosser, Harold M.

DATE: September 25, 2008

PHYSICIAN: Sarah O. Mendenhall, MD

HISTORY

HISTORY OF PRESENT ILLNESS

This is a 71-year-old white male who came to the office today with a chief complaint of nausea, decreased appetite, stomach upset, a little bit of dizziness, and what he believed were dark stools. The patient never had any similar problem. He has an interesting past medical history. He is a nonsmoker. He occasionally drinks but not very often. The patient had an appendectomy in 1950. He had an undescended testicle, which later had to be removed because of testicular cancer being diagnosed, and he has had injections of testosterone since that time. He did have postsurgical irradiation. He has also had diffuse arthritis for years.

MEDICATIONS

Tagamet 400 mg per day, allopurinol 300 mg per day for presumed gout, and Feldene 20 mg once a day.

FAMILY MEDICAL HISTORY

His father died of rheumatoid complications; his mother of died old age. The patient is regularly seen by his doctor up north. He had a physical this summer, which was unremarkable. His laboratory data is generally unremarkable. His hemoglobin and hematocrit were 15.1 and 43.8, respectively. When seen today, the patient said that he did not feel well. He did not have much to eat or drink and complained of a mild upset stomach but no vomiting. He states he gets a little dizzy upon standing.

PHYSICAL

VITAL SIGNS: Blood pressure lying down approximately 140/80; when he stands it goes to about 128/80. Pulse is 128 and regular.

SKIN: Skin is somewhat pale. Turger is good.

HEENT: There does appear to be capillary blood in the conjunctivae. Funduscopic examination was benign. Ears normal. Cranial nerves intact. Throat normal.

NECK: No adenopathy. No carotid bruits.

LUNGS: Clear with no crackles or wheezes.

HEART: The heart is tachycardic at about 130 and is regular with no ectopy noted.

UPPER EXTREMITIES: No tremor. Active reflexes. Good pulses and sensations.

ABDOMEN: Soft. There is no organomegaly noted. No rebound, tenderness, or masses, although he says that diffusely he feels bad with palpation of the stomach.

GENITALIA: He has only one testicle because of the previous surgery.

RECTAL EXAMINATION: Reveals that the prostate appears to be slightly enlarged. No stool blockages or growths are noted, but he has a dark sticky-type stool which is almost black and tested heme-positive.

LOWER EXTREMITIES: Active reflexes in the patellar tendon areas. Sensation is normal in the lower extremities with no edema.

OVERALL IMPRESSION

1. Gastrointestinal bleeding, probably gastric duodenal in location. Rule out nonsteroidal anti-inflammatory drug induced.
2. Diffuse osteoarthritis.
3. History of gout.
4. Status post excision of left testicle for testicular cancer with postradiation.
5. Nonsteroidal anti-inflammatory drug therapy.

OVERALL ASSESSMENT/PLAN

He is to be referred to David Childs, MD, a gastroenterologist, at Quali-Care Clinic.

_____

Sarah O. Mendenhall, MD

SOM/si

D:10/25/08

T:10/25/08

Douglasville Medicine Associates

5076 Brand Boulevard, Suite 401 • Douglasville, NY 01234 • (123) 456-7890

Sarah O. Mendenhall, MD—Family Practice

L.D. Heath, MD—Family Practice

D.J. Schwartz, MD—Family Practice

PATIENT: Alvarez, Francisco B.

DATE: February 8, 2009

PHYSICIAN: Sarah O. Mendenhall, MD

HISTORY

Had bleeding duodenal ulcer in October. Off all medications. Now on Zantac one o.d. and Tylenol p.r.n. is permitted.

PHYSICAL

VITALS

WEIGHT: 165; blood pressure: 140/70; pulse: 96 w/PC's; temperature: 98.6.

HEENT: Having dental work.

EYES: Normal. Fundi benign.

NECK: Thyroid not palpable.

LUNGS: Clear.

HEART: Not enlarged. Irregular. No murmur.

ABDOMEN: Fullness RUQ. Lumbar laminectomy scar.

GENITALIA: Normal male. Circumcised.

RECTAL: Normal. Prostate Normal.

EXTREMITIES: Atrophy left shoulder. Frozen left wrist. Contracture left 5th finger.

NEURO: Absent DTR's LE's. Pulses full and equal.

HISTORY AND PHYSICAL
ALVAREZ, FRANCISCO B.
PAGE 2
FEBRUARY 8, 2009

IMPRESSIONS

1. Cardiac arrhythmia.
2. Post lumbar laminectomy.
3. Respiratory allergies.
4. Post bleeding duodenal ulcer.
5. Renal colic history.

RX

1. PE EKG, lab.
2. Zantac 150 mg one o.d.
3. Tylenol p.r.n.

Sarah O. Mendenhall, MD

SOM/si
D: 02/08/09
T: 02/08/09

Douglasville Medicine Associates

5076 Brand Boulevard, Suite 401 • Douglasville, NY 01234 • (123) 456-7890

Sarah O. Mendenhall, MD—Family Practice
L.D. Heath, MD—Family Practice
D.J. Schwartz, MD—Family Practice

PATIENT: Wittmer, John J.
DATE: February 15, 2010
PHYSICIAN: Sarah O. Mendenhall, MD

HISTORY

This 53-year-old white male came to the office with a complaint of chest pain and gastrointestinal discomfort. The history is that the patient was feeling well and went out Saturday night to have seafood. On Sunday he was out eating at a restaurant and suddenly felt somewhat weak-legged and queasy and like his legs might give out. He went into the bathroom and felt a little bit better but decided to start for home. While he was in the car, the nausea became worse, and he experienced some epigastric discomfort. The discomfort apparently did not start at the restaurant but after he had been riding in the car. He said he felt a fullness in the epigastric area. There was no radiation to the neck, jaw, or arm. When he got home, he vomited. He said he felt a little bit better, but because of these symptoms he decided that he would call the office this morning. He had never had a symptom of this type before. No exertionally induced substernal chest pain or pressure with exertion or at rest, PND or orthopnea, cardiac arrhythmia, palpitations or rapid heart action; no syncope, dizziness, or near syncope. He has had no history of peptic ulcer or gastrointestinal disease per se.

He denies any sudden loss of vision or slurred speech. No difficulty chewing or swallowing. No focal, motor, or sensory deficits or difficulty with gait or balance.

He had a questionable history of hypertension and was treated with medication and then apparently was placed on garlic he apparently started taking garlic pills and does not take any antihypertensive now. He has no idea what his cholesterol level is. There is a very positive family history of coronary disease. His father died at 70 years of age, probably from a heart attack. His mother died from heart failure. Also, he had three brothers, all of whom are deceased at a relatively young age with apparent coronary artery disease. He does not smoke cigarettes.

He has had no temperature, chills, fever, nausea, or vomiting. No upper respiratory infections. No hematuria, dysuria, urgency, or frequency. He did have several bowel movements after this event started with the nausea.

PHYSICAL

The physical examination revealed a 52-year-old white male with a pectus excavatum. His heart rate and rhythm were regular. There was a questionable midsystolic click. His lungs are mostly vesicular. The abdomen was soft. The liver and spleen were not enlarged. There was no pretibial edema. The peripheral pulses were 2+. His facial symmetry was normal. The extraocular muscle movement was conjugate. His hearing was intact. Cranial nerves II through XII were intact.

IMPRESSIONS

1. Atypical chest pain.
2. Very positive family history of coronary artery disease.
3. Acute enteritis, food related.

RECOMMENDATIONS

It sounds very much like this patient had a vasovagal reaction after he became nauseated and vomited. He said he was lightheaded, diaphoretic, and pale. He had some epigastric discomfort, but again, this does not definitely relate to a heart problem. It is curious that he did have some nonspecific ST and T wave changes on his cardiogram, which could be related to the excess vagotonia. This was in the precordial leads, and they are not definitely ischemic changes. More-over, the serial enzymes at this point show no heart attack.

Medicate on nitrate therapy and aspirin. Will complete thallium stress test. If thallium stress test shows any abnormality, may prescribe cardiac catheterization.

Sarah O. Mendenhall, MD

SOM/si
D: 02/15/10
T: 02/16/10

Douglasville Medicine Associates

5076 Brand Boulevard, Suite 401 • Douglasville, NY 01234 • (123) 456-7890

PATIENT INFORMATION FORM

DATE 10/13/2010

Section A

LAST NAME .... Furtaw   FIRST NAME .... Thomas   MI ... M

SS# .. 798-45-6321 .   GENDER ☑ MALE ☐ FEMALE   DATE OF BIRTH 7/17/1954

MARITAL STATUS

☐ Single   ☐ Divorced   ☑ Married   ☐ Other (separated, widowed)

HOME ADDRESS .... 780 Spring Lane
                              Street   Apt./Unit

CITY .... Vance   STATE .... NY   ZIP CODE 25894

HOME PHONE .... (123) 556-4819   WORK PHONE .... (123) 556-7737 EXT ....

EMPLOYMENT STATUS   EMPLOYER/SCHOOL Mountain View Automotive

☑ Employed   ☐ Full-time student   ☐ Unemployed   ☐ Retired   ☐ Part-time student

EMPLOYER ADDRESS .... 829 Maple Ave   Vance   NY   25894
                                   Street   City   State   Zip Code

REFERRAL SOURCE ....   RESPONSIBLE PARTY ☑ SELF ☐ GUARANTOR

Section B – Spouse Information

LAST NAME .... Furtaw   FIRST NAME .... Jane   MI ....

GENDER ☐ MALE ☑ FEMALE   DATE OF BIRTH 2/27/1956

SS# ....   Is your spouse the guarantor of the account? ☐ Y ☑ N

Section C – Health Insurance Information

NAME OF INSURANCE PLAN .... FlexiHealth PPO In-Network

PATIENT RELATIONSHIP TO THE POLICYHOLDER ☑ Self ☐ Spouse ☐ Child ☐ Other

POLICYHOLDER INFORMATION: (If same as patient, check box and skip to ID#, If not, complete all
information beginning with Last Name.)

☑ Same as patient

LAST NAME .... Furtaw   FIRST NAME .... Thomas   MI ... M

GENDER ☑ MALE ☐ FEMALE   DATE OF BIRTH 7/17/1954

ID# 999901475   POLICY# (If different from ID#) ....

GROUP # .... MVA475   EMPLOYER NAME .. Mountain View Automotive

Do you have a secondary insurance plan? If yes, complete information below. ☐ Y ☑ N

NAME OF INSURANCE PLAN ....   ID # ....

POLICY # ....   GROUP # ....

PATIENT RELATIONSHIP TO THE POLICYHOLDER ☐ Self ☐ Spouse ☐ Child ☐ Other

Are you seeing a doctor due to a work-related injury? ☐ Y ☑ N If yes, date of injury ....

Are you seeing a doctor due to the result of an auto accident? ☐ Y ☑ N If yes, date of accident ....

Section D – Assignment of Benefits

I hereby authorize the physicians at Douglasville Medicine Associates to release all information necessary concerning my medical condition to secure proper payment, and I hereby assign the physicians payment for services rendered. I understand that I am responsible for all charges whether or not paid by my insurance. This assignment will remain in effect until revoked by me in writing.

SIGNATURE .... *Thomas Furtaw*   DATE 10/13/2010

Douglasville Medicine Associates

5076 Brand Boulevard, Suite 401 • Douglasville, NY 01234 • (123) 456-7890

PATIENT INFORMATION FORM   DATE 10/13/2010

Section A

LAST NAME .... Perez   FIRST NAME .... Raul   MI ..... J

SS# .. 999-70-0700   GENDER ☑ MALE ☐ FEMALE   DATE OF BIRTH 3/2/1971

MARITAL STATUS

☐ Single   ☐ Divorced   ☑ Married   ☐ Other (separated, widowed)

HOME ADDRESS .... 818 Liberty Court
                            Street   Apt./Unit

CITY .... Douglasville   STATE ..... NY   ZIP CODE 01234

HOME PHONE .... (123) 456-8280   WORK PHONE .. (123) 457-2244 EXT ....

EMPLOYMENT STATUS   EMPLOYER/SCHOOL Sheen, Marks, Thompson Law

☑ Employed   ☐ Full-time student   ☐ Unemployed   ☐ Retired   ☐ Part-time student

EMPLOYER ADDRESS ..... 19215 Commerce Drive   Douglasville   NY   01234
                        Street   City   State   Zip Code

REFERRAL SOURCE .... RESPONSIBLE PARTY ☑ SELF ☐ GUARANTOR

Section B – Spouse Information

LAST NAME .... Perez   FIRST NAME .... Maria   MI ....

GENDER ☐ MALE ☑ FEMALE   DATE OF BIRTH 12/18/1972

SS# .... Is your spouse the guarantor of the account? ☐ Y ☑ N

Section C – Health Insurance Information

NAME OF INSURANCE PLAN .... Signal HMO

PATIENT RELATIONSHIP TO THE POLICYHOLDER ☑ Self ☐ Spouse ☐ Child ☐ Other

POLICYHOLDER INFORMATION: (If same as patient, check box and skip to ID#, If not, complete all
information beginning with Last Name.)
☑ Same as patient

LAST NAME .... FIRST NAME .... MI ....

GENDER ☐ MALE ☐ FEMALE   DATE OF BIRTH ....

ID# 07007099   POLICY# (If different from ID#) ....

GROUP # .... SMT099   EMPLOYER NAME ....

Do you have a secondary insurance plan? If yes, complete information below. ☐ Y ☑ N

NAME OF INSURANCE PLAN .... ID # ....

POLICY # .... GROUP # ....

PATIENT RELATIONSHIP TO THE POLICYHOLDER ☐ Self ☐ Spouse ☐ Child ☐ Other

Are you seeing a doctor due to a work-related injury? ☐ Y ☑ N If yes, date of injury ....

Are you seeing a doctor due to the result of an auto accident? ☐ Y ☑ N If yes, date of accident ....

Section D – Assignment of Benefits

I hereby authorize the physicians at Douglasville Medicine Associates to release all information necessary concerning my medical condition to secure proper payment, and I hereby assign the physicians payment for services rendered. I understand that I am responsible for all charges whether or not paid by my insurance. This assignment will remain in effect until revoked by me in writing.

SIGNATURE ... Raul Perez .... DATE 10/13/2010

Douglasville Medicine Associates

5076 Brand Boulevard, Suite 401 • Douglasville, NY 01234 • (123) 456-7890

PATIENT INFORMATION FORM

DATE 10/12/2010

Section A

LAST NAME .... Freno   FIRST NAME .... Elmer   MI .... J

SS# 999-40-3333   GENDER ☑ MALE ☐ FEMALE   DATE OF BIRTH 1/20/1953

MARITAL STATUS

☑ Single   ☐ Divorced   ☐ Married   ☐ Other (separated, widowed)

HOME ADDRESS .... 23 Copper Street
Street   Apt./Unit

CITY .... Douglasville   STATE .... NY   ZIP CODE 01234

HOME PHONE .... (123) 456-8041   WORK PHONE .... (123) 457-4008   EXT 41886

EMPLOYMENT STATUS   EMPLOYER/SCHOOL .... Douglasville High School

☑ Employed   ☐ Full-time student   ☐ Unemployed   ☐ Retired   ☐ Part-time student

EMPLOYER ADDRESS .... 734 Creek Road   Douglasville   NY   01234
Street   City   State   Zip Code

REFERRAL SOURCE ....   RESPONSIBLE PARTY ☑ SELF ☐ GUARANTOR

Section B – Spouse Information

LAST NAME ....   FIRST NAME ....   MI ....

GENDER ☐ MALE ☐ FEMALE   DATE OF BIRTH ....

SS# ....   Is your spouse the guarantor of the account? ☐ Y ☐ N

Section C – Health Insurance Information

NAME OF INSURANCE PLAN .... FlexiHealth PPO In-Network

PATIENT RELATIONSHIP TO THE POLICYHOLDER ☑ Self ☐ Spouse ☐ Child ☐ Other

POLICYHOLDER INFORMATION: (If same as patient, check box and skip to ID#, If not, complete all information beginning with Last Name.)

☐ Same as patient

LAST NAME ....   FIRST NAME ....   MI ....

GENDER ☑ MALE ☐ FEMALE   DATE OF BIRTH ....

ID# 999403333   POLICY# (If different from ID#) ....

GROUP # .... DHS9433   EMPLOYER NAME ....

Do you have a secondary insurance plan? If yes, complete information below. ☐ Y ☑ N

NAME OF INSURANCE PLAN ....   ID # ....

POLICY # ....   GROUP # ....

PATIENT RELATIONSHIP TO THE POLICYHOLDER ☐ Self ☐ Spouse ☐ Child ☐ Other

Are you seeing a doctor due to a work-related injury? ☐ Y ☑ N If yes, date of injury ....

Are you seeing a doctor due to the result of an auto accident? ☐ Y ☑ N If yes, date of accident ....

Section D – Assignment of Benefits

I hereby authorize the physicians at Douglasville Medicine Associates to release all information necessary concerning my medical condition to secure proper payment, and I hereby assign the physicians payment for services rendered. I understand that I am responsible for all charges whether or not paid by my insurance. This assignment will remain in effect until revoked by me in writing.

SIGNATURE .... Elmer Freno   DATE 10/12/2010

Douglasville Medicine Associates

5076 Brand Boulevard, Suite 401 • Douglasville, NY 01234 • (123) 456-7890

PATIENT INFORMATION FORM

DATE .... 10/12/2010 ....

Section A

LAST NAME .... Boyd .... FIRST NAME .... Karen .... MI ...... E

SS# .. 999132583 ..   GENDER ☐ MALE ☑ FEMALE   DATE OF BIRTH .... 5/26/1986 ....

MARITAL STATUS

☐ Single   ☐ Divorced   ☑ Married   ☐ Other (separated, widowed)

HOME ADDRESS .... 18 Creekview Road ....
Street   Apt./Unit

CITY .... Douglasville ....   STATE .... NY ....   ZIP CODE 01234

HOME PHONE .... (123) 457-8992 ....   WORK PHONE .... (123) 456-4500 ...   EXT ....

EMPLOYMENT STATUS   EMPLOYER/SCHOOL .... Jefferson Charter School ....

☑ Employed   ☐ Full-time student   ☐ Unemployed   ☐ Retired   ☐ Part-time student

EMPLOYER ADDRESS .... 10267 Main Street .... Douglasville .... NY 01234
                            Street   City   State   Zip Code

REFERRAL SOURCE ....   RESPONSIBLE PARTY ☑ SELF   ☐ GUARANTOR

Section B – Spouse Information

LAST NAME .... Boyd ....   FIRST NAME .... Nick ....   MI ....

GENDER ☑ MALE ☐ FEMALE   DATE OF BIRTH .... 3/7/1985 ....

SS# .... 997-24-8331 ....   Is your spouse the guarantor of the account? ☑ Y ☐ N

Section C – Health Insurance Information

NAME OF INSURANCE PLAN .... Aetna ....

PATIENT RELATIONSHIP TO THE POLICYHOLDER ☐ Self ☑ Spouse ☐ Child ☐ Other

POLICYHOLDER INFORMATION: (If same as patient, check box and skip to ID#, If not, complete all information beginning with Last Name.)

☐ Same as patient

LAST NAME .... Boyd ....   FIRST NAME .... Nick ....   MI ....

GENDER ☑ MALE ☐ FEMALE   DATE OF BIRTH .... 3/7/1985 ....

ID# .... ZCW999180524 ....   POLICY# (If different from ID#) ....

GROUP # .... BSC0524 ....   EMPLOYER NAME .... Boyd & Sons Constructions ....

Do you have a secondary insurance plan? If yes, complete information below. ☐ Y ☑ N

NAME OF INSURANCE PLAN ....   ID # ....

POLICY # ....   GROUP # ....

PATIENT RELATIONSHIP TO THE POLICYHOLDER ☐ Self ☐ Spouse ☐ Child ☐ Other

Are you seeing a doctor due to a work-related injury? ☐ Y ☑ N   If yes, date of injury ....

Are you seeing a doctor due to the result of an auto accident? ☐ Y ☑ N   If yes, date of accident ....

Section D – Assignment of Benefits

I hereby authorize the physicians at Douglasville Medicine Associates to release all information necessary concerning my medical condition to secure proper payment, and I hereby assign the physicians payment for services rendered. I understand that I am responsible for all charges whether or not paid by my insurance. This assignment will remain in effect until revoked by me in writing.

SIGNATURE .... Karen Boyd ....   DATE .... 10/12/2010 ....

Douglasville Medicine Associates

5076 Brand Boulevard, Suite 401 • Douglasville, NY 01234 • (123) 456-7890

PATIENT INFORMATION FORM

DATE *10/12/2010*

Section A

LAST NAME .... *Brewer*   FIRST NAME .... *Edward*   MI .... *D.*

SS# .. *999-10-1010* ..   GENDER ☑ MALE ☐ FEMALE   DATE OF BIRTH *04/04/1991*

MARITAL STATUS

☑ Single ☐ Divorced ☐ Married ☐ Other (separated, widowed)

HOME ADDRESS .... *10 Pine Street*
                     Street   Apt./Unit

CITY .... *Vance*   STATE .... *NY*   ZIP CODE *25894*

HOME PHONE .... *(123) 404-8223 (Cell)*   WORK PHONE .... EXT ....

EMPLOYMENT STATUS   EMPLOYER/SCHOOL ....

☐ Employed ☑ Full-time student ☐ Unemployed   ☐ Retired ☐ Part-time student

EMPLOYER ADDRESS ....
                       Street   City   State   Zip Code

REFERRAL SOURCE ....   RESPONSIBLE PARTY ☑ SELF ☐ GUARANTOR

Section B – Spouse Information

LAST NAME ....   FIRST NAME .... MI ....

GENDER ☐ MALE ☐ FEMALE   DATE OF BIRTH ....

SS# ....   Is your spouse the guarantor of the account? ☐ Y ☐ N

Section C – Health Insurance Information

NAME OF INSURANCE PLAN .... *Self-Pay*

PATIENT RELATIONSHIP TO THE POLICYHOLDER ☐ Self ☐ Spouse ☐ Child ☐ Other

POLICYHOLDER INFORMATION: (If same as patient, check box and skip to ID#, If not, complete all information beginning with Last Name.)

☐ Same as patient

LAST NAME ....   FIRST NAME .... MI ....

GENDER ☐ MALE ☐ FEMALE   DATE OF BIRTH ....

ID# ....   POLICY# (If different from ID#) ....

GROUP # ....   EMPLOYER NAME ....

Do you have a secondary insurance plan? If yes, complete information below. ☐ Y ☐ N

NAME OF INSURANCE PLAN ....   ID # ....

POLICY # ....   GROUP # ....

PATIENT RELATIONSHIP TO THE POLICYHOLDER ☐ Self ☐ Spouse ☐ Child ☐ Other

Are you seeing a doctor due to a work-related injury? ☐ Y ☑ N   If yes, date of injury ....

Are you seeing a doctor due to the result of an auto accident? ☐ Y ☑ N   If yes, date of accident ....

Section D – Assignment of Benefits

I hereby authorize the physicians at Douglasville Medicine Associates to release all information necessary concerning my medical condition to secure proper payment, and I hereby assign the physicians payment for services rendered. I understand that I am responsible for all charges whether or not paid by my Insurance. This assignment will remain in effect until revoked by me in writing.

SIGNATURE *Edward Brewer* ....   DATE *10/12/2010*

AUTHORIZATION TO RELEASE MEDICAL INFORMATION

I, _____, authorize Douglasville Medicine Associates, 5076 Brand Boulevard, Suite 401, Douglasville, NY, 01234, to release the records specified to the provider(s) listed below.

Provider Name:	Provider Address:
	Phone#: Fax#:
Records Authorized to be Released: ❏ History & Physical ❏ Chart notes (from _____to_____) ❏ Lab reports (from _____ to _____) ❏ X-rays (from _____ to _____) ❏ Other imaging studies (MRI/CT scans) (from_____ to _____) ❏ Consultation notes or reports (from _____ to _____) ❏ Other (please specify)_____ **Information related to HIV, drug/alcohol, or psychiatric/psychotherapy notes requires a separate release.**	**This Information Will Be Used for the Purposes of:** ❏ Continuity of care ❏ Legal services/representation ❏ Personal information ❏ Other **Method of Release:** ❏ US Mail ❏ In person ❏ Fax with coversheet

I understand that I am entitled to a copy of this authorization and that a copy of this form can serve as the original. Additionally, I understand I may, at any time, revoke in writing this authorization; however, any disclosures made previous to the time of the revocation will not be affected.

This authorization will expire six (6) months from the date of signature below.

_____   _____
Patient or Representative   Date
(If signing as representative, please state relationship to patient)

_____   _____
Witness   Date

MESSAGE

TO _Dr. Heath_

DATE _10/15_ TIME _12:30_

WHILE YOU WERE OUT

M rs. Nancy Coleman

OF _____

PHONE _____

✓	Telephoned		Will Call Again
✓	Please Phone		Returned Your Call
	Came To See You		IMPORTANT

MESSAGE _Father, Francois Blanc, is pt at_
Retirement Inn nursing home. Has questions
about his medication.

TAKEN BY _____

MESSAGE

TO _Dr. Mendenhall_

DATE _10/15_ TIME _12:40_

WHILE YOU WERE OUT

M rs. Julia Richard

OF _____

PHONE _457-7701_

✓	Telephoned		Will Call Again
✓	Please Phone		Returned Your Call
	Came To See You	✓	IMPORTANT

MESSAGE _Wants to speak with you_
immediately.

TAKEN BY _____

MESSAGE

TO _Dr. Mendenhall_

DATE _10/15_ TIME _12:53_

WHILE YOU WERE OUT

M r. Santana

OF _____

PHONE _457-7124_

✓	Telephoned		Will Call Again
✓	Please Phone		Returned Your Call
	Came To See You		IMPORTANT

MESSAGE _Thinks he may be having an_
allergic reaction to his antibiotic.

TAKEN BY _____

MESSAGE

TO _Mrs. Fleet_

DATE _____ TIME _12:59_

WHILE YOU WERE OUT

M _Paula Shektar_

OF _____

PHONE _456-1118_

✓	Telephoned		Will Call Again
✓	Please Phone		Returned Your Call
	Came To See You		IMPORTANT

MESSAGE _Demanding to be seen by_
Dr. Schwartz today. Was "no-show" yesterday
and 2 other times this month.

TAKEN BY _____

QUALI-CARE CLINIC

TELEPHONE REFERRAL INFORMATION FORM

- Identify yourself.
- Identify your office.
- Identify procedure.
- State the patient's name, address, and telephone number.
- State the patient's date of birth.
- State the patient's Social Security number.
- State the patient's insurance coverage ID number, and group number (if appropriate).
- State the patient's primary diagnosis.
- State the name of the referring physician.
- Assist the person on the other end in making the appointment. (Ask patient ahead of time what days of the week are best, and whether morning or afternoon is preferable.)
- Reaffirm the date and time of appointment.
- Ask if there are any specific instructions for the patient in preparation for the appointment.
- Ask for directions to the office (if patient does not know where the office is located).
- End call politely.
- Notify patient of the date, time, instructions, and directions. (If patient is present when you make the call, fill out an appointment card and make sure patient understands instructions. If patient is not present, call him or her with the information.)
- Document that patient has an appointment with Dr. on _____(date) at _____ (time). Document that the patient was given specific instructions to do _____ and that patient understood instructions (PUI).

Sample progress note

Name: _John Doe_____

| Date | | | Progress Note |
MO.	DAY	YR.	
11	16	10	10 a.m. Pt. scheduled with Family Gastroenterology Associates on Friday, Nov. 16, 2010, at 10 a.m. Pt. given
			instructions for upper GI Prep. PUI. DMiller, CMA ——————————————————————

Douglasville Medicine Associates

5076 Brand Boulevard, Suite 401 • Douglasville, NY 01234 • (123) 456-7890

Fax

To: _____   From: _____

Fax: _____   Phone of Sender: _____

Phone of Receiver: _____   Pages (including this one): _____

Re: _____   Date: _____

☐ Urgent   ☐ For Review   ☐ Please Comment   ☐ Please Reply   ☐ Please Recycle

Comments:

Confidentiality Note: These documents may contain privileged and confidential information. They are intended only for the addressee. Please be aware that if you are not the intended recipient, any disclosure, copying, distribution, or other use of the data contained herein is strictly prohibited. If you have received this fax in error, please notify us by telephone so that we may make arrangements for the return of the original documents at no cost to you.

Name: _____

DATE			PROGRESS NOTES
MO.	DAY	YR.	

Douglasville Medicine Associates

5076 Brand Boulevard, Suite 401 • Douglasville, NY 01234 • (123) 456-7890

Sarah O. Mendenhall, MD—Family Practice
L.D. Heath, MD—Family Practice
D.J. Schwartz, MD—Family Practice

PATIENT: Richard, Julia T.
DATE: October 19, 2010
PHYSICIAN: Sarah O. Mendenhall, MD

HISTORY

CHIEF COMPLAINT
Lamp in the left breast detected on Self-breast exam.

HISTORY OF PRESENT ILLNESS
This 64-Year-old female presented today with concern over the finding of a dime-sige lump in the left breast. she states that her mother died at age 65 of breast cancer.

PAST MEDICAL HISTORY
The patient had T&A in the Past.

ALLERGIES
There is no history of drug allergies.

MEDICATIONS
The patient is taking a daily Multivitamin and calcium supplement.

PHYSICAL

GENERAL: A moderately developed, cooperative, alert, white female in no distress.
VITAL SIGNS: Blood pressure was 122/84; temperature, 98.6; pulse, 72; respirations, 20.
HEAD AND NECK: Head, eyes, ears, nose, and throat examination is grossly normal. Neck is supple; no lymphadenopathy.
CHEST: Chest is symmetrical. Breasts: well-defined mass palpable on left breast in upper outer quadrant . Lungs are clear to percussion and auscultation

HEART: Normal sinus rhythm without murmur.
ABDOMEN: Soft; flat; no tenderness.
RECTAL: Unremarkable.
EXTREMITIES: Unremarkable.

IMPRESSION
Tumor, left breast.
Ruleout Plan
1. Mammgraphy today.

Sarah O. Mendenhall, MD

SOM/si
D: 10/19/2010
T: 10/19/2010

Douglasville Medicine Associates
5076 Brand Boulevard, Suite 401
Douglasville, NY 01234
(123) 456-7890

_____
has an appointment with

Dr. _____

_____
Date

At _____a.m. _____p.m.

If unable to keep appointment,
please give 24 hours notice. Thank you.

DRAFT

PROCEDURE: VASECTOMY

Italics ~an~

You and your doctor are considering an operation called (vasectomy). The operation

consists of making two small surgical cuts in the scrotal sac (the bag that contains the

testicles) and cutting and typing up the tubes that carry the sperm or "seed. ~Today this~

that

operation is usually performed to sterilize the patient. A man who has been sterilized is

un

able to make a woman pregnant; he is unable to father a child. This operation (ordinarily)

e *the* *or his* (tr)

does not have any affect on a man's enjoyemnt of ~intercourse~ of ability to have

~age~ *Psychological* *had*

intercourse. A small percent of patients do have ~mental~ difficulties after having a

mental *interfere*

vasectomy. These difficul ties could ~result in interference~ with normal sexual function

cannot *a*

and normal social behavior. Your doctor ~can make no~ gurantee ~as to~ the results that

might be obtained from this operation.

lc

The Vasectomy operation is quite simple, and the vast majority of patients do not

is

have any problems during or after surgery The operation is usually done under a "local"

tic *tic* *rare*

anesthesia ~to "deaden" the skin there~. This anesthesia is very safe although ~there have~

have appeared

~been some~ reports of severe allergic reactions in the medical literature. Conceivably, a

tic

person could have heart stoppage and stop breathing from the effects of this anesthesia.

However, it is not possible to advise you of every imaginable complication. ~The purpose~

negative effects

~of this form is not to frighten you or upset you.~ The ~bad complications~ referred to are

will *e* (Cap)

very unlikely. ~The purpose of~ this form ~is to~ merely insure that your decision to have a

A very small percentage of vasectomy operations are complicated by infection and damage to the testicles.

vasectomy is not made in ignorance of the risks and side effects of this kind of operation.

~~You should be advised that the vasectomy operation is not immediately effective.~~ Until

the doctor tests you after the operation and finds that you are sterile, you cannot engage in

intercourse without the risk of making the woman pregnant usually, vasectomy results in

permanent sterility. ~~In a very small percentage of patients the tubes that carry the sperm~~

~~of "seed" open up again all by themselves. This result in an unexpected or unwanted~~

~~pregnancy.~~ If you decide after the operation that you do want to father a child, you will

need to have ~~a second~~ another operation. Only about 30% of patients who have this second

operation can father children again. Because of this you should ~~consider~~ assume that the

vasectomy will make you permanently unable to father children.

I certify: I have read or had read to me the contents of this consent form. I understand the

risks and side effects of this operation; all blanks or statements requiring ~~insertion of~~

completion were filled in or crossed out before I singed. I hereby request and authorize (tr)

(double space to allow for signature)
Dr. _____ to perform a vasec operation on me

(quadruple space)

Date _____

Patients signature

(quadruple space)

_____

Witness

Additional Risk: This sterilization operation cannot be guaranteed 100%. Although the failure rate is less than 1%, there is always the possibility that you will be able to father a child after the surgery is performed.

Douglasville Medicine Associates

5076 Brand Boulevard, Suite 401 • Douglasville, NY 01234 • (123) 456-7890

Sarah O. Mendenhall, MD—Family Practice
L.D. Heath, MD—Family Practice
D.J. Schwartz, MD—Family Practice

OCCUPATIONAL EXPOSURE INCIDENT REPORT

Definition of occupational exposure: An occupational exposure is defined as a percutaneous injury (e.g., needlestick or cut with a sharp object); contact of mucous membranes; human bite; or contact of skin (especially chapped, abraded, or having dermatitis) with blood, body fluids or tissues.

Body fluids or substances linked to transmission of HBV and/of HIV include: blood, blood products, semen, vaginal secretions, pericardial fluid, cerebrospinal fluid, synovial fluid, pleural fluid, peritoneal fluid, saliva in dental settings, and any body fluid that is visibly contaminated with blood.

Employee: _____ **Job Title:** _____

Employee Social Security Number: _____ **Date of Birth:** _____

Date of Incident: _____

Time of Exposure: _____

Location of Incident: _____ **Telephone (Business):** _____

Nature of Employee Duties: _____

Information which documents the route(s) of exposure and the circumstances under which the exposure incident occurred:

_____

What body fluid(s) were you exposed to?

_____

At the time of exposure, was any personal protective equipment being used? If yes, describe.

_____

Exposed employee's Hepatitis B vaccination or immunity status, if known:

_____

PHYSICIAN'S CERTIFICATION OF EXPOSURE

Based on the information concerning the exposure incident described on this report, I hereby certify that the exposure was:

(Circle response)

Significant

Not significant

Attested to by: _____ (MD/DO)

_____
Print or Type Name

Date of certification: _____

FOLLOW-UP MANAGEMENT OF EXPOSED EMPLOYEE

Hepatitis B vaccination status:

Hepatitis C vaccination status:

Follow-up serologic testing:

Anti-Hbs

HIV antibody status:

Clinical illness reports:

Douglasville Medicine Associates

5076 Brand Boulevard, Suite 401 • Douglasville, NY 01234 • (123) 456-7890

PURCHASE ORDER

To:

Order No.: 0462

Date:

Terms:

Shipped Via:

Quantity	Stock No./Description	Unit Price	Amount

By _____

Douglasville Medicine Associates
5076 Brand Boulevard, Suite 401
Douglasville, NY 01234
(123) 456-7890

_____

has an appointment with

Dr. _____

_____
Date

At _____ a.m. _____ p.m.

If unable to keep appointment,
please give 24 hours notice. Thank you.

Douglasville Medicine Associates
5076 Brand Boulevard, Suite 401
Douglasville, NY 01234
(123) 456-7890

_____

has an appointment with

Dr. _____

_____
Date

At _____ a.m. _____ p.m.

If unable to keep appointment,
please give 24 hours notice. Thank you.

Douglasville Medicine Associates
5076 Brand Boulevard, Suite 401
Douglasville, NY 01234
(123) 456-7890

_____

has an appointment with

Dr. _____

_____
Date

At _____ a.m. _____ p.m.

If unable to keep appointment,
please give 24 hours notice. Thank you.

Douglasville Medicine Associates
5076 Brand Boulevard, Suite 401
Douglasville, NY 01234
(123) 456-7890

_____
has an appointment with

Dr. _____

_____
Date

At _____ a.m. _____ p.m.

If unable to keep appointment,
please give 24 hours notice. Thank you.

Douglasville Medicine Associates
5076 Brand Boulevard, Suite 401
Douglasville, NY 01234
(123) 456-7890

_____
has an appointment with

Dr. _____

_____
Date

At _____ a.m. _____ p.m.

If unable to keep appointment,
please give 24 hours notice. Thank you.

Douglasville Medicine Associates
5076 Brand Boulevard, Suite 401
Douglasville, NY 01234
(123) 456-7890

_____
has an appointment with

Dr. _____

_____
Date

At _____ a.m. _____ p.m.

If unable to keep appointment,
please give 24 hours notice. Thank you.

October 29

	Heath	Schwartz	Mendenhall
8:00			
:15			OFF
:30			
:45			
9:00	Bradley, A.		
:15	↓ (PE)		
:30			
:45	Camille, E.		
10:00		Leighton, L.	
:15	Herbert, N.		
:30	Suggs, R.	Gordon, E.	
:45			
11:00	Yamagata, N.	Lagasse, E.	
:15			
:30	Jefferson, A.	Pinkston, A.	
:45		↓ (PE)	
12:00			
:15			
:30			
:45			
1:00		Wittmer, J.	
:15			
:30	Furtaw, T.		
:45			
2:00	Perez, R.	Guest, D.	
:15		(NP)	
:30		↓	
:45			
3:00	Freno, E.	Boyd, K.	
:15			
:30	Santana, E.		
:45			
4:00			
:15	Brewer, E.		
:30			
:45			
5:00			
:15			
:30			
:45			
6:00			

PLEASE RETURN THIS FORM TO RECEPTIONIST

NAME John Wittmer

Receipt No: 21937

PLACE OF SERVICE:
(✓) OFFICE
( ) NEW YORK COUNTY HOSPITAL
( ) COMMUNITY GENERAL HOSPITAL
( ) RETIREMENT INN NURSING HOME
( ) _____

DATE OF SERVICE 10/29/2010

A. OFFICE VISITS - New Patient

Code	History	Exam	Dec.	Time	
99201	Prob. Foc.	Prob. Foc.	Straight	10 min.	
99202	Ex. Prob. Foc.	Ex. Prob. Foc.	Straight	20 min.	
99203	Detail	Detail	Low	30 min.	
99204	Comp.	Comp.	Mod.	45 min.	
99205	Comp.	Comp.	High	60 min.	

B. OFFICE VISIT - Established Patient

Code	History	Exam	Dec.	Time	
99211	Minimal	Minimal	Minimal	5 min.	
99212	Prob. Foc.	Prob. Foc.	Straight	10min.	
99213	Ex. Prob. Foc.	Ex. Prob. Foc.	Low	15 min.	
(99214)	Detail	Detail	Mod.	25 min.	X
99215	Comp.	Comp.	High	40 min.	

C. HOSPITAL CARE   Dx Units

1. Initial Hospital Care (30 min) ____ ____ 99221 ____
2. Subsequent Care ____ ____ 99231 ____
3. Critical Care (30-74 min) ____ ____ 99291 ____
4. each additional 30 min. ____ ____ 99292 ____
5. Discharge Services ____ ____ 99238 ____
6. Emergency Room ____ ____ 99282 ____

D. NURSING HOME CARE   Dx Units

Initial Care - New Pt.
1. Expanded ____ ____ 99322
2. Detailed ____ ____ 99323

Subsequent Care - Estab. Pt.
3. Problem Focused ____ ____ 99307
4. Expanded ____ ____ 99308
5. Detailed ____ ____ 99309
5. Comprehensive ____ ____ 99310

E. PROCEDURES

1. Arthrocentesis, Small Jt. ____ 20600 ____
2. Colonoscopy ____ 45378 ____
3. EKG w/interpretation 1 (93000) ____ X
4. X-Ray Chest, PA/LAT ____ 71020 ____

F. LAB

1. Blood Sugar ____ 82947 ____
2. CBC w/differential ____ 85031 ____
3. Cholesterol ____ 82465 ____
4. Comprehensive Metabolic Panel ____ 80053 ____
5. ESR ____ 85651 ____
6. Hematocrit ____ 85014 ____
7. Mono Screen ____ 86308 ____
8. Pap Smear ____ 88150 ____
9. Potassium ____ 84132 ____
10. Preg. Test, Quantitative ____ 84702 ____
11. Routine Venipuncture ____ 36415 ____

F. Cont'd   Dx Units

12. Strep Screen ____ 87081 ____
13. UA, Routine w/Micro ____ 81000 ____
14. UA, Routine w/o Micro ____ 81002 ____
15. Uric Acid ____ 84550 ____
16. VDRL ____ 86592 ____
17. Wet Prep ____ 82710 ____
18. _____ ____ ____ ____

G. INJECTIONS

1. Influenza Virus Vaccine ____ 90658 ____
2. Pneumoccocal Vaccine ____ 90772 ____
3. Tetanus Toxoids ____ 90703 ____
4. Therapeutic Subcut/IM ____ 90732 ____
5. Vaccine Administration ____ 90471 ____
6. Vaccine - each additional ____ 90472 ____

H. MISCELLANEOUS

1. _____ ____ ____
2. _____ ____ ____

AMOUNT PAID $ Ø

Mark diagnosis with
(1=Primary, 2=Secondary, 3=Tertiary)

DIAGNOSIS NOT LISTED BELOW _____

DIAGNOSIS	ICD-9-CM 1, 2, 3	DIAGNOSIS	ICD-9-CM 1, 2, 3	DIAGNOSIS	ICD-9-CM 1, 2, 3
Abdominal Pain	789.0_	Dehydration	276.51	Otitis Media, Acute NOS	382.9
Allergic Rhinitis, Unspec.	477.9	Depression, NOS	311	Peptic Ulcer Disease	536.9
Angina Pectoris, Unspec.	(413.9) 1	Diabetes Mellitus, Type II Controlled	250.00	Peripheral Vascular Disease NOS	443.9
Anemia, Iron Deficiency, Unspec.	280.9	Diabetes Mellitus, Type II Controlled	250.02	Pharyngitis, Acute	462
Anemia, NOS	285.9	Drug Reaction, NOS	995.29	Pneumonia, Organism Unspec.	486
Anemia, Pernicious	281.0	Dysuria	788.1	Prostatitis, NOS	601.9
Asthma w/ Exacerbation	493.92	Eczema, NOS	692.2	PVC	427.69
Asthmatic Bronchitis, Unspec.	493.90	Edema	782.3	Rash, Non Specific	782.1
Atrial Fibrillation	427.31	Fever, Unknown Origin	780.6	Seizure Disorder NOS	780.39
Atypical Chest Pain, Unspec.	786.59	Gastritis, Acute w/o Hemorrhage	535.00	Serous Otitis Media, Chronic, Unspec.	381.10
Bronchiolitis, due to RSV	466.11	Gastroenteritis, NOS	558.9	Sinusitis, Acute NOS	461.9
Bronchitis, Acute	466.0	Gastroesophageal Reflux	530.81	Tonsillitis, Acute	463.
Bronchitis, NOS	490	Hepatitis A, Infectious	070.1	Upper Respiratory Infection, Acute NOS	465.9
Cardiac Arrest	427.5	Hypercholesterolemia, Pure	272.0	Urinary Tract Infection, Unspec.	599.0
Cardiopulmonary Disease, Chronic, Unspec.	(416.9) 2	Hypertension, Unspec.	401.9	Urticaria, Unspec.	708.9
Cellulitis, NOS	682.9	Hypoglycemia NOS	251.2	Vertigo, NOS	780.4
Congestive Heart Failure, Unspec.	428.0	Hypokalemia	276.8	Viral Infection NOS	079.99
Contact Dermatitis NOS	692.9	Impetigo	684	Weakness, Generalized	780.79
COPD NOS	496	Lymphadenitis, Unspec.	289.3	Weight Loss, Abnormal	783.21
CVA, Acute, NOS	434.91	Mononucleosis	075		
CVA, Old or Healed	438.9	Myocardial Infarction, Acute, NOS	410.9		
Degenerative Arthritis (Specify Site)	715.9	Organic Brain Syndrome	310.9		
		Otitis Externa, Acute NOS	380.10		

ABN: I UNDERSTAND THAT MEDICARE PROBABLY WILL NOT COVER THE SERVICES LISTED BELOW

A. _____ B. _____ C. _____

Patient

Date _____ Signature _____

Doctor's Signature L.D. Heath _____

RETURN:_____ Days _____ Weeks _____ Months

DOUGLASVILLE MEDICINE ASSOCIATES
5076 BRAND BLVD., SUITE 401
DOUGLASVILLE, NY 01234
PHONE No. (123) 456-7890
EIN# 00-1234560

☐ L.D. HEATH, M.D.   ☒ D.J. SCHWARTZ, M.D.
NPI# 9995010111   NPI# 9995020212
☐ SARAH O. MENDENHALL, M.D.
NPI# 9995030313

PLEASE RETURN THIS FORM TO RECEPTIONIST

NAME _Thomas Furtaw_

Receipt No: _21938_

PLACE OF SERVICE:
(✓) OFFICE
( ) NEW YORK COUNTY HOSPITAL
( ) COMMUNITY GENERAL HOSPITAL
( ) RETIREMENT INN NURSING HOME
( ) _____

DATE OF SERVICE _10/29/2010_

A. OFFICE VISITS - New Patient

Code	History	Exam	Dec.	Time	
99201	Prob. Foc.	Prob. Foc.	Straight	10 min.	
99202	Ex. Prob. Foc.	Ex. Prob. Foc.	Straight	20 min.	
99203	Detail	Detail	Low	30 min.	
99204	Comp.	Comp.	Mod.	45 min.	
99205	Comp.	Comp.	High	60 min.	

B. OFFICE VISIT - Established Patient

Code	History	Exam	Dec.	Time	
(99211)	Minimal	Minimal	Minimal	5 min.	X
99212	Prob. Foc.	Prob. Foc.	Straight	10min.	
99213	Ex. Prob. Foc.	Ex. Prob. Foc.	Low	15 min.	
99214	Detail	Detail	Mod.	25 min.	
99215	Comp.	Comp.	High	40 min.	

C. HOSPITAL CARE

		Dx	Units	
1.	Initial Hospital Care (30 min)			99221
2.	Subsequent Care			99231
3.	Critical Care (30-74 min)			99291
4.	each additional 30 min.			99292
5.	Discharge Services			99238
6.	Emergency Room			99282

D. NURSING HOME CARE

	Dx	Units	
Initial Care - New Pt.			
1. Expanded			99322
2. Detailed			99323
Subsequent Care - Estab. Pt.			
3. Problem Focused			99307
4. Expanded			99308
5. Detailed			99309
5. Comprehensive			99310

E. PROCEDURES

		Dx	
1.	Arthrocentesis, Small Jt.		20600
2.	Colonoscopy		45378
3.	EKG w/interpretation		93000
4.	X-Ray Chest, PA/LAT		71020

F. LAB

		Dx	
1.	Blood Sugar		82947
2.	CBC w/differential		85031
3.	Cholesterol		82465
4.	Comprehensive Metabolic Panel		80053
5.	ESR		85651
6.	Hematocrit		85014
7.	Mono Screen		86308
8.	Pap Smear		88150
9.	Potassium		84132
10.	Preg. Test, Quantitative		84702
11.	Routine Venipuncture		36415

F. Cont'd

		Dx	Units	
12.	Strep Screen			87081
13.	UA, Routine w/Micro			81000
14.	UA, Routine w/o Micro			81002
15.	Uric Acid			84550
16.	VDRL			86592
17.	Wet Prep			82710
18.	_____			

G. INJECTIONS

		Dx	Units	
1.	Influenza Virus Vaccine			90658
2.	Pneumococcal Vaccine			90772
3.	Tetanus Toxoids			90703
4.	Therapeutic Subcut/IM			90732
5.	Vaccine Administration			90471
6.	Vaccine - each additional			90472

H. MISCELLANEOUS

1. _____
2. _____

AMOUNT PAID $ _10.00_
Cash

Mark diagnosis with
(1=Primary, 2=Secondary, 3=Tertiary)

DIAGNOSIS NOT LISTED BELOW _____

DIAGNOSIS	ICD-9-CM 1, 2, 3	DIAGNOSIS	ICD-9-CM 1, 2, 3	DIAGNOSIS	ICD-9-CM 1, 2, 3
Abdominal Pain	789.0_	Dehydration	276.51	Otitis Media, Acute NOS	382.9
Allergic Rhinitis, Unspec.	477.9	Depression, NOS	311	Peptic Ulcer Disease	536.9
Angina Pectoris, Unspec.	413.9	Diabetes Mellitus, Type II Controlled	250.00	Peripheral Vascular Disease NOS	443.9
Anemia, Iron Deficiency, Unspec.	280.9	Diabetes Mellitus, Type II Controlled	250.02	Pharyngitis, Acute	462
Anemia, NOS	285.9	Drug Reaction, NOS	995.29	Pneumonia, Organism Unspec.	486
Anemia, Pernicious	281.0	Dysuria	788.1	Prostatitis, NOS	601.9
Asthma w/ Exacerbation	493.92	Eczema, NOS	692.2	PVC	427.69
Asthmatic Bronchitis, Unspec.	493.90	Edema	782.3	Rash, Non Specific	782.1
Atrial Fibrillation	427.31	Fever, Unknown Origin	780.6	Seizure Disorder NOS	780.39
Atypical Chest Pain, Unspec.	786.59	Gastritis, Acute w/o Hemorrhage	535.00	Serous Otitis Media, Chronic, Unspec.	381.10
Bronchiolitis, due to RSV	466.11	Gastroenteritis, NOS	558.9	Sinusitis, Acute NOS	461.9
Bronchitis, Acute	466.0	Gastroesophageal Reflux	530.81	Tonsillitis, Acute	463.
Bronchitis, NOS	490	Hepatitis A, Infectious	070.1	Upper Respiratory Infection, Acute NOS	465.9
Cardiac Arrest	427.5	Hypercholesterolemia, Pure	272.0	Urinary Tract Infection, Unspec.	599.0
Cardiopulmonary Disease, Chronic, Unspec.	416.9	Hypertension, Unspec.	(401.9) 1	Urticaria, Unspec.	708.9
Cellulitis, NOS	682.9	Hypoglycemia NOS	251.2	Vertigo, NOS	780.4
Congestive Heart Failure, Unspec.	428.0	Hypokalemia	276.8	Viral Infection NOS	079.99
Contact Dermatitis NOS	692.9	Impetigo	684	Weakness, Generalized	780.79
COPD NOS	496	Lymphadenitis, Unspec.	289.3	Weight Loss, Abnormal	783.21
CVA, Acute, NOS	434.91	Mononucleosis	075		
CVA, Old or Healed	438.9	Myocardial Infarction, Acute, NOS	410.9		
Degenerative Arthritis		Organic Brain Syndrome	310.9		
(Specify Site) _____	715.9	Otitis Externa, Acute NOS	380.10		

ABN: I UNDERSTAND THAT MEDICARE PROBABLY WILL NOT COVER THE SERVICES LISTED BELOW

A. _____ B. _____ C. _____

Patient

Date _____ Signature _____

Doctor's Signature _L.D. Heath_

RETURN: _____ Days _____ Weeks _1_ Months

DOUGLASVILLE MEDICINE ASSOCIATES
5076 BRAND BLVD., SUITE 401
DOUGLASVILLE, NY 01234
PHONE No. (123) 456-7890
EIN# 00-1234560

☒ L.D. HEATH, M.D.   ☐ D.J. SCHWARTZ, M.D.
NPI# 9995010111   NPI# 9995020212
☐ SARAH O. MENDENHALL, M.D.
NPI# 9995030313

PLEASE RETURN THIS FORM TO RECEPTIONIST

NAME Raul Perez

Receipt No: 21939

PLACE OF SERVICE:
(✓) OFFICE
( ) NEW YORK COUNTY HOSPITAL
( ) COMMUNITY GENERAL HOSPITAL
( ) RETIREMENT INN NURSING HOME
( ) _____

⊛ Previous Balance: $15.00

DATE OF SERVICE 10/29/2010

A. OFFICE VISITS - New Patient

Code	History	Exam	Dec.	Time	
99201	Prob. Foc.	Prob. Foc.	Straight	10 min.	
99202	Ex. Prob. Foc.	Ex. Prob. Foc.	Straight	20 min.	
99203	Detail	Detail	Low	30 min.	
99204	Comp.	Comp.	Mod.	45 min.	
99205	Comp.	Comp.	High	60 min.	

B. OFFICE VISIT - Established Patient

Code	History	Exam	Dec.	Time	
99211	Minimal	Minimal	Minimal	5 min.	
(99212)	Prob. Foc.	Prob. Foc.	Straight	10min.	✗
99213	Ex. Prob. Foc.	Ex. Prob. Foc.	Low	15 min.	
99214	Detail	Detail	Mod.	25 min.	
99215	Comp.	Comp.	High	40 min.	

C. HOSPITAL CARE

		Dx	Units	
1. Initial Hospital Care (30 min)			99221	
2. Subsequent Care			99231	
3. Critical Care (30-74 min)			99291	
4. each additional 30 min.			99292	
5. Discharge Services			99238	
6. Emergency Room			99282	

D. NURSING HOME CARE

	Dx	Units
Initial Care - New Pt.		
1. Expanded		99322
2. Detailed		99323
Subsequent Care - Estab. Pt.		
3. Problem Focused		99307
4. Expanded		99308
5. Detailed		99309
5. Comprehensive		99310

E. PROCEDURES

1. Arthrocentesis, Small Jt.		20600
2. Colonoscopy		45378
3. EKG w/interpretation		93000
4. X-Ray Chest, PA/LAT		71020

F. LAB

1. Blood Sugar		82947		
2. CBC w/differential		85031		
3. Cholesterol		82465		
4. Comprehensive Metabolic Panel		80053		
5. ESR		85651		
6. Hematocrit		85014		
7. Mono Screen	1	(86308)	✗	
8. Pap Smear		88150		
9. Potassium		84132		
10. Preg. Test, Quantitative		84702		
11. Routine Venipuncture	1	(36415)	✗	

F. Cont'd

	Dx	Units	
12. Strep Screen		87081	
13. UA, Routine w/Micro		81000	
14. UA, Routine w/o Micro		81002	
15. Uric Acid		84550	
16. VDRL		86592	
17. Wet Prep		82710	
18. _____			

G. INJECTIONS

1. Influenza Virus Vaccine		90658
2. Pneumoccocal Vaccine		90772
3. Tetanus Toxoids		90703
4. Therapeutic Subcut/IM		90732
5. Vaccine Administration		90471
6. Vaccine - each additional		90472

H. MISCELLANEOUS

1. _____
2. _____

AMOUNT PAID $ 15.00

Visa

Mark diagnosis with (1=Primary, 2=Secondary, 3=Tertiary)

DIAGNOSIS NOT LISTED BELOW _____

DIAGNOSIS	ICD-9-CM 1, 2, 3	DIAGNOSIS	ICD-9-CM 1, 2, 3	DIAGNOSIS	ICD-9-CM 1, 2, 3
Abdominal Pain	789.0_	Dehydration	276.51	Otitis Media, Acute NOS	382.9
Allergic Rhinitis, Unspec.	477.9	Depression, NOS	311	Peptic Ulcer Disease	536.9
Angina Pectoris, Unspec.	413.9	Diabetes Mellitus, Type II Controlled	250.00	Peripheral Vascular Disease NOS	443.9
Anemia, Iron Deficiency, Unspec.	280.9	Diabetes Mellitus, Type II Controlled	250.02	Pharyngitis, Acute	(462) 2
Anemia, NOS	285.9	Drug Reaction, NOS	995.29	Pneumonia, Organism Unspec.	486
Anemia, Pernicious	281.0	Dysuria	788.1	Prostatitis, NOS	601.9
Asthma w/ Exacerbation	493.92	Eczema, NOS	692.2	PVC	427.69
Asthmatic Bronchitis, Unspec.	493.90	Edema	782.3	Rash, Non Specific	782.1
Atrial Fibrillation	427.31	Fever, Unknown Origin	780.6	Seizure Disorder NOS	780.39
Atypical Chest Pain, Unspec.	786.59	Gastritis, Acute w/o Hemorrhage	535.00	Serous Otitis Media, Chronic, Unspec.	381.10
Bronchiolitis, due to RSV	466.11	Gastroenteritis, NOS	558.9	Sinusitis, Acute NOS	461.9
Bronchitis, Acute	466.0	Gastroesophageal Reflux	530.81	Tonsillitis, Acute	463.9
Bronchitis, NOS	490	Hepatitis A, Infectious	070.1	Upper Respiratory Infection, Acute NOS	465.9
Cardiac Arrest	427.5	Hypercholesterolemia, Pure	272.0	Urinary Tract Infection, Unspec.	599.0
Cardiopulmonary Disease, Chronic, Unspec.	416.9	Hypertension, Unspec.	401.9	Urticaria, Unspec.	708.9
Cellulitis, NOS	682.9	Hypoglycemia NOS	251.2	Vertigo, NOS	780.4
Congestive Heart Failure, Unspec.	428.0	Hypokalemia	276.8	Viral Infection NOS	079.99
Contact Dermatitis NOS	692.9	Impetigo	684	Weakness, Generalized	780.79
COPD NOS	496	Lymphadenitis, Unspec.	289.3	Weight Loss, Abnormal	783.21
CVA, Acute, NOS	434.91	(Mononucleosis)	(075) 1		
CVA, Old or Healed	438.9	Myocardial Infarction, Acute, NOS	410.9		
Degenerative Arthritis		Organic Brain Syndrome	310.9		
(Specify Site) _____	715.9	Otitis Externa, Acute NOS	380.10		

ABN: I UNDERSTAND THAT MEDICARE PROBABLY WILL NOT COVER THE SERVICES LISTED BELOW

A. _____ B. _____ C. _____
                         Patient

Date _____ Signature _____

Doctor's Signature L.D. Heath

RETURN: _____ Days _____ Weeks _____ Months

DOUGLASVILLE MEDICINE ASSOCIATES
5076 BRAND BLVD., SUITE 401
DOUGLASVILLE, NY 01234
PHONE No. (123) 456-7890
EIN# 00-1234560

☒ L.D. HEATH, M.D.   ☐ D.J. SCHWARTZ, M.D.
NPI# 9995010111   NPI# 9995020212
☐ SARAH O. MENDENHALL, M.D.
NPI# 9995030313

PLEASE RETURN THIS FORM TO RECEPTIONIST

NAME _Denise Guest_

Receipt No: 21940

PLACE OF SERVICE:
(✓) OFFICE
( ) NEW YORK COUNTY HOSPITAL
( ) COMMUNITY GENERAL HOSPITAL
( ) RETIREMENT INN NURSING HOME
( ) _____

DATE OF SERVICE _10/29/2010_

A. OFFICE VISITS - New Patient

Code	History	Exam	Dec.	Time	
99201	Prob. Foc.	Prob. Foc.	Straight	10 min.	
99202	Ex. Prob. Foc.	Ex. Prob. Foc.	Straight	20 min.	
99203	Detail	Detail	Low	30 min.	
(99204)	Comp.	Comp.	Mod.	45 min.	X
99205	Comp.	Comp.	High	60 min.	

B. OFFICE VISIT - Established Patient

Code	History	Exam	Dec.	Time
99211	Minimal	Minimal	Minimal	5 min.
99212	Prob. Foc.	Prob. Foc.	Straight	10min.
99213	Ex. Prob. Foc.	Ex. Prob. Foc.	Low	15 min.
99214	Detail	Detail	Mod.	25 min.
99215	Comp.	Comp.	High	40 min.

C. HOSPITAL CARE

		Dx	Units	
1.	Initial Hospital Care (30 min)		99221	
2.	Subsequent Care		99231	
3.	Critical Care (30-74 min)		99291	
4.	each additional 30 min.		99292	
5.	Discharge Services		99238	
6.	Emergency Room		99282	

D. NURSING HOME CARE

		Dx	Units
Initial Care - New Pt.			
1.	Expanded		99322
2.	Detailed		99323
Subsequent Care - Estab. Pt.			
3.	Problem Focused		99307
4.	Expanded		99308
5.	Detailed		99309
5.	Comprehensive		99310

E. PROCEDURES

		Dx	Units
1.	Arthrocentesis, Small Jt.		20600
2.	Colonoscopy		45378
3.	EKG w/interpretation		93000
4.	X-Ray Chest, PA/LAT		71020

F. LAB

		Dx	Units	
1.	Blood Sugar		82947	
2.	CBC w/differential	1	(85031)	X
3.	Cholesterol		82465	
4.	Comprehensive Metabolic Panel	1,2	(80053)	X
5.	ESR		85651	
6.	Hematocrit		85014	
7.	Mono Screen		86308	
8.	Pap Smear		88150	
9.	Potassium		84132	
10.	Preg. Test, Quantitative	2	84702	
11.	Routine Venipuncture	2	(36415)	X

F. Cont'd

		Dx	Units	
12.	Strep Screen		87081	
13.	UA, Routine w/Micro		81000	
14.	UA, Routine w/o Micro		81002	
15.	Uric Acid		84550	
16.	VDRL		86592	
17.	Wet Prep		82710	
18.	Urine culture	4	87086	X

G. INJECTIONS

		Dx	Units
1.	Influenza Virus Vaccine		90658
2.	Pneumoccoccal Vaccine		90772
3.	Tetanus Toxoids		90703
4.	Therapeutic Subcut/IM		90732
5.	Vaccine Administration		90471
6.	Vaccine - each additional		90472

H. MISCELLANEOUS

1. _____
2. _____

AMOUNT PAID $ _20.00_
Visa

Mark diagnosis with (1=Primary, 2=Secondary, 3=Tertiary)

DIAGNOSIS NOT LISTED BELOW _____

DIAGNOSIS	ICD-9-CM 1, 2, 3	DIAGNOSIS	ICD-9-CM 1, 2, 3	DIAGNOSIS	ICD-9-CM 1, 2, 3
Abdominal Pain	789.0	Dehydration	276.51	Otitis Media, Acute NOS	382.9
Allergic Rhinitis, Unspec.	477.9	Depression, NOS	(311) 3	Peptic Ulcer Disease	536.9
Angina Pectoris, Unspec.	413.9	Diabetes Mellitus, Type II Controlled	250.00	Peripheral Vascular Disease NOS	443.9
Anemia, Iron Deficiency, Unspec.	280.9	Diabetes Mellitus, Type II Controlled	250.02	Pharyngitis, Acute	462
Anemia, NOS	285.9	Drug Reaction, NOS	995.29	Pneumonia, Organism Unspec.	486
Anemia, Pernicious	281.0	Dysuria	788.1	Prostatitis, NOS	601.9
Asthma w/ Exacerbation	493.92	Eczema, NOS	692.2	PVC	427.69
Asthmatic Bronchitis, Unspec.	493.90	Edema	782.3	Rash, Non Specific	782.1
Atrial Fibrillation	427.31	Fever, Unknown Origin	780.6	Seizure Disorder NOS	780.39
Atypical Chest Pain, Unspec.	786.59	Gastritis, Acute w/o Hemorrhage	535.00	Serous Otitis Media, Chronic, Unspec.	381.10
Bronchiolitis, due to RSV	466.11	Gastroenteritis, NOS	558.9	Sinusitis, Acute NOS	461.9
Bronchitis, Acute	466.0	Gastroesophageal Reflux	530.81	Tonsillitis, Acute	463.
Bronchitis, NOS	490	Hepatitis A, Infectious	070.1	Upper Respiratory Infection, Acute NOS	465.9
Cardiac Arrest	427.5	Hypercholesterolemia, Pure	272.0	Urinary Tract Infection, Unspec.	(599.0) 4
Cardiopulmonary Disease, Chronic, Unspec.	416.9	Hypertension, Unspec.	401.9	Urticaria, Unspec.	708.9
Cellulitis, NOS	682.9	Hypoglycemia NOS	251.2	Vertigo, NOS	780.4
Congestive Heart Failure, Unspec.	428.0	Hypokalemia	276.8	Viral Infection NOS	079.99
Contact Dermatitis NOS	692.9	Impetigo	684	Weakness, Generalized	(780.79) 1
COPD NOS	496	Lymphadenitis, Unspec.	289.3	Weight Loss, Abnormal	(783.21) 2
CVA, Acute, NOS	434.91	Mononucleosis	075		
CVA, Old or Healed	438.9	Myocardial Infarction, Acute, NOS	410.9		
Degenerative Arthritis (Specify Site)	715.9	Organic Brain Syndrome	310.9		
		Otitis Externa, Acute NOS	380.10		

ABN: I UNDERSTAND THAT MEDICARE PROBABLY WILL NOT COVER THE SERVICES LISTED BELOW

A. _____
B. _____
C. _____

Patient Signature _____

Date _____

Doctor's Signature _L.D. Heath_

RETURN: _____ Days __2__ Weeks _____ Months _____

DOUGLASVILLE MEDICINE ASSOCIATES
5076 BRAND BLVD., SUITE 401
DOUGLASVILLE, NY 01234
PHONE No. (123) 456-7890
EIN# 00-1234560

☐ L.D. HEATH, M.D.   ☒ D.J. SCHWARTZ, M.D.
   NPI# 9995010111   NPI# 9995020212
   ☐ SARAH O. MENDENHALL, M.D.
      NPI# 9995030313

PLEASE RETURN THIS FORM TO RECEPTIONIST

NAME *Elmer Freno*

Receipt No: *21941*

PLACE OF SERVICE:
(✓) OFFICE
( ) NEW YORK COUNTY HOSPITAL
( ) COMMUNITY GENERAL HOSPITAL
( ) RETIREMENT INN NURSING HOME
( ) _____

⊙Previous Balance: $50.00

DATE OF SERVICE ___*10/29/2010*___

A. OFFICE VISITS - New Patient

Code	History	Exam	Dec.	Time	
___ 99201	Prob. Foc.	Prob. Foc.	Straight	10 min.	___
___ 99202	Ex. Prob. Foc.	Ex. Prob. Foc.	Straight	20 min.	___
___ 99203	Detail	Detail	Low	30 min.	___
___ 99204	Comp.	Comp.	Mod.	45 min.	___
___ 99205	Comp.	Comp.	High	60 min.	___

B. OFFICE VISIT - Established Patient

Code	History	Exam	Dec.	Time	
___ 99211	Minimal	Minimal	Minimal	5 min.	___
___ 99212	Prob. Foc.	Prob. Foc.	Straight	10min.	___
(99213)	Ex. Prob. Foc.	Ex. Prob. Foc.	Low	15 min.	X
___ 99214	Detail	Detail	Mod.	25 min.	___
___ 99215	Comp.	Comp.	High	40 min.	___

C. HOSPITAL CARE

		Dx	Units	
1. Initial Hospital Care (30 min)	___	___	99221	___
2. Subsequent Care	___	___	99231	___
3. Critical Care (30-74 min)	___	___	99291	___
4. each additional 30 min.	___	___	99292	___
5. Discharge Services	___	___	99238	___
6. Emergency Room	___	___	99282	___

D. NURSING HOME CARE

	Dx	Units	
Initial Care - New Pt.			
1. Expanded	___ ___	99322	
2. Detailed	___ ___	99323	
Subsequent Care - Estab. Pt.			
3. Problem Focused	___ ___	99307	
4. Expanded	___ ___	99308	
5. Detailed	___ ___	99309	
5. Comprehensive	___ ___	99310	

E. PROCEDURES

1. Arthrocentesis, Small Jt.	___	20600	
2. Colonoscopy	___	45378	
3. EKG w/interpretation	1	(93000)	X
4. X-Ray Chest, PA/LAT	___	71020	

F. LAB

1. Blood Sugar	___	82947	
2. CBC w/differential	1	(85031)	X
3. Cholesterol	___	82465	
4. Comprehensive Metabolic Panel	___	80053	
5. ESR	___	85651	
6. Hematocrit	___	85014	
7. Mono Screen	___	86308	
8. Pap Smear	___	88150	
9. Potassium	___	84132	
10. Preg. Test, Quantitative	___	84702	
11. Routine Venipuncture	1	(36415)	X

F. Cont'd

	Dx	Units	
12. Strep Screen	___	87081	___
13. UA, Routine w/Micro	___	81000	___
14. UA, Routine w/o Micro	___	81002	___
15. Uric Acid	___	84550	___
16. VDRL	___	86592	___
17. Wet Prep	___	82710	___
18. _____			___

G. INJECTIONS

1. Influenza Virus Vaccine	___	90658	
2. Pneumoccocal Vaccine	___	90772	
3. Tetanus Toxoids	___	90703	
4. Therapeutic Subcut/IM	___	90732	
5. Vaccine Administration	___	90471	
6. Vaccine - each additional	___	90472	

H. MISCELLANEOUS

1. _____
2. _____

AMOUNT PAID $ ___*20.00*___

Check # 443

Mark diagnosis with (1=Primary, 2=Secondary, 3=Tertiary)

DIAGNOSIS NOT LISTED BELOW _____

DIAGNOSIS	ICD-9-CM 1, 2, 3	DIAGNOSIS	ICD-9-CM 1, 2, 3	DIAGNOSIS	ICD-9-CM 1, 2, 3
Abdominal Pain	789.0_	Dehydration	276.51	Otitis Media, Acute NOS	382.9
Allergic Rhinitis, Unspec.	477.9	Depression, NOS	311	Peptic Ulcer Disease	536.9
Angina Pectoris, Unspec.	413.9	Diabetes Mellitus, Type II Controlled	250.00	Peripheral Vascular Disease NOS	443.9
Anemia, Iron Deficiency, Unspec.	280.9	Diabetes Mellitus, Type II Controlled	250.02	Pharyngitis, Acute	462
Anemia, NOS	285.9	Drug Reaction, NOS	995.29	Pneumonia, Organism Unspec.	486
Anemia, Pernicious	281.0	Dysuria	788.1	Prostatitis, NOS	601.9
Asthma w/ Exacerbation	493.92	Eczema, NOS	692.2	PVC	427.69
Asthmatic Bronchitis, Unspec.	493.90	Edema	782.3	Rash, Non Specific	782.1
Atrial Fibrillation	(427.31) 1	Fever, Unknown Origin	780.6	Seizure Disorder NOS	780.39
Atypical Chest Pain, Unspec.	786.59	Gastritis, Acute w/o Hemorrhage	535.00	Serous Otitis Media, Chronic, Unspec.	381.10
Bronchiolitis, due to RSV	466.11	Gastroenteritis, NOS	558.9	Sinusitis, Acute NOS	461.9
Bronchitis, Acute	466.0	Gastroesophageal Reflux	530.81	Tonsillitis, Acute	463.
Bronchitis, NOS	490	Hepatitis A, Infectious	070.1	Upper Respiratory Infection, Acute NOS	465.9
Cardiac Arrest	427.5	Hypercholesterolemia, Pure	272.0	Urinary Tract Infection, Unspec.	599.0
Cardiopulmonary Disease, Chronic, Unspec.	416.9	Hypertension, Unspec.	401.9	Urticaria, Unspec.	708.9
Cellulitis, NOS	682.9	Hypoglycemia NOS	251.2	Vertigo, NOS	780.4
Congestive Heart Failure, Unspec.	428.0	Hypokalemia	276.8	Viral Infection NOS	079.99
Contact Dermatitis NOS	692.9	Impetigo	684	Weakness, Generalized	780.79
COPD NOS	496	Lymphadenitis, Unspec.	289.3	Weight Loss, Abnormal	783.21
CVA, Acute, NOS	434.91	Mononucleosis	075		
CVA, Old or Healed	438.9	Myocardial Infarction, Acute, NOS	410.9		
Degenerative Arthritis (Specify Site)	715.9	Organic Brain Syndrome	310.9		
		Otitis Externa, Acute NOS	380.10		

ABN: I UNDERSTAND THAT MEDICARE PROBABLY WILL NOT COVER THE SERVICES LISTED BELOW

A. _____ B. _____ C. _____

Patient

Date _____ Signature _____

Doctor's Signature *L.D. Heath*

RETURN: _____ Days _____ Weeks ___*1*___ Months

Refer To: Joseph Reed MD   @ *Midway Specialty Associates*

DOUGLASVILLE MEDICINE ASSOCIATES
5076 BRAND BLVD., SUITE 401
DOUGLASVILLE, NY 01234
PHONE No. (123) 456-7890
EIN# 00-1234560

☒ L.D. HEATH, M.D.   ☐ D.J. SCHWARTZ, M.D.
NPI# 9995010111   NPI# 9995020212
☐ SARAH O. MENDENHALL, M.D.
NPI# 9995030313

PLEASE RETURN THIS FORM TO RECEPTIONIST

NAME _Ernesto Santana_

Receipt No: _21942_

PLACE OF SERVICE:
(✓) OFFICE
( ) NEW YORK COUNTY HOSPITAL
( ) COMMUNITY GENERAL HOSPITAL
( ) RETIREMENT INN NURSING HOME
( ) _____

DATE OF SERVICE _10/29/2010_

A. OFFICE VISITS - New Patient

Code	History	Exam	Dec.	Time	
99201 Prob. Foc.	Prob. Foc.	Straight	10 min.	___
99202 Ex. Prob. Foc.	Ex. Prob. Foc.	Straight	20 min.	___
99203 Detail	Detail	Low	30 min.	___
99204 Comp.	Comp.	Mod.	45 min.	___
99205 Comp.	Comp.	High	60 min.	___

B. OFFICE VISIT - Established Patient

Code	History	Exam	Dec.	Time	
99211 Minimal	Minimal	Minimal	5 min.	___
99212 Prob. Foc.	Prob. Foc.	Straight	10min.	___
(99213) Ex. Prob. Foc.	Ex. Prob. Foc.	Low	15 min.	X
99214 Detail	Detail	Mod.	25 min.	___
99215 Comp.	Comp.	High	40 min.	___

C. HOSPITAL CARE   Dx Units

1. Initial Hospital Care (30 min) ___ ___ 99221
2. Subsequent Care ___ ___ 99231
3. Critical Care (30-74 min) ___ ___ 99291
4. each additional 30 min. ___ ___ 99292
5. Discharge Services ___ ___ 99238
6. Emergency Room ___ ___ 99282

D. NURSING HOME CARE   Dx Units

Initial Care - New Pt.
1. Expanded ___ ___ 99322
2. Detailed ___ ___ 99323

Subsequent Care - Estab. Pt.
3. Problem Focused ___ ___ 99307 ___
4. Expanded ___ ___ 99308 ___
5. Detailed ___ ___ 99309 ___
5. Comprehensive ___ ___ 99310 ___

E. PROCEDURES

1. Arthrocentesis, Small Jt. ___ 20600 ___
2. Colonoscopy ___ 45378 ___
3. EKG w/interpretation ___ 93000 ___
4. X-Ray Chest, PA/LAT ___ 71020 ___

F. LAB

1. Blood Sugar ___ 82947 ___
2. CBC w/differential ___ 85031 ___
3. Cholesterol ___ 82465 ___
4. Comprehensive Metabolic Panel ___ 80053 ___
5. ESR ___ 85651 ___
6. Hematocrit ___ 85014 ___
7. Mono Screen ___ 86308 ___
8. Pap Smear ___ 88150 ___
9. Potassium ___ 84132 ___
10. Preg. Test, Quantitative ___ 84702 ___
11. Routine Venipuncture ___ 36415 ___

F. Cont'd   Dx Units

12. Strep Screen ___ 87081 ___
13. UA, Routine w/Micro ___ 81000 ___
14. UA, Routine w/o Micro ___ 81002 ___
15. Uric Acid ___ 84550 ___
16. VDRL ___ 86592 ___
17. Wet Prep ___ 82710 ___
18. _____ ___ ___

G. INJECTIONS

1. Influenza Virus Vaccine ___ 90658 ___
2. Pneumoccocal Vaccine ___ 90772 ___
3. Tetanus Toxoids ___ 90703 ___
4. Therapeutic Subcut/IM ___ 90732 ___
5. Vaccine Administration ___ 90471 ___
6. Vaccine - each additional ___ 90472 ___

H. MISCELLANEOUS

1. _____ ___ ___
2. _____ ___ ___

AMOUNT PAID $ _10.00_ _Cash_

Mark diagnosis with (1=Primary, 2=Secondary, 3=Tertiary)

DIAGNOSIS NOT LISTED BELOW _____

DIAGNOSIS	ICD-9-CM 1, 2, 3	DIAGNOSIS	ICD-9-CM 1, 2, 3	DIAGNOSIS	ICD-9-CM 1, 2, 3
Abdominal Pain	789.0_	Dehydration	276.51	Otitis Media, Acute NOS	382.9
Allergic Rhinitis, Unspec.	477.9	Depression, NOS	311	Peptic Ulcer Disease	536.9
Angina Pectoris, Unspec.	413.9	Diabetes Mellitus, Type II Controlled	250.00	Peripheral Vascular Disease NOS	443.9
Anemia, Iron Deficiency, Unspec.	280.9	Diabetes Mellitus, Type II Controlled	250.02	Pharyngitis, Acute	462
Anemia, NOS	285.9	Drug Reaction, NOS	995.29	Pneumonia, Organism Unspec.	486
Anemia, Pernicious	281.0	Dysuria	788.1	Prostatitis, NOS	601.9
Asthma w/ Exacerbation	493.92	Eczema, NOS	692.2	PVC	427.69
Asthmatic Bronchitis, Unspec.	493.90	Edema	782.3	Rash, Non Specific	782.1
Atrial Fibrillation	427.31	Fever, Unknown Origin	780.6	Seizure Disorder NOS	780.39
Atypical Chest Pain, Unspec.	786.59	Gastritis, Acute w/o Hemorrhage	535.00	Serous Otitis Media, Chronic, Unspec.	381.10
Bronchiolitis, due to RSV	466.11	Gastroenteritis, NOS	558.9	Sinusitis, Acute NOS	461.9
Bronchitis, Acute	466.0	Gastroesophageal Reflux	530.81	Tonsillitis, Acute	(463.) 1
Bronchitis, NOS	490	Hepatitis A, Infectious	070.1	Upper Respiratory Infection, Acute NOS	465.9
Cardiac Arrest	427.5	Hypercholesterolemia, Pure	272.0	Urinary Tract Infection, Unspec.	599.0
Cardiopulmonary Disease, Chronic, Unspec.	416.9	Hypertension, Unspec.	401.9	Urticaria, Unspec.	708.9
Cellulitis, NOS	682.9	Hypoglycemia NOS	251.2	Vertigo, NOS	780.4
Congestive Heart Failure, Unspec.	428.0	Hypokalemia	276.8	Viral Infection NOS	079.99
Contact Dermatitis NOS	692.9	Impetigo	684	Weakness, Generalized	780.79
COPD NOS	496	Lymphadenitis, Unspec.	289.3	Weight Loss, Abnormal	783.21
CVA, Acute, NOS	434.91	Mononucleosis	075		
CVA, Old or Healed	438.9	Myocardial Infarction, Acute, NOS	410.9		
Degenerative Arthritis (Specify Site)	715.9	Organic Brain Syndrome	310.9		
		Otitis Externa, Acute NOS	380.10		

ABN: I UNDERSTAND THAT MEDICARE PROBABLY WILL NOT COVER THE SERVICES LISTED BELOW

A. _____ B. _____ C. _____

Patient

Date _____ Signature _____

Doctor's Signature _L.D. Heath_

RETURN: ___ Days ___ Weeks _3_ Months ___

DOUGLASVILLE MEDICINE ASSOCIATES
5076 BRAND BLVD., SUITE 401
DOUGLASVILLE, NY 01234
PHONE No. (123) 456-7890
EIN# 00-1234560

☒ L.D. HEATH, M.D.   ☐ D.J. SCHWARTZ, M.D.
NPI# 9995010111   NPI# 9995020212
☐ SARAH O. MENDENHALL, M.D.
NPI# 9995030313

PLEASE RETURN THIS FORM TO RECEPTIONIST

NAME *Karen Boyd*

Receipt No: 21943

PLACE OF SERVICE:
(✓) OFFICE
( ) NEW YORK COUNTY HOSPITAL
( ) COMMUNITY GENERAL HOSPITAL
( ) RETIREMENT INN NURSING HOME
( ) _____

⊕ Previous Balance: $30.00

DATE OF SERVICE *10/29/2010*

A. OFFICE VISITS - New Patient

Code	History	Exam	Dec.	Time	
____ 99201	Prob. Foc.	Prob. Foc.	Straight	10 min.	_____
____ 99202	Ex. Prob. Foc.	Ex. Prob. Foc.	Straight	20 min.	_____
____ 99203	Detail	Detail	Low	30 min.	_____
____ 99204	Comp.	Comp.	Mod.	45 min.	_____
____ 99205	Comp.	Comp.	High	60 min.	_____

B. OFFICE VISIT - Established Patient

Code	History	Exam	Dec.	Time	
(99211)	Minimal	Minimal	Minimal	5 min.	X
____ 99212	Prob. Foc.	Prob. Foc.	Straight	10min.	_____
____ 99213	Ex. Prob. Foc.	Ex. Prob. Foc.	Low	15 min.	_____
____ 99214	Detail	Detail	Mod.	25 min.	_____
____ 99215	Comp.	Comp.	High	40 min.	_____

C. HOSPITAL CARE

		Dx	Units	
1.	Initial Hospital Care (30 min)	____ ____	99221	_____
2.	Subsequent Care	____ ____	99231	_____
3.	Critical Care (30-74 min)	____ ____	99291	_____
4.	each additional 30 min.	____ ____	99292	_____
5.	Discharge Services	____ ____	99238	_____
6.	Emergency Room	____ ____	99282	_____

D. NURSING HOME CARE

Dx Units

Initial Care - New Pt.
1.	Expanded	____ ____	99322	_____
2.	Detailed	____ ____	99323	_____

Subsequent Care - Estab. Pt.
3.	Problem Focused	____ ____	99307	_____
4.	Expanded	____ ____	99308	_____
5.	Detailed	____ ____	99309	_____
5.	Comprehensive	____ ____	99310	_____

E. PROCEDURES

1.	Arthrocentesis, Small Jt.	____	20600	_____
2.	Colonoscopy	____	45378	_____
3.	EKG w/interpretation	____	93000	_____
4.	X-Ray Chest, PA/LAT	____	71020	_____

F. LAB

1.	Blood Sugar	____	82947	_____
2.	CBC w/differential	____	85031	_____
3.	Cholesterol	____	82465	_____
4.	Comprehensive Metabolic Panel	____	80053	_____
5.	ESR	____	85651	_____
6.	Hematocrit	____	85014	_____
7.	Mono Screen	____	86308	_____
8.	Pap Smear	____	88150	_____
9.	Potassium	____	84132	_____
10.	Preg. Test, Quantitative	1	(84702)	X
11.	Routine Venipuncture	1	(36415)	X

F. Cont'd

		Dx	Units	
12.	Strep Screen		87081	_____
13.	UA, Routine w/Micro	____	81000	_____
14.	UA, Routine w/o Micro	____	81002	_____
15.	Uric Acid		84550	_____
16.	VDRL		86592	_____
17.	Wet Prep		82710	_____
18.	_____			_____

G. INJECTIONS

1.	Influenza Virus Vaccine	____	90658	_____
2.	Pneumoccocal Vaccine	____	90772	_____
3.	Tetanus Toxoids	____	90703	_____
4.	Therapeutic Subcut/IM	____	90732	_____
5.	Vaccine Administration	____	90471	_____
6.	Vaccine - each additional	____	90472	_____

H. MISCELLANEOUS

1. _____ ____ _____
2. _____ ____ _____

AMOUNT PAID $ 20.00

Check # 105

Mark diagnosis with (1=Primary, 2=Secondary, 3=Tertiary)

DIAGNOSIS NOT LISTED BELOW   *Pregnancy Test, Positive Result*   V72.42   (1)

DIAGNOSIS	ICD-9-CM 1, 2, 3	DIAGNOSIS	ICD-9-CM 1, 2, 3	DIAGNOSIS	ICD-9-CM 1, 2, 3
Abdominal Pain	789.0 ____	Dehydration	276.51 ____	Otitis Media, Acute NOS	382.9 ____
Allergic Rhinitis, Unspec.	477.9 ____	Depression, NOS	311 ____	Peptic Ulcer Disease	536.9 ____
Angina Pectoris, Unspec.	413.9 ____	Diabetes Mellitus, Type II Controlled	250.00 ____	Peripheral Vascular Disease NOS	443.9 ____
Anemia, Iron Deficiency, Unspec.	280.9 ____	Diabetes Mellitus, Type II Controlled	250.02 ____	Pharyngitis, Acute	462 ____
Anemia, NOS	285.9 ____	Drug Reaction, NOS	995.29 ____	Pneumonia, Organism Unspec.	486 ____
Anemia, Pernicious	281.0 ____	Dysuria	788.1 ____	Prostatitis, NOS	601.9 ____
Asthma w/ Exacerbation	493.92 ____	Eczema, NOS	692.2 ____	PVC	427.69 ____
Asthmatic Bronchitis, Unspec.	493.90 ____	Edema	782.3 ____	Rash, Non Specific	782.1 ____
Atrial Fibrillation	427.31 ____	Fever, Unknown Origin	780.6 ____	Seizure Disorder NOS	780.39 ____
Atypical Chest Pain, Unspec.	786.59 ____	Gastritis, Acute w/o Hemorrhage	535.00 ____	Serous Otitis Media, Chronic, Unspec.	381.10 ____
Bronchiolitis, due to RSV	466.11 ____	Gastroenteritis, NOS	558.9 ____	Sinusitis, Acute NOS	461.9 ____
Bronchitis, Acute	466.0 ____	Gastroesophageal Reflux	530.81 ____	Tonsillitis, Acute	463. ____
Bronchitis, NOS	490 ____	Hepatitis A, Infectious	070.1 ____	Upper Respiratory Infection, Acute NOS	465.9 ____
Cardiac Arrest	427.5 ____	Hypercholesterolemia, Pure	272.0 ____	Urinary Tract Infection, Unspec.	599.0 ____
Cardiopulmonary Disease, Chronic, Unspec.	416.9 ____	Hypertension, Unspec.	401.9 ____	Urticaria, Unspec.	708.9 ____
Cellulitis, NOS	682.9 ____	Hypoglycemia NOS	251.2 ____	Vertigo, NOS	780.4 ____
Congestive Heart Failure, Unspec.	428.0 ____	Hypokalemia	276.8 ____	Viral Infection NOS	079.99 ____
Contact Dermatitis NOS	692.9 ____	Impetigo	684 ____	Weakness, Generalized	780.79 ____
COPD NOS	496 ____	Lymphadenitis, Unspec.	289.3 ____	Weight Loss, Abnormal	783.21 ____
CVA, Acute, NOS	434.91 ____	Mononucleosis	075 ____		
CVA, Old or Healed	438.9 ____	Myocardial Infarction, Acute, NOS	410.9 ____		
Degenerative Arthritis (Specify Site) _____	715.9 ____	Organic Brain Syndrome	310.9 ____		
		Otitis Externa, Acute NOS	380.10 ____		

ABN: I UNDERSTAND THAT MEDICARE PROBABLY WILL NOT COVER THE SERVICES LISTED BELOW

A. _____ B. _____ C. _____

Patient

Date _____ Signature _____

Doctor's Signature *L.D. Heath* _____

RETURN: _____ Days _____ Weeks _____ Months

DOUGLASVILLE MEDICINE ASSOCIATES
5076 BRAND BLVD., SUITE 401
DOUGLASVILLE, NY 01234
PHONE No. (123) 456-7890
EIN# 00-1234560

☐ L.D. HEATH, M.D.   ☒ D.J. SCHWARTZ, M.D.
NPI# 9995010111   NPI# 9995020212
☐ SARAH O. MENDENHALL, M.D.
NPI# 9995030313

PLEASE RETURN THIS FORM TO RECEPTIONIST

NAME *Edward Brewer*

Receipt No: *21944*

PLACE OF SERVICE:

(✓) OFFICE
( ) NEW YORK COUNTY HOSPITAL
( ) COMMUNITY GENERAL HOSPITAL

( ) RETIREMENT INN NURSING HOME

( ) _____

DATE OF SERVICE *10/29/2010*

A. OFFICE VISITS - New Patient

Code	History	Exam	Dec.	Time	
____ 99201	Prob. Foc.	Prob. Foc.	Straight	10 min.	_____
____ 99202	Ex. Prob. Foc.	Ex. Prob. Foc.	Straight	20 min.	_____
____ 99203	Detail	Detail	Low	30 min.	_____
____ 99204	Comp.	Comp.	Mod.	45 min.	_____
____ 99205	Comp.	Comp.	High	60 min.	_____

B. OFFICE VISIT - Established Patient

Code	History	Exam	Dec.	Time	
____ 99211	Minimal	Minimal	Minimal	5 min.	_____
(99212)	Prob. Foc.	Prob. Foc.	Straight	10min.	✗
____ 99213	Ex. Prob. Foc.	Ex. Prob. Foc.	Low	15 min.	_____
____ 99214	Detail	Detail	Mod.	25 min.	_____
____ 99215	Comp.	Comp.	High	40 min.	_____

C. HOSPITAL CARE   Dx Units

1. Initial Hospital Care (30 min)	____ ___	99221	_____
2. Subsequent Care	____ ___	99231	_____
3. Critical Care (30-74 min)	____ ___	99291	_____
4. each additional 30 min.	____ ___	99292	_____
5. Discharge Services	____ ___	99238	_____
6. Emergency Room	____ ___	99282	_____

D. NURSING HOME CARE

Dx Units

Initial Care - New Pt.

1. Expanded	____ ___	99322	_____
2. Detailed	____ ___	99323	_____

Subsequent Care - Estab. Pt.

3. Problem Focused	____ ___	99307	_____
4. Expanded	____ ___	99308	_____
5. Detailed	____ ___	99309	_____
5. Comprehensive	____ ___	99310	_____

E. PROCEDURES

1. Arthrocentesis, Small Jt.	____	20600	_____
2. Colonoscopy	____	45378	_____
3. EKG w/interpretation	____	93000	_____
4. X-Ray Chest, PA/LAT	____	71020	_____

F. LAB

1. Blood Sugar	____	82947	_____
2. CBC w/differential	____	85031	_____
3. Cholesterol	____	82465	_____
4. Comprehensive Metabolic Panel	____	80053	_____
5. ESR	____	85651	_____
6. Hematocrit	____	85014	_____
7. Mono Screen	____	86308	_____
8. Pap Smear	____	88150	_____
9. Potassium	____	84132	_____
10. Preg. Test, Quantitative	____	84702	_____
11. Routine Venipuncture	____	36415	_____

F. Cont'd   Dx Units

12. Strep Screen	____	87081	_____
13. UA, Routine w/Micro	____	81000	_____
14. UA, Routine w/o Micro	____	81002	_____
15. Uric Acid	____	84550	_____
16. VDRL	____	86592	_____
17. Wet Prep	____	82710	_____
18. _____	____	____	_____

G. INJECTIONS

1. Influenza Virus Vaccine	____	90658	_____
2. Pneumoccocal Vaccine	____	90772	_____
3. Tetanus Toxoids	____	90703	_____
4. Therapeutic Subcut/IM	____	90732	_____
5. Vaccine Administration	____	90471	_____
6. Vaccine - each additional	____	90472	_____

H. MISCELLANEOUS

1. _____ _____ _____
2. _____ _____ _____

AMOUNT PAID $ *10.00*
Cash

Mark diagnosis with (1=Primary, 2=Secondary, 3=Tertiary)

DIAGNOSIS NOT LISTED BELOW _____

DIAGNOSIS	ICD-9-CM 1, 2, 3	DIAGNOSIS	ICD-9-CM 1, 2, 3	DIAGNOSIS	ICD-9-CM 1, 2, 3
Abdominal Pain	789.0_	Dehydration	276.51	Otitis Media, Acute NOS	382.9
Allergic Rhinitis, Unspec.	477.9	Depression, NOS	311	Peptic Ulcer Disease	536.9
Angina Pectoris, Unspec.	413.9	Diabetes Mellitus, Type II Controlled	250.00	Peripheral Vascular Disease NOS	443.9
Anemia, Iron Deficiency, Unspec.	280.9	Diabetes Mellitus, Type II Controlled	250.02	Pharyngitis, Acute	462
Anemia, NOS	285.9	Drug Reaction, NOS	995.29	Pneumonia, Organism Unspec.	486
Anemia, Pernicious	281.0	Dysuria	788.1	Prostatitis, NOS	601.9
Asthma w/ Exacerbation	493.92	Eczema, NOS	692.2	PVC	427.69
Asthmatic Bronchitis, Unspec.	493.90	Edema	782.3	Rash, Non Specific	782.1
Atrial Fibrillation	427.31	Fever, Unknown Origin	780.6	Seizure Disorder NOS	780.39
Atypical Chest Pain, Unspec.	786.59	Gastritis, Acute w/o Hemorrhage	535.00	Serous Otitis Media, Chronic, Unspec.	381.10
Bronchiolitis, due to RSV	466.11	Gastroenteritis, NOS	558.9	Sinusitis, Acute NOS	(461.9) 1
Bronchitis, Acute	466.0	Gastroesophageal Reflux	530.81	Tonsillitis, Acute	463.
Bronchitis, NOS	490	Hepatitis A, Infectious	070.1	Upper Respiratory Infection, Acute NOS	465.9
Cardiac Arrest	427.5	Hypercholesterolemia, Pure	272.0	Urinary Tract Infection, Unspec.	599.0
Cardiopulmonary Disease, Chronic, Unspec.	416.9	Hypertension, Unspec.	401.9	Urticaria, Unspec.	708.9
Cellulitis, NOS	682.9	Hypoglycemia NOS	251.2	Vertigo, NOS	780.4
Congestive Heart Failure, Unspec.	428.0	Hypokalemia	276.8	Viral Infection NOS	079.99
Contact Dermatitis NOS	692.9	Impetigo	684	Weakness, Generalized	780.79
COPD NOS	496	Lymphadenitis, Unspec.	289.3	Weight Loss, Abnormal	783.21
CVA, Acute, NOS	434.91	Mononucleosis	075		
CVA, Old or Healed	438.9	Myocardial Infarction, Acute, NOS	410.9		
Degenerative Arthritis (Specify Site) ____	715.9	Organic Brain Syndrome	310.9		
		Otitis Externa, Acute NOS	380.10		

ABN: I UNDERSTAND THAT MEDICARE PROBABLY WILL NOT COVER THE SERVICES LISTED BELOW

A. _____ B. _____ C. _____

Patient

Date _____ Signature _____

Doctor's Signature *L.D. Heath*

RETURN: _____ Days _____ Weeks _____ Months

DOUGLASVILLE MEDICINE ASSOCIATES
5076 BRAND BLVD., SUITE 401
DOUGLASVILLE, NY 01234
PHONE No. (123) 456-7890
EIN# 00-1234560

☑ L.D. HEATH, M.D.   ☐ D.J. SCHWARTZ, M.D.
NPI# 9995010111   NPI# 9995020212
☐ SARAH O. MENDENHALL, M.D.
NPI# 9995030313

DEPOSIT SLIP

Record of checks for deposit

	Dollars	Cents
Cash	.	
Checks	.	
	.	
	.	
	.	
	.	
	.	
	.	
	.	
	.	
	.	
	.	
	.	
	.	
	.	

Enter total $

DATE _____

⑈606121504⑈   162715943⑈

State Bank
3550 Commerce Blvd.
Douglasville, NY 01234

Douglasville Medicine Associates

5076 Brand Boulevard, Suite 401 • Douglasville, NY 01234 • (123) 456-7890

PATIENT INFORMATION FORM

DATE *10/29/2010*

Section A

LAST NAME .... *Guest*   FIRST NAME .... *Denise*   MI *R*

SS# *999-09-0288*   **GENDER** ☐ MALE ☑ FEMALE   DATE OF BIRTH *11/30/1980*

MARITAL STATUS

☐ Single   ☑ Divorced   ☐ Married   ☐ Other (separated, widowed)

HOME ADDRESS .... *1003 South Garfield Street*
            Street   Apt./Unit

CITY .... *Douglasville*   STATE .... *NY*   ZIP CODE *01234*

HOME PHONE .... *(123) 457-6606*   WORK PHONE *(123) 555-2587*   EXT ....

EMPLOYMENT STATUS   EMPLOYER/SCHOOL .... *Community General Hospital*

☑ Employed   ☐ Full-time student   ☐ Unemployed   ☐ Retired   ☐ Part-time student

EMPLOYER ADDRESS .... *4000 Brand Boulevard*   *Douglasville*   *NY*   *01234*
            Street   City   State   Zip Code

REFERRAL SOURCE ....   **RESPONSIBLE PARTY** ☑ SELF   ☐ GUARANTOR

Section B – Spouse Information

LAST NAME ....   FIRST NAME ....   MI ....

GENDER ☐ MALE ☐ FEMALE   DATE OF BIRTH ....

SS# ....   Is your spouse the guarantor of the account? ☐ Y ☐ N

Section C – Health Insurance Information

NAME OF INSURANCE PLAN .... *FlexiHealth PPO In-Network*

PATIENT RELATIONSHIP TO THE POLICYHOLDER ☑ Self   ☐ Spouse   ☐ Child   ☐ Other

POLICYHOLDER INFORMATION: (If same as patient, check box and skip to ID#, If not, complete all information beginning with Last Name.)

☑ Same as patient

LAST NAME ....   FIRST NAME ....   MI ....

GENDER ☐ MALE ☐ FEMALE   DATE OF BIRTH ....

ID# .... *999098880*   POLICY# (If different from ID#) ....

GROUP # .... *CGH880*   EMPLOYER NAME .... *Community General Hospital*

Do you have a secondary insurance plan? If yes, complete information below. ☐ Y ☑ N

NAME OF INSURANCE PLAN ....   ID # ....

POLICY # ....   GROUP # ....

PATIENT RELATIONSHIP TO THE POLICYHOLDER ☐ Self   ☐ Spouse   ☐ Child   ☐ Other

Are you seeing a doctor due to a work-related injury? ☐ Y ☐ N   If yes, date of injury ....

Are you seeing a doctor due to the result of an auto accident? ☐ Y ☐ N   If yes, date of accident ....

Section D – Assignment of Benefits

I hereby authorize the physicians at Douglasville Medicine Associates to release all information necessary concerning my medical condition to secure proper payment, and I hereby assign the physicians payment for services rendered. I understand that I am responsible for all charges whether or not paid by my insurance. This assignment will remain in effect until revoked by me in writing.

SIGNATURE *Denise Guest*   DATE *10/29/2010*

Work Record   For Week Ending   October 22, 2010

Employee	Hourly Rate	S	M	T	W	Th	F	S	Reg Hours	OT Hours	Total Hours	Regular Earnings	Overtime Earnings	Total Earnings	Taxable Earnings This Year
Fleet, F.	20	-	8	9	9	8	8	3	40	5	45	800	150	950	34,550
Balash, W.	17	-	8	8	8	8	8	-	40	-	40	680		680	29,240
Hasara, J.	10	-	8	8	8	4	4	-	32	-	32	320		320	16,820
Chun, M.	10	-	8	-	-	-	8	-	24 / 16 sick	-	40	400		400	17,220
Parker, E.	9	-	8	8	8	8	8	-	40	-	40	360		360	15,480
Student	7	-	8	8	8	8	8	-	40	-	40	280		280	1,064

H - Paid Holiday   I - Illness   V - Vacation   E - Other

Payroll Register   For Period Ending   October 22, 2010

Employee	Marital Status	No. W/H Allow.	Total Earnings	FICA Tax	Federal Income Tax	State Income Tax	Group Insurance	Other Deductions	Total Deductions	Amount	Check No.
Fleet, F.	M	1	950	72 68	95	46 25	50 -		263 93	686 07	
Balash, W.	S	1	680	52 02	78	28 41	25 -		183 43	496 57	
Hasara, J	M	3	320	24 48	0	4 90	50 -		79 38	240 62	
Chun, M.	M	2	400	30 60	12	9 30	50 -		101 90	298 10	
Parker, E.	M	0	360	27 54	21	9 30	50 -		107 84	252 16	
Student	S	1	280	21 42	18	5 30	0 -		44 72	235 28	
Totals			2990	228 74	224	103 46	225 -		781 20	2208 80	

Work Record

For Week Ending October 29, 2010

Employee	Hourly Rate	Time Record S	M	T	W	Th	F	S	Reg Hours	OT Hours	Total Hours	Regular Earnings	Overtime Earnings	Total Earnings	Taxable Earnings This Year
Fleet, F.	20	-	8	8	8	8	8	-							
Balash, W.	17	-	8	8	8	8	8	4							
Hasara, J.	10	-	I	8	8	8	8	-							
Chun, M.	10	-	8	8	E	8	8	-							
Parker, E.	9 50	-	8	8	V	V	V	-							
Student	7	-	8	8	8	8	8	-							

H-Paid Holiday   I - Illness   V - Vacation   E - Other

Payroll Register

For Period Ending October 29, 2010

Employee	Marital Status	No. W/H Allow.	Total Earnings	Deductions FICA Tax	Federal Income Tax	State Income Tax	Group Insurance	Other Deductions	Total Deductions	Amount	Check No.

PROCEDURAL AND DIAGNOSTIC CODING
PRACTICE WORKSHEET

Directions: For each of the following sections, you will be asked to identify either a procedure/diagnostic code or its description. Utilize the correct CPT or ICD-9 manual or the internet site provided to find the information. Your instructor will assist you in the proper use of the CPT and ICD-9 manuals.

Reference site for ICD-9 codes: www.icd9data.com

A. Complete the shaded section first by matching the ICD-9 code with the diagnosis. Then match the ICD-9 code to the procedure in the examples below.

_____80061 (lipid panel)

_____84550 (uric acid)

_____83550 (iron, TIBC, & % sat)

_____86900 (blood typing ABO) and 86901 (blood typing Rh)

_____84443 (TSH – thyroid stimulating hormone)

274	_____	a.	weight loss, abnormal
783.21	_____	b.	pregnancy
382.9	_____	c.	pure hypercholesterolemia
272.0	_____	d.	gout
V22.2	_____	e.	iron-deficiency anemia secondary to inadequate dietary intake

B. Insert the correct ICD-9 codes for the descriptions below.

1. _____ bronchial status asthmaticus

2. _____ autistic disorder, active

3. _____ elevated PSA (prostatic specific antigen)

4. _____ viral hepatitis B

5. _____ open wound to the ear drum, uncomplicated

6. _____ congestive heart failure

7. _____ left-sided congestive heart failure

8. _____ congestive heart failure in the immediate postoperative period

9. _____ migraine headache (menstrual)

10. _____ strep throat

JOB 31

Pre-Admission Questionnaire

1. What is the patient's full name?

2. What is the patient's date of birth?

3. What is the patient's address, including zip code?

4. What is the patient's SS#?

5. Is the patient married? (If yes, complete #6)

6. What is the patient's spouse's name and address?

7. What is and patient's admitting diagnosis?

8. What procedure will he/she be admitted for?

9. What is the expected length of stay?

10. Who will be performing the surgery?

11. What is the telephone number of the physician?

12. What is the expected date of admission?

13. Does the patient have an emergency contact? If yes, what is the name and relationship to the patient?

14. What is the telephone number of the patient's emergency contact?

15. Does the patient have insurance?

16. What is the name of the patient's insurance?

17. Who is the subscriber?

18. What is the relationship of the patient to the subscriber?

19. What is the ID#?

20. What is the group#?

21. Is this admission a result of Workman's Compensation?

22. Who is referring this patient for this admission?

"Thank you for this information. The patient is scheduled for _____. We will call him/her the day before with an exact time. His/her pre-operative instructions are as follows:........"

Name: _____

DATE			PROGRESS NOTES
MO.	DAY	YR.	

Douglasville Medicine Associates

5076 Brand Boulevard, Suite 401 • Douglasville, NY 01234 • (123) 456-7890

DISCHARGE SUMMARY

Patient: Gormann, Edward

Date: October 29, 2010

Physician: Lee Westfail, MD

OPERATION: Modified putti-platt procedure, left sholder

HISTORY: Unremarkable. No known allergies. This 41 year old white male suffered a disloka-
tion of theleft sholder while participating in sports 3 years ago Following that he had reorcur-
rent dislokations of the sholder, which the patient was able to reducehimself. He was admitted
at this time for surgecal correction.

PHYICAL EXAMINATION

VITAL SIGNS: Afebrile. Pulse 70.

SKIN: Clear. HEENT: Head and neck unremarkable. LUNGS: Clear. HEART: Cardiovascular
examination normal.

ABDOMEN: Soft nontender, with no masses.

EXTREMETIES: Good range of motion of left sholder with no focaltenderness. There was vol-
untery guarding on abduction and external rotation of the left sholder. Flexors were normal.

LABATORY DATA: x-ray of the chestwas normal

OTHER: Urinalysis was;normal. Electrolighs, BUM normal. Hematocrit 42, WBC 7,700.
Platelets adequate. Prothrombin time was normal.

OUTPATIENT CLINC COURSE: On October 29, 2010, the patient was taken to the operating room where a modified Putti Platt reconstruction of the left sholder was performed.
The patient tolerated the procedurewell.

OPERATIVE PROCEDURE: Modified putti-platt procedure, left sholder.

PROGNOSIS: The Patient should have gradual recovery of full function with limitation of
external rotation

_____
Lee Westfail, MD

:   D. J. Schwartz, MD

D: November 3, 2009

T: November 3, 2009

DJM/si

Douglasville Medicine Associates

5076 Brand Boulevard, Suite 401 • Douglasville, NY 01234 • (123) 456-7890

HISTORY AND PHYSICAL EXAMINATION RECORD

Patient: DELGADO, Manuel M.

Date: November 3, 2010

Physician: Sarah O. Mendenhall, MD

CHIEF COMPLAINT: Congestive heart failure, pulmonary emfysema, diabetes melletus, and xanthomas over a rather large area of his body in a period of 2 months.

PRESENT ILLNESS: His last hospitalization, in July of 2010 was for pulmonary emfysema, artieriosclerotic heart disease, decompensated state and diabetes melletus. Duringf his hospitalization the patient has pulmonary function studies done, which showed a generalized decompensation in all measurements since 2007. A gall bladder and upper GI study at that time were normal. A lipid panel source showed hyperuricemia and Tkpe IV huperlipidemia. The patient had an uneventful hospital course and was discharged on digoxin, 0.25 mg daily, Lasix, 40 mg daily. Since that time the patient states he has been "drugging."

HISTORY – –

ALLERGIES: The patient denies any allergies to food or medicine.

MEDICATIONS: His present medication include Digoxin, 0.25 mg daily, Lasic, 40 mg daily, Pronestyl, 250 mg ocassionally for abnormal heart rhythm.

SURGICAL: Negative.

SOCIAL: The patient is a prominent businessman in Douglasville and has been for the past 30 years. He states that his activities are the same now as two to three years ago. The patient was a two pack a day smoker until his hospitalization in July, 2010, when he dicided to quit smoking. He admits to an occasional drink, and there is some question regareding an ethanol history. He does not admit to any trouble with sleeping or eating.

FAMILY HISTORY: The patient's mother is 86 years old and has empfysema and high blood pressure. His father died at age 35 from tubercluosis. The patient has one sister, age 55, who is a known asthmetic. There is no family history of cancer, heart disease, diabetes, kidney disease, allergies.

JOB 34

REVIEW OF SYSTEMS

GI: Complains of polydipsi, polyuria, polyphagia. He has been on a diet to control his hyper-triglyceridemi and hypercholesterolemia and states that he is chronically hungry.

CR: Denies ankly edema, paroxysmal mocturnal dyspnea, but he does admit toi two pillow orthopnea. He denies any chest pain.

GU: Denies urinarytrac complaints.

Skin: Approximately 2 months ago the patient noticed a gradual on set of xanthomas over the lower thighs anteriorly and in the knee areas. This spread to the extensor surfaces of the lower arms and elbows, followed by the voar surface of the left index finger, and, finally, the entire buttock area.

_____
Sarah O. Mendenhall, MD

SOM/si
D: October 28, 2010
T: October 28, 2010

Glossary of Medical Terms

acromion (ah-kro'me-on)—lateral triangular projection of the spine of the scapula that forms the point of the shoulder.

adenoid (ad'ĕ-noid)—resembling a gland; in the plural, lymphoid tissue that normally exists in the nasopharynx of children and is known as the pharyngeal tonsil.

adenopathy (ad"e-nŏp'ah-the)—enlargement of the glands, especially of the lymphatic glands.

adipose (ad'ĭ-po–s)—of a fatty nature, fatty; fat present in the cells of adipose tissue.

afebrile (a-feb'ril)—without fever.

allergy (al'er-je)—acquired hypersensitivity to a substance (allergen) that does not normally cause a reaction. The reaction is caused by the release of a histamine or histamine-like substances from injured cells.

allopurinol (al"o-pūr'ĭ-nōl)—used in the treatment of hyperuricemia of gout and of that secondary to blood dyscrasias or cancer chemotherapy.

antihypertensive (an'tĭ-hi"per-ten'siv)—counteracting high blood pressure.

anti-inflammatory (an"tĭ-in-flam'ah'-to"re)—an agent that counteracts or suppresses the inflammatory process.

arrhythmia (ah-rith'me-ah)—irregularity or loss of rhythm, especially of the heartbeat.

arterial (ar-te're-al)—pertaining to an artery.

arteriosclerotic (ar-te"re-o"-skle-rot'ik)—pertaining to the hardening of the walls of the arteries.

asymptomatic (a"simp"to-mat'ik)—without symptoms; no complaints by the patient.

auscultation (aws'kul-ta'shun)—the act of listening for sounds within the body.

Betadine (ba'tah-dī n)—trade name for providone-iodine, a topical anti-infective; kills germs.

bilateral (bi-lat'er-al)—pertaining to two sides.

bimanual palpation (bi-man'u-al pal-pa'shun)—act of feeling with both hands.

bruit (brwe)—a sound or murmur heard in auscultation, especially an abnormal one.

buccal (buk'al)—pertaining to or directed towards the cheek.

BUN (bun)—blood urea nitrogen.

bursitis (ber-si'tis)—inflammation of a bursa, occasionally accompanied by a calcific deposit in the underlying supraspinatus tendon.

cardiorespiratory (kar"de-o-re-spi'rah-to"re)—pertaining to the cardiac and respiratory systems.

carotid (kah-rot'id)—pertaining to the right and left common carotid arteries, both of which arise from the aorta and are the principal blood supply to the head and neck.

Catapres (kat"ah-pres)—trade name for clonidine hydrochloride (an antihypertensive agent).

catheterization (kath"ĕ-ter-i-za'shun)—the employment or passage of a catheter.

CBC (CBC)—complete blood count.

cecum (se'kum)—any blind pouch or cul-de-sac; part of the intestines.

Cetacaine (set'a-cane")—topical anesthetic.

cholecystectomy (ko"le-sis-tek'to-me)—surgical removal of the gallbladder.

cholesterol (ko-les'ter-ol)—a sterol contained in animal tissue.

cholesterol/HDL—cholesterol/high density lipoprotein (lip"o-pro'te-in).

colonoscope (ko-lon'o-skōp)—an elongated flexible endoscope that permits visual examination of the colon.

colonoscopy (ko"lon-os'ko-pe)—examination by means of colonoscope.

conjunctiva (kon"junk'ti'vah)—the delicate membrane that lines the eyelid.

contracture (kon-trak'tūr)—an abnormal shortening of muscle(s) usually resulting in a deformity of the part and rendering the part resistant to movement.

Corgard (kor'gard)—trade name for a beta-blocking agent, which is a medication for heart circulatory problems.

costal (kos'tal)—pertaining to the ribs.

crepitus (krep'ĭ-tus)—noise of gas discharged from the intestines; joint c., the grating sensation caused by the rubbing together of the dry synovial surfaces of joints.

C-section—cesarean section.

cyanosis (si"ah-no'sis)—a bluish discoloration applied especially to skin and mucous membranes.

cystoscopy (sis-tos'ko-pe)—direct visual examination of the urinary tract with a cystoscope.

Cytotec (sī-tō-tĕc)—trade name for misoprostol; indicated for the prevention of nonsteroidial anti-inflammatory drug-induced gastric ulcer.

Demerol (dem'er-ol)—trade name for preparations of meperidine, opiate agonist.

diabetes mellitus (di"ah-be'tēz melli'tus)—a chronic syndrome of impaired carbohydrate, protein, and fat metabolism secondary to insufficient secretion of insulin or to target tissue insulin resistance.

dorsalis (dor-sa'lis)—a term denoting closer to the back surface.

DTR—deep tendon reflex.

duodenal (du"o-de'nal)—pertaining to or situated in the duodenum (first portion of the small intestines).

Dyazide (dye-uh-zid')—trade name for preparations of triamterene with hydrochlorothiazide, a diuretic combination product.

dysphasia (dis-fa'ze-ah)—impairment of speech, consisting in lack of coordination and failure to arrange words in the proper order.

dyspnea (disp'ne-ah)—difficulty breathing.

dysuria (dĭsū're-ah)—difficult or painful urination.

ecchymosis (ek"ĭ-mo'sis)—bleeding into skin or mucous membranes producing blue-black discoloration.

echocardiogram (ek"o-kar'de-o-gram")—the record produced by echocardiography.

ectopy (ek'to-pe)—ectopia; displacement or malposition, especially if congenital.

edema (ĕ-de'mah)—the presence of abnormally large amounts of fluid in the intracellular tissue spaces of the body.

electrocoagulation (e-lek"tro-ko-ag"u-la'shun)—coagulation of tissue by means of a high-frequency electric current.

electrolyte (e-lek'tro-līt)—a substance capable of conducting electricity.

emphysema (em"fi-se'mah)—a pathological accumulation of air in tissues or organs; applied especially to such a condition of the lungs.

endoscopy (en-dos'ko-pe)—visual inspection of any cavity of the body by means of an endoscope.

endotracheal (en"do-tra'ke-al)—within or through the trachea.

enteritis (en"ter-i'tis)—inflammation of the intestine; applied chiefly to inflammation of the small intestine.

epigastric (ep"ĭ-gas'trik)—pertaining to above the stomach.

epinephrine (ep"ĭ-nef rin)—chemical name; secreted by the adrenal medulla. Stimulator of the sympathetic nervous system.

esophagitis (ĕ-sof"ah-ji'tis)—inflammation of the esophagus.

esophagogastroduodenoscopy (ĕ-sof"ah-go-gas-tro-du"o-de-nos'ko-pe)—visual examination of the esophagus, stomach, and duodenum.

excavatum (eks"kah-va'tum)—pertaining to hollowing out.

extraocular (eks"trah-ok'u-lar)—situated outside of the eye.

exudate (eks'u-dāt)—cellular material that has passed through vessel walls into adjacent tissues or surfaces usually as a result of inflammation.

FBS (FBS)—fasting blood sugar.

Feldene (fel'dēn)—nonsteroidal anti-inflammatory agent, used in the treatment of rheumatoid and osteoarthritis. Trade name for piroxicam.

femoral (fem'or-al)—pertaining to the femur, or to the thigh.

Feosol (fe'o-sol)—iron preparation.

fibrocystic (fi"bro-sis'tik)—characterized by the development of cystic spaces, especially in relation to some duct or gland.

fossa (fos'ah)—general term for a hollow or depressed space.

funduscopic (fund'dus-skōp-ic) **device**—(an ophthalmoscope) (of-thal'mo-skōp) for examining the fundus of the eye.

gastrointestinal (gas"tro-in-tes'tĭ-nal)—pertaining to the stomach and the intestine.

genitourinary (jen"ĭ-to-u'rĭ-nar-e)—pertaining to the genital and urinary organs.

GI—gastrointestinal; pertaining to the stomach and the intestine.

GU—genitourinary tract.

HDL—high-density lipoproteins (lip"o-pro'te-ins).

health care clearinghouse—a public or private entity that processes or facilitates the processing of nonstandard data elements of health information into standard data elements.

HEENT—Head, Eyes, Ears, Nose, and Throat.

hematocrit (he-mat'o-krit)—volume percentage of cells in a whole blood sample.

hematolytic (hem"ah-to-lit'-ik)—pertaining to the destruction of red blood cells.

hematuria (hem"ah-tu're-ah)—blood in the urine.

heme (hēm)—blood.

hemi-pelvis (hem"e-pel'vis)—pertaining to half the pelvis.

hemoglobin (he'mo-glo"bin)—the oxygen carrying pigment of the red blood cells.

hemostasis (he'mo-sta'sis)—stopping of bleeding, stagnation of blood in one area.

hepatosplenomegaly (hep'ah-to-sple"no-meg'ah-le)—enlargement of the liver and spleen.

HIV—human immuno-deficiency (im"u-no-dĕ-fish'en-se) virus; identified as the AIDS virus.

Holter monitor—a portable device used to record electrocardiograms of ambulatory patients.

HPI—history of present illness.

hypercholesterolemia (hi"per-ko-les"ter-e'me-ah)—excessive amount of cholesterol in the blood.

hyperlipidemia (hi"per-lip"ĭde'me-ah)—a general term for elevated concentrations of any or all of the lipids in the plasma.

hyperplasia (hi"per-pla'ze-ah)—the abnormal multiplication or increase in the number of normal cells in normal arrangement in a tissue.

hyperplastic (hi"per-plas'tik)—pertaining to an extra growth of normal tissue.

hypertriglyceridemia (hi"per-tri-glis"er-i-de'me-ah)—an excess of triglycerides in the blood.

hyperuricemia (hi"per-u"rĭ-se'me-ah)—excess of uric acid in the blood.

ileocecal (il"e-o-se'kal)—pertaining to the ileum and cecum.

immunodeficiency (im"u-no-dĕ-fish'en-se)—a deficiency of immune response or a disorder characterized by deficient immune response.

incontinence (in-kon"tĭ-nen"se)—unable to control excretory functions.

Indocin (in'do-sin)—nonsteroidal anti-inflammatory agent used in the treatment of rheumatoid and osteoarthritis, ankylosing spondylitis. Trade name for indomethacin.

infarction (in-fark'shun)—the formation of an area of coagulation necroses in a tissue caused by local ischemia.

intercostal (in"ter-kos'tal)—situated between the ribs.

intraductal (in"trah-duk'tal)—situated or occurring within the duct of a gland.

intraluminal (in"trah-lu'mĭ-nal)—within the lumen of a tube, as of a blood vessel.

io.d. (one o.d.)—prescription instruction meaning take one pill every day. Used with caution in transcription due to high possibility of misinterpretation with other similar abbreviations.

irradiation (i-ra"de-a'-shun)—treatment by photons, electrons, neutrons, or other forms of ionizing radiations.

ischemia (is-ke'me-ah)—local and temporary deficiency of blood supply caused by obstruction of the blood flow to the part.

IV—intravenous.

labile (la'bĭl)—gliding; moving from point to point over the surface; unstable; fluctuating.

laminectomy (lam"ĭ-nek'to-me)—excision of the posterior care arch of a vertebra.

Lasix (la'siks)—trade name for preparations of furosemide.

lavage (lah-vahzh')—the irrigation or washing out of an organ, such as the stomach or bowel.

LE—lower extremities.

leukoplakia (loo"ko-pla'ke-ah)—formation of white spots or patches on the mucous membrane of the tongue or cheek.

lobulated (lob'u-lăt"ed)—made up of or divided into lobules.

lumbar (lum'bar)—pertaining to the loins; the part of the back between the thorax and the pelvis.

lumbosacral (lum"bo-sa'kral)—pertaining to the loins and sacrum.

lumpectomy (lum-pek'to-me)—surgical removal of a mass.

lymph (limf)—a transparent slightly yellow liquid of alkaline reaction, found in the lymphatic vessels and derived from the tissue fluids.

lymphadenopathy (lim-fad"ĕ-nop'ah-the)—disease of the lymph nodes.

lymphatic (lim-fat'ik)—pertaining to lymph or a lymph vessel.

mammography (mam-og'rah-fe)—roentgenography (x-ray) of the mammary gland.

metaplasia (met"ah-pla'ze-ah)—the change in the type of adult cells in a tissue to a form that is not normal for the tissue.

microcyst (mi-kro-sist)—a very small cyst.

midsternal (mid-ster'nal)—middle of sternum.

mucosa (mu-ko'sah)—a mucous membrane.

mucosal (mu-ko'sal)—pertaining to the mucous membrane.

musculoskeletal (mus"ku-lo-skel'ĕ-tal)— pertaining to or comprising the skeleton and the muscles.

Mutamycin (mu"tah-mi'sin)—trade name for a preparation of mitomycin.

Mylanta (my-lan'ta)—trade name of an antacid.

myocardial (mi"o-kar'de-al)—pertaining to the myocardium (the middle layer of the walls of the heart, composed of cardiac muscle).

nasogastric (na"zo-gas'trik)—pertaining to the nose and stomach.

nasopharynx (na"zo-far'inks)—the part of the pharynx that lies above the level of the soft palate.

neuro (nu"ro)—nerve.

neurologic (nu-ro-loj'ik)—pertaining to neurology or to the nervous system.

Nitro-Dur (nītra-dur)—nitroglycerin agent; antianginal.

NKA—no known allergies.

Nolvadex (nol'va-dex")—antineoplastic agent; indicated in advanced premenopausal and postmenopausal breast cancer. Trade name for tamoxifen citrate.

nonsteroid (non"steer'oid)—pertaining to absence of steroids.

Ogen (o'jen)—estrogen; hormonal agent. Trade name for estropipate.

organomegaly (or"gah-no-meg'ah-le)—enlargement of visceral (abdominal) organs.

oropharynx (o"ro-far'inks)—that division of the pharynx that lies between the soft palate and the upper edge of the epiglottis.

orthopnea (or"thop-ne'ah)—respiratory condition in which there is discomfort in breathing except when in a sitting or standing position.

OSHA—Occupational Safety and Health Administration.

osteoarthritis (os"te-o-ar-thri'tis)—noninflammatory degenerative joint disease occurring chiefly in older persons, characterized by degeneration of the articular cartilage, hypertrophy of bone at the margins, and changes in the synovial membrane.

otopharynx (o"to-fah'inks)—pertaining to ear and throat.

panendoscope (pan-en'do-skōp)—a cystoscope that permits wide-angle viewing of the urinary bladder and urethra.

paravertebral (par"ah-ver'tĕ-bral)—beside the vertebral column.

Parkinson's (par'kin-sunz) **disease**—a disease marked by slowing and weakness of voluntary movement, muscular rigidity, and tremors.

pectus (pek'tus)—the breast, the chest thorax.

percussion (per-kush'un)—act of striking a part with short, sharp blows as an aid in diagnosing the condition of the underlying parts by the sound obtained.

peritonsillar (per"ĭ-ton'sĭ-lar)—situated around a tonsil.

PND—**paroxysmal** (par"ok-siz'mal) **nocturnal dyspnea** (disp'ne-ah)—a form of respiratory distress related to posture (especially reclining at night) and usually attributed to congestive heart failure with pulmonary edema.

polyp (pol'ip)—a morbid excrescence or protruding growth, from mucous membrane.

popliteal (pop-lit'e-al)—pertaining to the posterior surface (back) of the knee.

precordial (pre-kor'de-al)—pertaining to the precordium (the region over the heart and lower part of the thorax).

Prilosec—trade name for omeprazole; used in the short-term treatment of active duodenal ulcer.

p.r.n.—as needed.

prothrombin (pro-throm'bin)—coagulation factor II.

Provera (pro-ver'ah)—Progestin (pro-jes'tin); indicated in abnormal uterine bleeding caused by hormonal imbalance. Trade name for medroxyprogesterone acetate.

pulmonary (pul'mo-ner"e)—pertaining to the lungs.

Putti-Platt—capsulorrhaphy (suture of joint capsule or of a tear in a capsule) of shoulder for recurrent dislocation; an orthopedic procedure.

pylorus (pi-lo'rus)—the distal aperture of the stomach.

pyorrhea (pi"or-re'ah)—a discharge of pus.

rale (rahl)—abnormal rattle or scraping sound heard on auscultation of the chest—in the lungs or air passages.

respiration (res"pĭ-ra'shun)—the exchange of oxygen and carbon dioxide between the atmosphere and cells of the body.

resuscitation (re-sus" ĭ-ta'shun)—the restoration of life or consciousness of one apparently dead; it includes such measures as artificial respiration and cardiac massage.

RUQ (RUQ)—right upper quadrant.

Rx—prescription.

sclerosed (skle-rōst')—affected with sclerosis (an induration, or hardening).

sclerotherapy (skle"ro-ther'ah-pe)—the injection of sclerosing solutions in the treatment of hemorrhoids, varicose veins, or esophageal varices.

scrotal (skro'tal)—pertaining to the scrotum.

sesamoid (ses'ah-moid)—denoting a small nodular bone embedded in a tendon or joint capsule.

SGOT—serum (se'rum) glutamic (gloo-tam'ik) oxaloacetic (oks" al-o-ah-se'tik) transaminase (trans-am'ĭ-nās); an enzyme present in high concentrations in muscle, liver, and brain).

SGPT—serum (se'rum) glutamic (gloo-tam'ik) pyruvic (pi-roo'vik) transaminase (trans-am'ĭ-nās); an enzyme similar to SGOT).

sigmoid (sig'moid)—shaped like the letter S or the letter C; the sigmoid colon.

slough (sluf)—necrotic tissue in the process of separating from viable portions of the body.

splenic (splen'ik)—pertaining to the spleen.

submucous (sub-mu'kus)—situated or performed beneath the mucous membrane.

substernal (sub-ster'nal)—situated beneath the sternum.

suture (su'chur)—fine thread, wire, or other material used in the operation of stitching parts of the body together.

syncope (sin'ko-pe)—a temporary suspension of consciousness caused by generalized cerebral ischemia.

T&A—tonsillectomy (ton"sĭ-lek'to-me) and adenoidectomy (ad"ě-noid-ek'to-me).

tachycardia (tak"e-kar'de-ah)—abnormal rapidity of heart action, usually defined as a heart rate over 100 beats per minute.

Tagamet (tag'ah-met)—trade name for preparations of cimetidine.

tenaculum (těnak'ulum)—a hooklike instrument for seizing and holding tissue.

tendonitis (ten"do-ni'tis)—inflammation of a tendon or tendons.

testicular (tes-tik'u-lar)—pertaining to the testis.

thyromegaly (thi"ro-meg'ah-le)—enlargement of the thyroid gland.

tibial (tib'e-al)—pertaining to the tibia (inner and larger bone of the leg).

tonsillectomy (ton"sĭ-lek-to-me)—surgical removal of a tonsil or tonsils.

tonsillitis (ton"sĭ-li'tis)—inflammation of the tonsils.

tortuous (tor'choo-us)—twisted; full of turns and twists.

triglyceride (tri-glis'er-īd)—a compound consisting of three molecules of fatty acid esterified to glycerol; it is a neutral fat synthesized from carbohydrates for storage in animal adipose cells.

turgor (tur'gor)—normal tension in a cell; resistance of the skin to deformation, especially to being grasped between the fingers.

ureteral (u-re'ter-al)—pertaining to or used upon the ureter.

urinalysis (u"rĭ-nal'ĭ-sis)—physical, chemical, or microscopic analysis or examination of urine.

urosepsis (u"ro-sep'sis)—septic poisoning from the absorption and decomposition of urinary substances in the tissues.

vagotonia (va"go-to'ne-ah)—hyperexcitability of the vagus nerve; a condition in which the vagus nerve dominates the general functioning of the body organs.

varicosity (var"ĭ-kos'ĭ-te)—a varicose condition; swollen or twisted.

vasculature (vas'ku-lah-tūr)—the vascular system of the body or any part of it.

vasectomy (vah-sek'to-me)—surgical removal of the ductus vas deferens or a portion of it; done in association with prostatectomy (pros"tah-tek'to-me) or to induce infertility.

vasovagal (vas"o-va'gal)—vascular and vagal.

Vistaril (vis'tah-ril)—antianxiety agent; indicated for anxiety and tension. Trade name for hydroxyzine pamoate.

vesicular (vě-sik'u-lar)—composed of or relating to small saclike bodies.

vital IVP—intravenous pyelogram.

WNL—within normal limits.

xanthoma (zan-tho'mah)—a papule, nodule, or plaque of a yellow color in skin caused by deposits of lipids.

Xylocaine (zi'lo-kān)—local anesthesia. Trade name for lidocaine.

Zantac (zan'tak)—trade name for ranitidine; indicated in the short-term treatment of duodenal ulcer.

Zyloprim (zi'lo-prim)—trade name for allopurinol (an anti-hyperuricemic, which is commonly used to treat gout and uric acid).